Smart Medical Imaging for Diagnosis and Treatment Planning

This book presents advanced research on smart health technologies, focusing on the innovative transformations in diagnosis and treatment planning using medical imaging and data analysed by data science techniques. It shows how smart health technologies leverage artificial intelligence (AI) and big data analytics to provide more accurate and efficient diagnosis and treatment planning. In search for innovative and novel methods and techniques for health technologies and medical data processing, the book

- Discusses applications of Artificial Intelligence, Data Science, Machine Learning, Deep Learning, the Internet of Things, Big Data, and Cloud Computing;
- Includes use of electronic patient records in healthcare, analysis of big data in medical diagnosis, reliability, and challenges of EPR and EHR in smart healthcare;
- Explores evolving techniques for smart healthcare, its application in medical imaging, and prediction in the fields of treatment planning;
- Provides recent studies in AI-driven healthcare technologies and medical imaging to outline insight into smart healthcare technologies;
- Discusses the role of big data in smart healthcare, computing techniques for healthcare for medical diagnosis and treatment planning;
- Encompasses the ethical and legal challenges of using smart healthcare and medical data.

This book serves as a valuable reference for researchers working on smart health technologies. Researchers of medical imaging, artificial intelligence, and data science along with healthcare domain will find it a great resource as well.

Smart Medical Imaging for Diagnosis and Treatment Planning

Edited by
Nilanjan Dey, Bitan Misra, and
Sayan Chakraborty

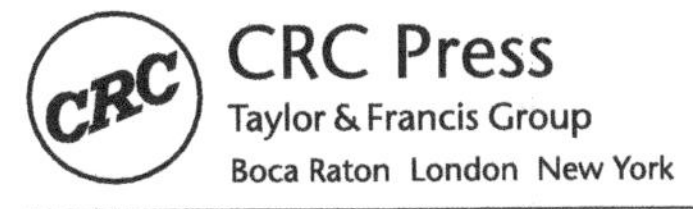

CRC Press
Taylor & Francis Group
Boca Raton London New York

CRC Press is an imprint of the
Taylor & Francis Group, an **informa** business

A CHAPMAN & HALL BOOK

Front cover image:toodtuphoto/Shutterstock

First edition published 2025
by CRC Press
2385 NW Executive Center Drive, Suite 320, Boca Raton, FL 33431

and by CRC Press
4 Park Square, Milton Park, Abingdon, Oxon, OX14 4RN

CRC Press is an imprint of Taylor & Francis Group, LLC

Library of Congress Cataloging-in-Publication Data
Names: Dey, Nilanjan, 1984- editor. | Misra, Bitan, editor. |
Chakraborty, Sayan, PhD, editor.
Title: Smart medical imaging for diagnosis and treatment planning / edited
by Nilanjan Dey, Bitan Misra, Sayan Chakraborty.
Description: First edition. | Boca Raton : C&H/CRC Press, 2025. | Includes
bibliographical references and index. | Identifiers: LCCN 2024010478 (print) |
LCCN 2024010479 (ebook) | ISBN 9781032735023 (hardback) | ISBN 9781032735788 (paperback) |
ISBN 9781003464884 (ebook)
Subjects: MESH: Image Interpretation, Computer-Assisted | Artificial
Intelligence | Medical Informatics Applications | Delivery of Health
Care--methods
Classification: LCC R859 (print) | LCC R859 (ebook) | NLM WN 182 |
DDC 610.285--dc23/eng/20240430
LC record available at https://lccn.loc.gov/2024010478
LC ebook record available at https://lccn.loc.gov/2024010479

ISBN: 978-1-032-73502-3 (hbk)
ISBN: 978-1-032-73578-8 (pbk)
ISBN: 978-1-003-46488-4 (ebk)

DOI: 10.1201/9781003464884

Typeset in Times
by Deanta Global Publishing Services, Chennai, India

Contents

Preface

Smart health medical imaging involves the use of cutting-edge tools and services in the medical imaging industry to identify, track, and manage a wide range of illnesses. It provides precise and thorough images of the human body by using cutting-edge imaging methods such as CT, MRI, and ultrasound scans. Medical experts may use these and precisely identify a range of medical disorders. Patients' individualized treatment regimens can be developed with the use of smart health medical imaging. Medical experts can correctly assess the degree of an injury or sickness and choose the best course of therapy by receiving detailed photographs of the affected area. This book highlights the basic role of smart health medical imaging in disease detection, diagnosis, and treatment planning. It includes various smart health imaging techniques that are applied in different domains of treatment planning and diagnosis. The book comprises ten chapters in which Chakraborty et al., in Chapter 1, provide information for researchers and scientists working in this domain regarding the enhancement of intelligent medical imaging to revolutionize healthcare. In addition, Gupta and Pandey highlight the role of artificial intelligence in smart health diagnosis and treatment in Chapter 2. In Chapter 3, Rangaswamy and Mathkunti analyse early-stage smart diagnosis and prediction of Alzheimer's disease using machine learning models. In Chapter 4, Bhattacharya and Polkowski discuss the impact of artificial intelligence in healthcare. The chapter focuses on predictors of multiple sclerosis. Roy et al. in Chapter 5, describe modality-based image registration in modern healthcare to enhance patient care.

In Chapter 6, Maji and Mondal describe fashionable and disposable electrochemical sensors as modern healthcare appliances. In Chapter 7, Moharana et al. present an analysis of the use of smart healthcare systems for combating infectious disease outbreaks. In Chapter 8, Das et al. present a study on facemask and hand glove detection using a hybrid deep learning model. In Chapter 9, Ghandorh present a comparative analysis on the utilization of machine learning and deep learning classifiers in predicting users' performance in augmented reality surgical environments. In the final chapter, Chapter 10, Acharya and Paul discuss the future of medical imaging with respect to ethical and legal compliance.

The editors are thankful to the outstanding authors and referees for their contributions and outcomes. Their diligence and collaboration led to this remarkable book. They also appreciate the members of the CRC team for their support.

About the Editors

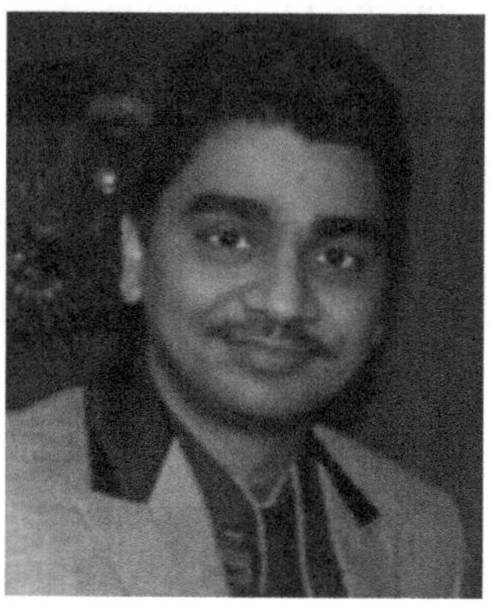

Nilanjan Dey is Associate Professor in the Department of Computer Science and Engineering, Techno International New Town, Kolkata, India. He is Visiting Fellow of the University of Reading, UK. He also holds a position of Adjunct Professor at Ton Duc Thang University, Ho Chi Minh City, Vietnam. Previously, he held an honorary position of Visiting Scientist at Global Biomedical Technologies Inc., CA, USA (2012–2015). He was awarded his Ph.D from Jadavpur University in 2015. He is Editor-in-Chief of the *International Journal of Ambient Computing and Intelligence*, IGI Global, USA. He is Series Co-Editor of *Springer Tracts in Nature-Inspired Computing* (SpringerNature), *Data-Intensive Research* (SpringerNature), *Advances in Ubiquitous Sensing Applications for Healthcare* (Elsevier). He was Associate Editor of *IET Image Processing* and Editorial Board Member of *Complex & Intelligent Systems*, SpringerNature. He is Editorial Board Member of *Applied Soft Computing*, Elsevier. He has authored 35 books and has over 300 publications in the area of medical imaging, machine learning, computer-aided diagnosis, data mining, etc. He is Fellow of *IETE* and Senior Member of *IEEE*.

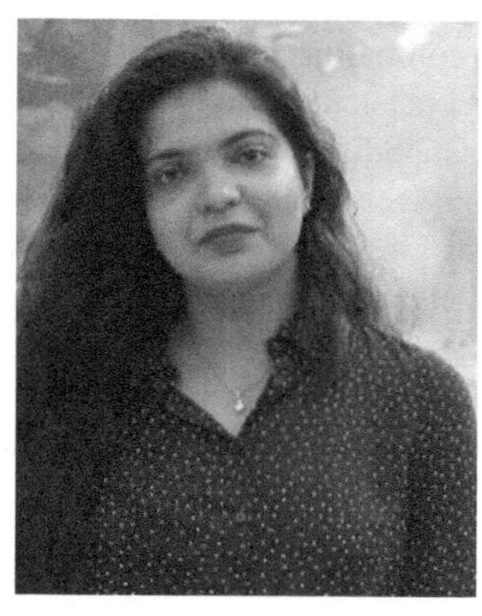

Bitan Misra is currently working as Assistant Professor in the Department of CSE, Techno International New Town, Kolkata, India. She received her B.Tech and M.Tech dual degrees in Electronics and Telecommunication Engineering from KIIT University, Bhubaneswar, India, in 2018. She received her Ph.D in 2022 from the National Institute of Technology, Durgapur, India. She received a Gold Medal during her U.G for securing the highest CGPA in the university. She has published almost 15 research papers in various international journals and conferences and has three copyrights. Her main research interests include optimization techniques, deep learning, evolutionary algorithms, and soft computing techniques. She has worked as a reviewer in several national and international journals and conferences. She is Associate Editor of *International Journal of Ambient Computing and Intelligence*, IGI Global. She is Member of *IEEE* and Internet Society.

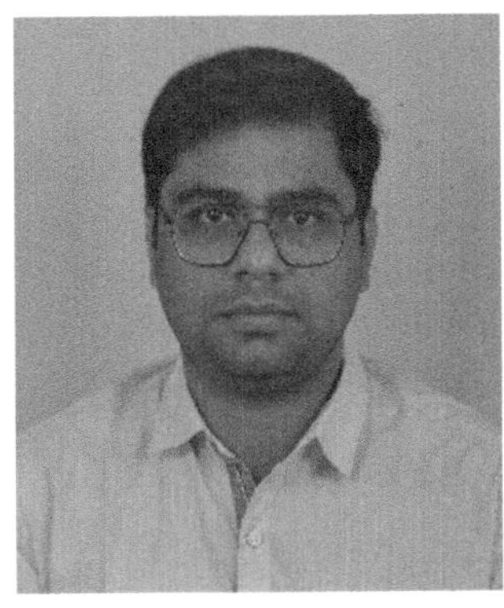

Sayan Chakraborty is currently working as Assistant Professor in the Department of Computer Science and Engineering at the Techno International New Town, West Bengal, India. He has completed his Ph.D in Image Registration from Sikkim Manipal University in the year 2023. He has completed M.Tech from Computer Science & Engineering, JIS College of Engineering. He has also completed his B.Tech. from the same college. He has academic experience of 10 years. His research area includes digital image processing, nature-inspired algorithms and machine learning. He has about 65 research papers published in international journals, book chapters, and conferences on various topics such as optimization, artificial intelligence, pattern recognition, and digital image processing. He has one book published in Springer. He is Associate Editor of *International Journal of Ambient Computing and Intelligence*, IGI Global, and is Editorial Board Member of *International Journal of Rough Sets and Data Analysis (IJRSDA)*, IGI Global. He is Senior Member of IEEE.

List of Contributors

Soubhik Acharya
Techno International New Town
Kolkata, India

Abhirup Bhattacharya
Techno International New Town
Kolkata, India

Sanjay Chakraborty
Techno International New Town
Kolkata, India

Sayan Chakraborty
Techno International New Town
Kolkata, India

Sraddha Roy Choudhury
Swami Vivekananda University
Kolkata, India

Akash Das
Techno International New Town
Kolkata, India

Sabyasachi Ganguly
Techno International New Town
Kolkata, India

Hamza Waleed Ghandorh
Taibah University
Saudi Arabia

Priyanka Gupta
Guru Ghasidas Central University
Bilaspur, India

Raj Kamal
Techno International New Town
Kolkata, India

Fahmida Khan
National Institute of Technology
Raipur, India

Prakash Chandra Maharana
Ericsson-AB
Stockholm, Sweden

Paramita Kundu Maji
Techno International New Town
Kolkata, India

Pranabi Maji
JIS University
Kolkata, India

Nivedita Manohar Mathkunti
Alliance University
Bengaluru, India

Bitan Misra
Techno International New Town
Kolkata, India

Dwaipayan Mistry
Techno International New Town
Kolkata, India

Anirban Mitra
Amity University
Kolkata, India

Maheswata Moharana
National Institute of Technology
Raipur, India

Shrabani Mondal
Kazi Nazrul University
West Bengal, India

Muhammad Firoz Mridha
American International University-
    Bangladesh (AIUB)
Dhaka, Bangladesh

Manoj Kumar Pandey
Pranveer Singh Institute of Technology
Kanpur, India

Subrat Kumar Pattanayak
National Institute of Technology
Raipur, India

Priti Paul
Techno International New Town
Kolkata, India

Sheng-Lung Peng
National Taipei University of Business
Taiwan

Zdzislaw Polkowski
WSG University
Poland

Shanta Rangaswamy
Rashtreeya Vidyalaya College of
    Engineering
Bengaluru, India

Abhisek Roy
Seacom Skills University
West Bengal, India

Pranab Kanti Roy
Seacom Skills University
West Bengal, India

Part I

Introduction

1 Enhancing Intelligent Medical Imaging to Revolutionize Healthcare

Sayan Chakraborty, Bitan Misra, and Muhammad Firoz Mridha

1.1 INTRODUCTION

Technological advancements have impacted all facets of human life, but the use of technology in the domain of healthcare has had a particularly positive impact on society. The ultimate goal of smart medicine is to offer precise diagnosis and individualized therapy so as to ensure the good health of humans. Recent advancements in smart healthcare and the use of artificial intelligence (AI) in radiology have demonstrated impressive advancements in image-recognition tasks to automatically identify various items in imaging data. Medical imaging is the practice of representing various human body tissues and organs visually in order to track both normal and pathological anatomy and physiology. X-rays, computed tomography (CT), positron emission tomography (PET), magnetic resonance imaging (MRI), single-photon emission computed tomography (SPECT), digital mammography, and diagnostic sonography are just a few of the medical imaging methods that are employed for this purpose [1–2]. Cardiac-related dangerous medical conditions, including cardiac diseases, cancer of various tissues, neurological disorders, congenital heart disease, stomach illnesses, complex bone fractures, and other maladies, can be diagnosed using these cutting-edge medical imaging techniques. Early disease detection can assist in controlling the spread of the disease and safeguard the vulnerable human body parts, including the blood, breast, lungs, and skin. Without prompt and proper diagnosis, illnesses and tumors can spread extremely infectiously, increasing the risk of fatality [3].

Medical imaging technology has altered the way healthcare was provided over the last 30 years. Medical imaging enables clinicians to identify diseases in their early stages, improving patient outcomes. Early diagnosis and treatment of diseases make them more manageable, making this cutting-edge technology genuinely life-changing. Radiographs were the only type of medical imaging for many years, but as new technologies emerged, three-dimensional imaging, four-dimensional imaging (three-dimensional imaging in real time), functional imaging, and molecular imaging gradually replaced two-dimensional flat images. Medical imaging has experienced

DOI: 10.1201/9781003464884-2

success over the past few decades due to both technological advancements and the digital revolution [2–4]. Films are increasingly being replaced by digital images on workstations, enabling multiplanar reconstruction of images. Radiologists can now analyze enormous volumes of data, compare new studies to old ones, and rebuild multiplanar and three-dimensional images thanks to improvements in workstations made possible by computer technology and software. Another significant outcome of technological advancement includes the electronic health record. While protocoling or reviewing an imaging study, radiologists can access medical history, test findings, clinical notes, and detailed medical data. Modern hospitals can now combine the radiological information system and hospital information system with coding and billing, workflow dashboards, and computerized order input with decision-assistance tools [5]. The fundamental concepts of medical imaging, its multiple varieties, limitations, difficulties, moral and legal concerns, and its potential for future research are briefly covered in this chapter.

1.2 MEDICAL IMAGING PRELIMINARIES

1.2.1 FUNDAMENTALS OF MEDICAL IMAGING

To determine the most effective course of treatment for a patient, a physician must first accurately diagnose the condition. To have a peek into the patient, numerous methods (Figure 1.1) have been devised. All of them rely on physical phenomena that allow signals to pass through patients directly, including sound waves or other forms of electromagnetic radiation that interact with the patient's tissues [6–8]. It is possible to create an internal image of the patient using sound waves or radiation that has been attenuated or released. This type of radiation is inappropriate since visible

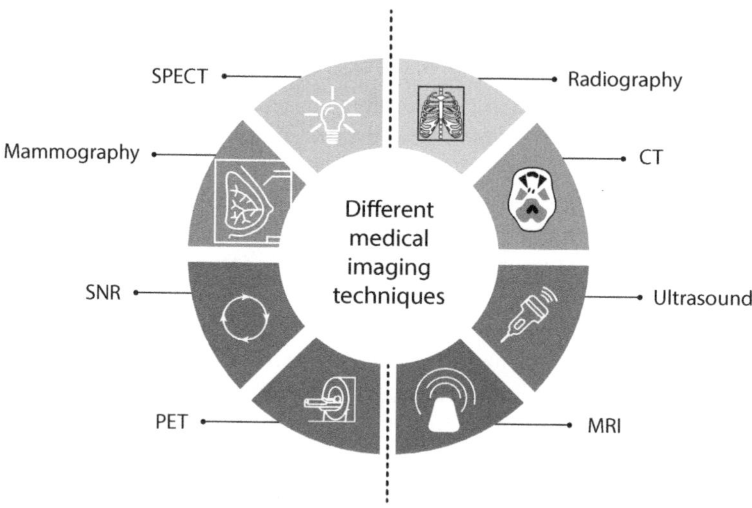

FIGURE 1.1 Different medical imaging techniques.

light waves cannot penetrate the molecules that make up the human body. Different physical approaches and, thus, different imaging instruments are required because different techniques measure distinct physical qualities that rely on the constituents of different tissues. For instance, bone fractures can be visible on CT slices or X-ray films, while soft tissues with a lot of water and fat are usually examined with MRIs. Comprehending the principles of image production is imperative for enhancing imaging methodologies, including contrast optimization and image signal-to-noise ratio (SNR) enhancement [9–11].

1.2.2 DIFFERENT MEDICAL IMAGING TECHNIQUES

Medical imaging comes in a variety of forms, and as technology develops, new methods are created. Magnetic resonance, X-ray transmission, acoustic or light reflection, and radiation emission are the four main types of medical imaging modalities [9, 10]. Although the many imaging modalities within a given category may have many variables that can be adjusted to measure distinct structures or occurrences, they all have the same basic idea. This technique's main benefits are its speed, accessibility, affordability, and ability to identify lung problems and fractures. Nevertheless, it exposes the user to ionizing radiation continuously and offers little information about soft tissues.

1.2.2.1 Radiography

With this imaging technique, images of the inside of the body are captured using electromagnetic radiation. X-rays are the most widely used and prevalent type of radiography. Electromagnetic waves, which have wavelengths ranging from 0.01 to 10 nanometers, are the type of radiation that includes X-rays. X-ray equipment projects high-energy waves onto the body throughout this imaging process [10, 11]. These waves are absorbed by hard tissues like bones, but not by soft tissues like skin and organs. The apparatus projects the images from the X-ray onto a film, showing the body portions that were absorbed in white and the unabsorbed material in black.

1.2.2.2 Computed Tomography (CT)

Radiologists, biologists, archaeologists, and many other scientists employ computed tomography (CT) scans to create cross-sectional images of various items they scan. CT is a noninvasive method that creates images of the body. The two types of CT scans are single-photon emission computed tomography (SPECT) and positron emission tomography (PET). CT is a useful tool for tracking different kinds of cancer and also detects distant metastases to the brain, liver, bones, and lungs. Compared to traditional X-rays, CT scans provide clearer, more accurate images of the body's soft tissue, internal organs, blood arteries, and bones [10]. A CT scan produces cross-sectional images that can be reformatted in several planes and even turned into three-dimensional images that can be saved to electronic devices, reproduced on film, or seen on a computer monitor. Four-dimensional (4D) computed tomography (CT) has recently been developed to address issues caused by breathing motions. Organ mobility information is produced by 4D CT in both temporal and spatial dimensions [11].

1.2.2.3 Ultrasound

In order to create images, medical ultrasonography uses sound waves with a frequency range of 118 MHz. These waves reflect off of tissues to differing degrees. A piezoelectric transducer, also known as a transmitter, creates sound waves by converting electrical signals into ultrasonic waves [9]. A separate transducer (receiver) or the same transducer (transceiver) receives the reflected soundwaves, and the vibrations the transducer detects are transformed into electrical signals. Compared to X-ray and magnetic resonance imaging, ultrasound usually offers less anatomic details because of its lower signal to noise and tissue contrast. However, it is inexpensive, portable, and very good at capturing moving structures in real time. Additionally, it can track actual material points of tissue with image speckles. Ultrasound is one of the most affordable and safest medical imaging methods available. It may be used for a variety of purposes and is considered to be completely safe [12].

1.2.2.4 Magnetic Resonance

Strong magnetic fields and radio waves are used in magnetic resonance imaging (MRI) to distinguish between different kinds of tissues and materials by obtaining contrasting signals. There is no known pain associated with an MRI examination, and there is no known tissue damage caused by the electromagnetic fields [8–10]. Compared to CT, MRI often employs nonionizing radiation, which is preferable. The majority of the time, soft tissue analysis uses MRI alone. Multiple sclerosis, CNS tumors, brain and spine infections, stroke, damage to ligaments and tendons, muscle degeneration, bone tumors, and blood vessel blockage are the most common conditions found on magnetic resonance imaging (MRI). Using precisely graded magnetic fields, MRI can visualize any arbitrary 2D slice of anatomy by stimulating it inside a 3D volume of space. A completely resolved 3D volumetric image can be created by stacking a sequential collection of these 2D slices together. MRI differs from previous diagnostic methods in that there is no ionizing radiation risk [12]. Unlike CT and PET scans, an MRI has no adverse effects. The process of scanning body target parts from many perspectives and angles does not result in any degradation in image quality.

1.2.2.5 Positron Emission Tomography (PET)

A nuclear medicine functional technology called positron emission tomography is utilized to produce crisp images that show the entire concentration of radioactively labeled materials in the body. The first PET machine was installed at Massachusetts General Hospital in 1953. Numerous more devices, including the PET scanner, tomographic positron camera, and other PET instruments, emerged after it in a sequential fashion. It is very useful for therapeutic applications and has the ability to diagnose biological processes within live organisms. The most widely used PET radiotracer is 18-fluorine, and the most often used PET agent is 18F-FDG (radioactive sugar), which is used to stage and restage a variety of malignancies. Accurate whole-body scans are now possible to examine early primary and metastatic diseases because of the advancements in PET technology [12, 13]. It is a novel diagnostic tool that can identify conditions including schizophrenia, cancer, aging, and atherosclerosis, while further advancements in modeling and technology are still needed.

1.2.2.6 Mammography

A form of radiological modality that's mostly employed for breast cancer diagnosis and detection. It includes taking pictures of the breast tissue using low-dose X-rays. Mammography is a commonly used technique for breast cancer screening [14]. The resulting picture, known as mammography, can be used to find any anomalies, like tumors or tissue alterations in the breast. For effective treatment and better results, breast cancer identification is essential early on. More positive outcomes are obtained when 3D mammography is utilized in addition to standard mammography. A problem with mammography is the high rate of false positives, which are abnormalities on a mammogram that turn out not to be malignant. This may cause the patient to get anxious and result in needless biopsies [10]. However, improvements in mammography technology and interpretation have led to a decrease in false positives.

1.2.2.7 Single-Photon Emission Computed Tomography (SPECT)

Using gamma rays, single-photon emission computed tomography (SPECT) is a sophisticated imaging method that produces very accurate three-dimensional (3D) images of things. SPECT is becoming a very useful medical imaging method for both clinical and research settings. Essentially, SPECT creates a three-dimensional representation of the distribution of a radioactive tracer, also known as a probe, that is injected into the circulation and then absorbed by certain organs. SPECT uses high-energy gamma rays to evaluate numerous two-dimensional (2D) pictures from various perspectives. A computer program creates 3D images of the desired body part by reconstructing and recording data [13]. These imaging modalities make it simpler to diagnose a variety of illnesses that are concealed inside the body or beneath the skin. Both patients and medical professionals need to be aware of the many radiology modalities. There are three primary considerations to consider: (1) what is visible, (2) what is necessary to observe, and (3) imaging danger. It's critical to convey that by choosing the right procedure and employing techniques to lower patient exposure without sacrificing clinical efficacy, risks can be managed, and benefits can be optimized. Every modality has distinct advantages and disadvantages, therefore selecting the best one will mostly depend on clear communication. X-ray radiology, positron emission tomography (PET), single-photon emission computed tomography (SPECT), computed tomography (CT), and mammography are examples of radiological imaging techniques that use high-energy X-rays, which can cause excessive radiation doses in certain people. Radiation exposure during radiotherapy can result in the development of cancer, genetic alterations, growth and developmental retardation in the fetus, and abnormalities of the cardiovascular system. Skin damage, redness, cataracts, and hair loss can all result from direct radiation exposure. Although radiographs are typically the first thing that people think of when they think of X-rays, they are also utilized in fluoroscopy and computed tomography (CT), two other significant modalities. Soft tissue contrast resolution is limited in X-ray imaging techniques and X-rays themselves include hazardous ionizing radiation that can cause cell damage [10, 14, 15]. Comparatively speaking, CT scans are less expensive and require a longer post-processing time than X-ray radiography. In addition, there were various adverse consequences of ultrasound, including hormonal changes, very low-frequency chromosomal breaks, chemical reactions, and other health issues. In the medical field, an ultrasound system's drawback is that it produces a lot of heat. Strong ultrasound waves cause tiny cavities to form in the aqueous environment. These cavities then grow, collapse into one another, and release heat. This state that generates heat causes the formation of an unneeded chemical environment. Finding the negative impacts of medical ultrasonography on human health will require ongoing investigation. Ionizing radiation is used in PET and SPECT procedures, rendering the patient radioactive for a variable amount of time. Extra care is required in handling radioactive materials, costly and relatively low spatial resolution [16].

1.3 SMART IMAGING TECHNIQUES FOR DIAGNOSIS

Smart imaging techniques for diagnosis have emerged as a result of recent notable technological developments in the medical imaging industry. These methods transform the way diseases are identified and managed by combining the strength of imaging [17, 18] technology with artificial intelligence (AI). These smart imaging approaches improve patient outcomes by using machine learning (ML) algorithms to provide faster, more accurate, and more tailored diagnosis. The process of visually representing the composition and operation of the various human tissues and organs for clinical purposes and scientific research into the normal and abnormal architecture and physiology of the body is known as medical imaging. Medical imaging methods are used to identify anomalies, cure illnesses, and reveal interior structures hidden behind the skin and bones. Healthcare science [19] has evolved from medical imaging. It's a crucial component of biological imaging and encompasses radiology, which makes use of imaging technologies like thermography, digital mammography, electrical source imaging (ESI), digital mammography, single-photon emission computed tomography (SPECT), endoscopy, magnetic resonance imaging (MRI), magnetic resonance spectroscopy (MRS), positron emission tomography (PET), tactile imaging, magnetic source imaging (MSI), medical optical imaging, and ultrasonic and electrical impedance tomography (EIT).

1.3.1 COMPUTER-AIDED DIAGNOSIS (CAD) SYSTEMS

Different systems for processing and interpreting different kinds of medical images have been created recently in an effort to make the diagnosis work as objectively as feasible. In particular, these technologies make it possible to define human tissues, questionable areas, diseases, etc. and to generate an automatic or semi-automated diagnostic. These systems are called computer-aided diagnosis (CAD). To develop the most accurate diagnosis possible, CAD systems [20] combine the most sophisticated image processing techniques with AI and ML. They have the benefit of being able to recognize pathological alterations that doctors are unable to recognize and of surpassing the boundaries of human memory. Their goal is to raise the standard of patient care. Smart imaging techniques for diagnosis rely heavily on computer-aided diagnosis (CAD) systems. These technologies [21, 22] improve the precision and effectiveness of diagnostic procedures by helping radiologists and physicians analyze medical pictures using sophisticated algorithms and machine learning models. CAD systems are intended to support the identification, description, and categorization of anomalies in medical imaging.

These systems are able to detect minute alterations or anomalies in the images that could point to the existence of illnesses or other problems by applying image processing techniques and pattern recognition algorithms. When it comes to early-stage cancers, such as breast or lung cancer, where early diagnosis is essential for better patient outcomes, CAD systems can be especially helpful. The scientific community has produced two primary types of CAD systems: (i) systems that function by extracting characteristics from human experts, and (ii) systems that autonomously learn the features necessary for pathology discrimination. Although they are not the focus of this work, there exist hybrid systems that rely on both automatically learned features and manually retrieved features from human specialists. Being able to provide radiologists a "second opinion" is one of the main benefits of CAD systems. CAD systems [23] can aid in lowering human error and improving diagnosis accuracy by offering automated analysis and exposing possible problem areas. By comparing their own interpretation with the CAD-generated results, radiologists can make more confident diagnoses and decrease the likelihood of missing problems. Moreover, by ranking cases according to severity or urgency, CAD systems can facilitate the diagnostic procedure. CAD systems can assist radiologists in concentrating their efforts on critical cases, guaranteeing prompt diagnosis and actions, by automatically highlighting worrisome findings. This maximizes the use of healthcare resources while simultaneously improving patient outcomes. It's crucial to remember that CAD systems [24] should be used in conjunction with human expertise, not as a substitute for it. Medical professionals with training still make the final diagnostic and treatment decisions after considering pertinent data such as the patient's clinical history. CAD systems give radiologists and other medical professionals more data and insights to help and improve the diagnostic process. CAD systems are a crucial part of diagnostic smart imaging methods. These technologies help radiologists and physicians understand medical pictures by using sophisticated algorithms and machine learning models. Medical imaging could undergo a revolution thanks to CAD systems' enhanced accuracy, efficiency, and workflow, which would result in more accurate diagnoses and better patient care.

1.3.2 Deep-Learning-Based Approaches for Diagnosis

The application of deep-learning-based techniques has shown great promise in a number of domains, including smart health diagnosis. Advances in computer power and the availability of more health data have made deep learning algorithms more promising in terms of correctly identifying and forecasting medical disorders. The capacity of deep learning [17, 18] to analyze vast volumes of data and spot intricate patterns that conventional approaches might miss is a major benefit for smart health diagnostics. Deep neural networks are trained on large datasets of patient information, medical records, and diagnostic imaging to enable these models to identify minute correlations [19] and generate precise predictions. For example, deep learning algorithms have been created in radiology to interpret medical pictures, including CT, MRI, and X-rays. These algorithms help radiologists diagnose patients more quickly and accurately by automatically spotting anomalies (Figure 1.2).

Deep learning models can learn to extract features from medical images and use those features to identify particular conditions or anomalies by utilizing the capability of convolutional neural networks. The examination of electronic health records (EHRs) is another area where deep-learning-based methods have demonstrated potential. Deep learning algorithms are able to evaluate a patient's medical history, test results, and other pertinent information in order to determine risk factors and forecast the probability of specific diseases. This can support medical professionals in taking proactive measures and offering individualized care. Deep learning models have also been used in mobile applications and wearable technology, allowing for ongoing vital sign monitoring and early health concern diagnosis. These models can notify consumers and healthcare professionals of potential concerns by evaluating real-time data from wearable sensors, enabling prompt intervention. While there are still obstacles to be solved, like protecting the confidentiality and integrity of private health information, deep-learning-based methods have enormous promise to transform smart health diagnosis. These strategies are expected to be extremely important in raising patient care and boosting healthcare outcomes as long as artificial intelligence is integrated and technological breakthroughs continue.

The topic of machine learning approaches in smart health was covered by Rayan et al. in 2019. In this work, they examined recently published articles in the field of smart health from 2011 to 2017 and conducted a systematic analysis [17]

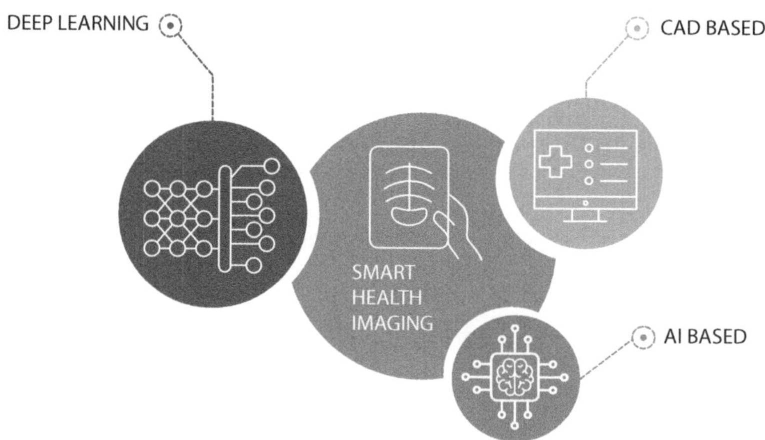

FIGURE 1.2 Smart imaging techniques for diagnosis.

of the various machine learning (ML) techniques used in s-Health. The findings demonstrated the widespread applicability of machine learning (ML) in the field of s-Health, including the diagnosis of glaucoma, Alzheimer's disease, bacterial sepsis, readmissions from the intensive care unit (ICU), and cataract identification. Ahsan et al. gave a summary of machine-learning-based illness diagnosis in 2022. In order to identify the most prolific writers, countries, organizations, and most referenced articles in ML-based disease diagnosis, this work presented a bibliometric analysis of 1216 publications. After that, the review provided an overview of the most current developments and methods in machine-learning-based disease diagnosis (MLBDD), taking into account the types of diseases, algorithms, data, applications, and assessment metrics. Finally, they summarized the main findings and offered insight into potential future trends and possibilities in the field of MLBDD in this study. Recently in 2023, Elseddik et al. (2023) suggested a unique method for predicting, diagnosing, and tracking the course of CTS. There are three primary layers in the suggested architecture. They used three different deep learning (DL) models [24] to diagnose CTS. Their results showed that the suggested method performs better on several evaluation criteria, including accuracy (0.969%), precision (0.982%), and recall (0.963%). In order to predict how the disease would advance while receiving therapy, the second layer employs machine learning (ML) models to estimate the cross-sectional area (CSA) at one, three, and six months. Rahman et al. examined federated learning-based (FL) artificial intelligence (AI) methods in smart healthcare in 2023. They provided a thorough review of FL utilizing AI for intelligent healthcare [25] applications in their work. They talked about the state of the healthcare system and modern conceptions of developing technologies like FL, AI, and explainable AI (XAI). They categorized and combined healthcare technology in many sectors utilizing FL–AI. They also addressed the issues that are now facing the healthcare industry, such as security, privacy, stability, and dependability.

1.3.3 AI IN SMART IMAGING DIAGNOSIS

In the area of smart imaging diagnosis, artificial intelligence (AI) has become a game-changing technology that is transforming healthcare by increasing patient outcomes, efficiency, and accuracy. Artificial intelligence (AI) algorithms can help medical personnel diagnose patients more quickly and accurately because of their capacity to evaluate large volumes of medical imaging data. Deep learning algorithms are used by AI-powered smart imaging diagnosis systems to process and interpret medical pictures, including X-rays, CT scans, and MRIs. Because these algorithms are trained on massive datasets, they may identify patterns and anomalies that might be hard for human eyes to notice. Artificial intelligence (AI) systems can offer important insights and help in the early diagnosis of diseases including cancer, cardiovascular ailments, and neurological disorders by comparing new photos to this acquired information.

The capacity of AI to supplement radiologists' and other healthcare professionals' experience is one of the technology's main benefits for smart imaging diagnosis. Artificial intelligence (AI) technologies can serve as a "second set of eyes," helping to decrease diagnostic errors and provide more reliable and impartial results. This helps save healthcare costs and optimize resource allocation in addition to improving patient care. AI is also making image analysis in smart imaging diagnostics faster and more effective. Radiologists typically take a long time to examine and analyze medical imaging. By automatically evaluating photos and identifying any anomalies for additional examination, AI algorithms can speed up this procedure. Radiologists can concentrate on more complex patients and give urgent diagnosis priority as a result of the time savings.

AI-enabled healthcare delivery was proposed by Reddy et al. in 2019. The study demonstrated [17] how artificial intelligence (AI)-enabled systems might be created by conducting a realistic evaluation of existing AI technology and anticipated advancements. A survey on the use of artificial intelligence in disease diagnostics was presented by Kumar et al. in 2022. They discussed the extensive survey that used artificial intelligence methods [19] to diagnose a wide range of illnesses, including diabetes, Alzheimer's, cancer, chronic heart disease, TB, stroke, cerebrovascular disease, hypertension, skin, and liver problems. Along with the medical imaging dataset they employed and their feature extraction and classification procedure for predictions, they also carried out a thorough survey. In their research published in 2022, Chen et al. addressed the role of data and AI in smart healthcare. In this article, information fusion research [26] for healthcare using artificial intelligence was described methodically and the state of the art was comprehended. To identify the main research subjects discussed in 351 pertinent articles, structural topic modeling was used. Even with all of the advantages, there are drawbacks to using AI in smart imaging diagnosis. Since sensitive patient information is contained in medical imaging data, data privacy and security must be guaranteed. To guarantee excellent accuracy and dependability, AI algorithms must also be carefully developed and validated. The use of AI in smart imaging diagnostics has improved patient outcomes, efficiency, and accuracy—a revolution in healthcare. AI systems may evaluate medical imagery, help medical practitioners diagnose patients, and speed up the decision-making process by utilizing deep learning algorithms. AI has the potential to further revolutionize the field of smart imaging diagnostics with future study and development, opening the door to more individualized and accurate treatment.

1.4 SMART IMAGING TECHNIQUES FOR TREATMENT PLANNING

1.4.1 IMAGE-GUIDED THERAPY AND INTERVENTION

In the sphere of healthcare, image-guided therapy and intervention has become a ground-breaking area that is transforming the planning and execution of medical procedures. Image-guided treatments allow medical practitioners to more accurately target and treat diseases with less invasiveness by fusing cutting-edge imaging technologies with real-time visualization and navigation systems. The idea behind image-guided therapy is to provide precise and detailed images of the patient's anatomy using medical imaging technologies [21, 22] including CT, MRI, and ultrasound. During surgical procedures, these images act as a guide for doctors, making it easier for them to precisely navigate through intricate anatomical systems. Physicians can accurately guide their instruments and make sure the treatment is administered to the appropriate region by seeing the target area in real time. The potential of image-guided therapy to enable minimally invasive procedures is one of its main advantages. Physicians can execute surgeries through small incisions with the help of imaging technologies, which lessens physical trauma to the patient and expedites their recovery. This method is very helpful for sensitive regions including the blood arteries, brain, and spine. Moreover, real-time monitoring and feedback are possible during operations with image-guided therapy. Doctors can monitor the treatment region in real time to see how the intervention is going and modify their strategy as needed. This prompt response reduces the possibility of problems or insufficient treatment, improving operation safety and effectiveness.

1.4.2 SURGICAL PLANNING AND NAVIGATION

The way surgical treatments are planned and carried [27, 28] out has been revolutionized by surgical planning and navigation, which have become essential tools in contemporary healthcare. Surgical planning and navigation improve accuracy, yield better results, and lower risks for patients undergoing complex surgical procedures by utilizing computer-aided systems and modern imaging technology. Obtaining comprehensive medical images, such as CT, MRI, or 3D reconstructions, is the first step in the surgical planning process. Surgeons are given a thorough insight into the anatomy of the patient as well as the particular area of interest by these photographs. Surgeons can plan the best course of action, practically mimic the procedure, and foresee any obstacles or issues with the use of specialist software. During this phase of preoperative preparation, surgeons can plan, choose the best surgical equipment, and streamline the surgical procedure. Surgical navigation systems become operational once the surgical plan is established. To assist surgeons throughout the process, these devices make use of real-time imaging [29] and tracking technologies. Surgeons can precisely visualize the placement of target areas and important structures by superimposing the patient's anatomy onto the operating field. This raises overall operation safety, increases precision, and lowers the possibility of damaging nearby tissues. Surgeons can track their progress and make any necessary adjustments thanks to real-time input from surgical navigation. In order to make sure surgical instruments are traveling along the intended course, these devices can track the position and orientation of the instruments. The surgeon can make quick adjustments and reduce mistakes by using the navigation system's notifications to notify them of deviations.

1.4.3 3D PRINTING AND BIOPRINTING FOR PATIENT-SPECIFIC TREATMENT

Rapidly developing technologies like bioprinting and 3D printing have enormous potential for patient-specific healthcare therapy. The field of personalized medicine is being revolutionized by these cutting-edge procedures that enable the fabrication of individualized implants, medicinal equipment, and even functional human tissues. The process of creating three-dimensional objects layer by layer using digital models is known as 3D printing. It permits the manufacturing of surgical equipment, prostheses, and implants customized for individual patients in the medical field. These devices can be customized to meet each patient's specific needs and anatomy by using imaging data from scans such as MRIs and CT scans. This personalization raises patient happiness and comfort levels, lowers problems, and improves treatment results. By employing bioinks—materials made of live cells—to construct functional human tissues and organs, bioprinting advances 3D printing. Bioprinting allows for the exact layer-by-layer creation of complex biological structures by depositing the bioinks. The lack of organ donors may be addressed by this technology, which also offers substitutes for organ transplants. Moreover, bioprinting creates opportunities for disease modeling, medication testing, and regenerative medicine. The fusion of 3D printing and bioprinting enables the production of tissues and implants tailored to each patient's own anatomy and physiology. This individualized strategy improves patient recovery, lowers the chance of rejection, and improves treatment outcomes. Furthermore, these technologies make it possible to produce medical equipment and tissues more quickly and affordably, increasing their accessibility to people who require them.

1.5   PRACTICAL, LEGAL, AND ETHICAL CONSIDERATIONS IN MEDICAL IMAGING

In many ways, the amount of data obtained by the new medical imaging techniques was greater than what we could have stored, transmitted, and used to create the images. The medical field has created network systems for the storing, processing, recall, and remote location of these diagnostic images thanks to advancements in computer technology and a decrease in the cost of memory and other hardware. This information covers a wide range of health-related topics, such as a patient's past, present, and future diagnoses, treatments, and prescriptions [30]. X-rays and mammograms are examples of electronic/digital images that could be included in this data. Gathering, storing, organizing, retrieving, using, disseminating, and consulting data are all included in data processing. Processing this data is essential since errors and misuse could have negative effects on patients, healthcare providers, and researchers. Medical personnel may be subject to legal repercussions for malpractice if their patient's medical records contain erroneous information, which may lead to a misdiagnosis. As a result, issues with confidentiality and access have grown in significance [31]. It is crucial to comprehend the ethical precepts that guide the medical field as well as the corresponding legal safeguards in order to preserve electronic medical data and keep patients, healthcare providers, and researchers safe. It's important to realize that different photos require different amounts of storage and retrieval. Large-scale imaging diagnostic studies may result in the storing of data that is never retrieved or put to use in a medical setting. More information that is relevant to diagnosis can be found in some photos than in others. The preservation of patient confidentiality and privacy is related to the security issue. Security levels are not the only factor that affects data integrity [30–32]. Safely stored data is more likely to retain its integrity because it is less susceptible to unauthorized or unintentional human intervention. To correctly recognize any health issues or to understand related and pertinent text, the image's material quality is undoubtedly crucial. Technical limitations on image expansion, reduction, or compression may improve the quality of the material in some cases, but they may negatively impact other areas of quality, usability, and accessibility. To lessen the need for additional technological adjustments and the possibility of changing the quality and content of the information, compatible file formats are crucial. The perspective and capacity for interpretation may be impacted by the various medical practices used by various cultures [32].

1.6 FUTURE DIRECTIONS AND CHALLENGES

Developments in artificial intelligence, machine learning, and technology integration are among the future paths that smart medical imaging will follow. Standardization, data protection, interoperability, and cost-effectiveness are among the difficulties.

1.6.1 EMERGING TRENDS IN SMART MEDICAL IMAGING

By increasing patient care, enabling more individualized therapies, and boosting diagnostic accuracy, emerging trends in smart medical imaging [33] are completely changing the healthcare industry. These trends make use of technological breakthroughs like cloud computing, machine learning, and artificial intelligence (AI) to improve the capabilities of medical imaging systems. The incorporation of artificial intelligence and machine learning algorithms is a significant rising trend in smart medical imaging. Medical imaging systems can learn to identify trends, spot anomalies, and help radiologists diagnose patients accurately by training these algorithms on big datasets. AI-powered picture analysis can offer important insights for treatment planning and assist in spotting early symptoms of diseases like cancer. The application of cloud computing to medical imaging [34] is another trend. Large volumes of medical imaging data can be securely and scalable stored on cloud platforms, giving healthcare providers in multiple places easy access to the data. Furthermore, real-time cooperation and distant consultations are made possible by cloud-based image analysis tools, which boost productivity and facilitate multidisciplinary decision-making. Another developing trend in smart medical imaging is the use of 3D and 4D imaging methods. These methods offer more thorough and in-depth knowledge of physiological functions and anatomical structures, which improves the visualization and comprehension of complicated illnesses. 3D and 4D imaging can help with precise treatment area targeting, surgical planning, and intervention guidance. Additionally, smart medical imaging is becoming more and more integrated with other technologies, such as augmented reality and robotics. More accurate and minimally invasive operations [35] are made possible by robotic-assisted interventions guided by real-time imaging. By superimposing medical pictures on the operating area, augmented reality helps surgeons by giving them real-time instruction and improving accuracy. Healthcare is being revolutionized by recent developments in smart medical imaging, including AI integration, cloud computing, better imaging techniques, and integration with other technology. These developments lead to more accurate diagnoses, more individualized treatments, and enhanced capabilities of medical imaging equipment. More breakthroughs and enhancements in smart medical imaging are probably in store as long as these fields continue to be researched and developed.

1.6.2 POTENTIAL IMPACT OF SMART IMAGING ON HEALTHCARE

There is a huge and broad potential influence of smart imaging on healthcare. The delivery of healthcare could be completely changed by smart imaging, which combines cutting-edge technology including cloud computing, machine learning, and artificial intelligence (AI). A major possible benefit of smart imaging is increased diagnostic precision. Smart imaging systems can scan enormous volumes of medical imaging [36, 37] data and spot patterns and abnormalities that might be challenging for human eyes to see by utilizing AI algorithms. As a result, patients may receive earlier and more precise diagnoses, which may allow for prompt interventions and better patient outcomes. Additionally, smart imaging may improve patient safety and care. Smart imaging technologies can help medical personnel precisely target treatment regions, lower the risk of problems, and minimize tissue damage by offering real-time imagery and navigation during procedures. Additionally, by customizing interventions to each patient's specific needs based on their anatomical features, smart imaging can support individualized treatment strategies. Further possible results of smart imaging are cost and efficiency savings.

Smart imaging technologies can optimize resource allocation and save healthcare workers' time by automating repetitive processes and optimizing workflows. Additionally, cloud computing integration makes it simple to access and share medical imaging data, which facilitates cooperation, remote consultations, and more effective healthcare delivery. Smart imaging has a huge potential impact on healthcare. Smart imaging has the ability to improve patient care, increase efficiency, and improve diagnostic accuracy, to name a few advantages for the healthcare sector. Smart imaging technology usage, research, and development hold enormous promise for revolutionizing healthcare and enhancing patient outcomes.

1.6.3 OVERCOMING CHALLENGES AND BARRIERS TO ADOPTION

The effective integration of cutting-edge technology, such as smart imaging, in healthcare, depends on overcoming obstacles and hurdles to acceptance. These technologies have a lot of potential uses, but there are a few issues that need to be resolved first. Within the healthcare sector, resistance to change is one of the main obstacles. A change in perspective, workflows, and conventional procedures is necessary for the adoption of new technology. As they are worried about trust, dependability, and possible interruptions to their daily routines, healthcare professionals [29, 38] could be reluctant to adopt new technologies. To overcome resistance and promote acceptance, it is imperative to address these issues through instruction, training, and transparent communication.

The integration and interoperability of smart imaging technologies with the current healthcare infrastructure present another challenge. For effective data interchange and decision-making, seamless integration with electronic health records (EHRs) and other healthcare information systems is essential. To tackle these interoperability issues, standardization initiatives, partnerships between technology developers and healthcare providers, and infrastructural expenditures are required. Adoption is also hampered by worries about data security and privacy. As medical imaging data is very sensitive, it needs to be shielded from breaches and unwanted access. Building confidence and tackling [39] these issues requires putting in place strong security measures, adhering to legislation, and making sure patient consent and privacy are protected. Financial factors may hinder the extensive integration of intelligent imaging technologies. Costs associated with implementation, equipment upgrades, and training can be major obstacles, especially in healthcare settings with limited resources. These financial obstacles can be addressed with the use of incentives, cooperation between technology companies and healthcare providers, and transparent cost-benefit evaluations. It is imperative that obstacles and hurdles to adoption are overcome before smart imaging technologies may be successfully incorporated into healthcare. Important stages toward wider acceptance include resolving resistance to change, guaranteeing interoperability, addressing concerns about data privacy and security, and weighing the financial ramifications. The successful use of smart imaging technology can be facilitated by stakeholder collaboration, education and training programs, and supporting legislation. This will ultimately improve patient care and results.

1.7   CONCLUSIONS

To sum up, the development of intelligent medical imaging has great promise for transforming healthcare in a variety of ways. More opportunities for precise diagnosis, individualized treatment regimens, and better patient outcomes have arisen with the integration of artificial intelligence and machine learning algorithms into medical imaging technologies. Enhancing early disease identification and diagnosis is one of the main advantages of intelligent medical imaging. Medical personnel can swiftly and reliably examine enormous amounts of imaging data with the use of AI algorithms, which can help identify diseases early on that may have gone undetected otherwise. The prognosis for patients and the likelihood of a successful course of treatment can both be greatly enhanced by this early identification. Personalized treatment plans can also be developed with the help of clever medical imaging.

AI algorithms can assist in customizing therapy options for specific patients by evaluating imaging data, medical history, genetic information, and other pertinent criteria. This increases the effectiveness of the medication while lowering the likelihood of side effects and unneeded procedures. Enhancing workflow efficiency in healthcare settings is another possible benefit of intelligent medical imaging. Medical personnel can focus on more important patient care aspects and save time by automating repetitive operations like picture interpretation and report generation. Patients may have shorter wait times as a result, and healthcare facilities may operate more efficiently overall. Nonetheless, it's critical to recognize the difficulties in putting intelligent medical imaging into practice. Obstacles that must be overcome include worries about privacy and security, ethical issues, and the requirement for medical practitioners to have continual training and education. To sum up, the development of intelligent medical imaging has enormous potential to completely transform healthcare. We may anticipate better patient outcomes, individualized treatment regimens, and more precise diagnoses thanks to the application of AI and machine learning. Even though there are obstacles to overcome, the advantages are too great to pass up. When intelligent medical imaging technologies are integrated, the future of healthcare appears more promising.

REFERENCES

1. Suetens, P. (2017). *Fundamentals of Medical Imaging.* Cambridge University Press.
2. Beutel, J. (2000). *Handbook of Medical Imaging* (Vol. 3). Spie Press.
3. Louis, A. K. (1992). Medical imaging: State of the art and future development. *Inverse Problems*, 8(5), 709.
4. Erickson, B. J., Korfiatis, P., Akkus, Z., & Kline, T. L. (2017). Machine learning for medical imaging. *Radiographics*, 37(2), 505–515.
5. Suzuki, K. (2017). Overview of deep learning in medical imaging. *Radiological Physics and Technology*, 10(3), 257–273.
6. Lin, E. C. (2010, December). Radiation risk from medical imaging. In *Mayo Clinic Proceedings*, H. P. Adams, Jr.(ed.), (Vol. 85, No. 12, pp. 1142–1146). Elsevier.
7. Dey, N., Ashour, A. S., & Bhatt, C. (2017). Internet of things driven connected healthcare. In *Internet of Things and Big Data Technologies for Next Generation Healthcare*, C. Bhatt, N. Dey, and , A. S. Ashour(eds.), (pp. 3–12).
8. Dey, N., Ashour, A. S., Shi, F., Fong, S. J., & Tavares, J. M. R. (2018). Medical cyber-physical systems: A survey. *Journal of Medical Systems*, 42(4), 1–13.
9. Pham, D. L., Xu, C., & Prince, J. L. (2000). Current methods in medical image segmentation. *Annual Review of Biomedical Engineering*, 2(1), 315–337.
10. Hussain, S., Mubeen, I., Ullah, N., Shah, S. S. U. D., Khan, B. A., Zahoor, M., ... Sultan, M. A. (2022). Modern diagnostic imaging technique applications and risk factors in the medical field: A review. *BioMed Research International*, 2022, 1–19.
11. Elhayatmy, G., Dey, N., & Ashour, A. S. (2018). Internet of Things based wireless body area network in healthcare. In *Internet of Things and Big Data Analytics Toward Next-Generation Intelligence*, N. Dey, A. Ella Hassanien, C. Bhatt, A. S. Ashour, and S. C. Satapathy(eds.),3–20. Springer.
12. Jaiswal, S. (2018). Applications and comparison of medical imaging modalities. *International Journal of Engineering and Science Invention*, 7(1), 94–100.
13. Malcius, D., Jonkus, M., Kuprionis, G., Maleckas, A., Monastyreckienė, E., Uktveris, R., ... Barauskas, V. (2009). The accuracy of different imaging techniques in diagnosis of acute hematogenous osteomyelitis. *Medicina*, 45(8), 624.
14. Kasban, H., El-Bendary, M. A. M., & Salama, D. H. (2015). A comparative study of medical imaging techniques. *International Journal of Information Science and Intelligent System*, 4(2), 37–58.
15. Chaki, J., Dey, N., & De, D. (Eds.). (2020). *Smart Biosensors in Medical Care.* Academic Press.

16. Guetari, R., Ayari, H., & Sakly, H. (2023). Computer-aided diagnosis systems: A comparative study of classical machine learning versus deep learning-based approaches. *Knowledge and Information Systems*, 65, 3881–3921. doi:10.1007/s10115-023-01894-7.

17. Rayan, Z., Alfonse, M., & Salem, A.-B. M. (2019). Machine learning approaches in smart health. *Procedia Computer Science*, 154, 361–368. doi:10.1016/j.procs.2019.06.052.

18. Ahsan, M. M., Luna, S. A., & Siddique, Z. (2022). Machine-learning-based disease diagnosis: A comprehensive review. *Healthcare*, 10(3), 541. doi:10.3390/healthcare10030541.

19. Kumar, Y., Koul, A., Singla, R., & Ijaz, M. F. (2023). Artificial intelligence in disease diagnosis: A systematic literature review, synthesizing framework and future research agenda. *Journal of Ambient Intelligence and Humanized Computing*, 14(7), 8459–8486. doi:10.1007/s12652-021-03612-z. Epub 2022 Jan 13. PMID: 35039756; PMCID: PMC8754556.

20. Fujita, H., Uchiyama, Y., Nakagawa, T., Fukuoka, D., Hatanaka, Y., Hara, T., Lee, G. N., Hayashi, Y., Ikedo, Y., Gao, X., & Zhou, X. (2008). Computer-aided diagnosis: The emerging of three CAD systems induced by Japanese health care needs. *Computer Methods and Programs in Biomedicine*, 92(3), 238–248.

21. Rizzi, M., D'Aloia, M., Guaragnella, C., & Castagnolo, B. (2012 October 12). Health care improvement: Comparative analysis of two CAD systems in mammographic screening. *IEEE Transactions on Systems, Man, and Cybernetics,-Part A: Systems and Humans*, 42(6), 1385–1395.

22. Rizzi, M., Matteo, D., & Castagnolo, B. (2012 June 1). Health care CAD systems for breast microcalcification cluster detection. *Journal of Medical and Biological Engineering*, 32(3), 147–156.

23. Reddy, S., Fox, J., & Purohit, M. P. (2019). Artificial intelligence-enabled healthcare delivery. *Journal of the Royal Society of Medicine*, 112(1), 22–28. doi:10.1177/0141076818815510.

24. Elseddik, M., Mostafa, R. R., Elashry, A., El-Rashidy, N., El-Sappagh, S., Elgamal, S., & El-Bakry, H. (2023). Predicting CTS diagnosis and prognosis based on machine learning techniques. *Diagnostics*, 13(3), 492.

25. Rahman, A., Hossain, M. S., Muhammad, G., Kundu, D., Debnath, T., Rahman, M., Khan, M. S. I., Tiwari, P., & Band, S. S. (2023). Federated learning-based AI approaches in smart healthcare: Concepts, taxonomies, challenges and open issues. *Cluster Computing*, 26(4), 2271–2311.

26. Chen, X., Xie, H., Li, Z., Cheng, G., Leng, M., & Wang, F. L. (2023). Information fusion and artificial intelligence for smart healthcare: A bibliometric study. *Information Processing and Management*, 60(1), 103113.

27. Mezger, U., Jendrewski, C., & Bartels, M. (2013). Navigation in surgery. *Langenbeck's Archives of Surgery*, 398(4), 501–514.

28. Shaikh, T. A., Dar, T. R., & Sofi, S. (2022). A data-centric artificial intelligent and extended reality technology in smart healthcare systems. *Social Network Analysis and Mining*, 12(1), 122.

29. Wang, D., Ma, D., Wong, M. L., & Wáng, Y. X. J. (2015). Recent advances in surgical planning & navigation for tumor biopsy and resection. *Quantitative Imaging in Medicine and Surgery*, 5(5), 640.

30. Davis, K. D., Flor, H., Greely, H. T., Iannetti, G. D., Mackey, S., Ploner, M., ... Wager, T. D. (2017). Brain imaging tests for chronic pain: Medical, legal and ethical issues and recommendations. *Nature Reviews. Neurology*, 13(10), 624–638.

31. Malone, J. (2020). X-rays for medical imaging: Radiation protection, governance and ethics over 125 years. *Physica Medica*, 79, 47–64.

32. Malone, J. F. (2008). New ethical issues for radiation protection in diagnostic radiology. *Radiation Protection Dosimetry*, 129(1–3), 6–12.

33. Ehrenhard, M., Kijl, B., & Nieuwenhuis, L. (2014). Market adoption barriers of multi-stakeholder technology: Smart homes for the aging population. *Technological Forecasting and Social Change*, 89, 306–315.
34. Umirzakova, S., Ahmad, S., Khan, L. U., & Whangbo, T. (2023). Medical image super-resolution for smart healthcare applications: A comprehensive survey. *Information Fusion*, 103(C), 102075.
35. Yan, F., Li, N., Iliyasu, A. M., Salama, A. S., & Hirota, K. (2023). Insights into security and privacy issues in smart healthcare systems based on medical images. *Journal of Information Security and Applications*, 78, 103621.
36. Mukherjee, A., Mukherjee, P., De, D., & Dey, N. (2021). QoS-aware 6G-enabled ultra low latency edge-assisted Internet of drone things for real-time stride analysis. *Computers and Electrical Engineering*, 95, 107438.
37. Misra, B., Roy, N. D., Dey, N., & Sherratt, R. S. (2023). Visualizing wearable medical device research trends: A co-occurrence network based bibliometric analysis. *Galician Medical Journal*, 30(3), 202–222.
38. Tripathi, G., Ahad, M. A., & Paiva, S. (2020, March). S2HS-A blockchain based approach for smart healthcare system. In *Healthcare*, J. Stevens(ed.), (Vol. 8, No. 1, p. 100391). Elsevier.
39. Alaiad, A., & Zhou, L. (2017). Patients' adoption of WSN-based smart home health-care systems: An integrated model of facilitators and barriers. *IEEE Transactions on Professional Communication*, 60(1), 4–23.

Part II

Impact of AI in Healthcare, Medical Diagnosis, and Treatment

2 Role of AI for Smart Health Diagnosis and Treatment

Priyanka Gupta and Manoj Kumar Pandey

2.1 INTRODUCTION

Medical diagnosis is one of the major areas of concern for everyone, and everyone wants to improve the medical diagnosis system. Technology plays an important role in medical diagnosis and integrating these technologies with medical diagnosis may lead to good results. Artificial intelligence (AI) is a field which has proven its extended capabilities for better medical diagnosis. AI techniques range from traditional models to deep learning models. The use of AI is to provide better medical care for society and the nation. AI uses a number of machine learning algorithms like support vector machine (SVM) [1], linear discriminate analysis (LDA) [2, 3], artificial neural network (ANN) [4], convolutional neural networks (CNNs) [5] etc. which have shown better results in terms of accuracy and speed. Medical image recognition is also an important tool for the early prediction of various diseases like brain tumours, cancers, etc. Medical treatments produce a large amount of data ranging from patient's heartbeat to scanning data. The amount of data produced during the diagnosis is huge, and therefore big data management is required so that clinical decisions can be made easily. Clinical data is also needed the most to train the given machine learning models, and the more the data available for training the more accurately ML model can predict diseases. Artificial intelligence (AI) has ushered in a transformative era in the medical field, empowering healthcare professionals with intelligent algorithms and machine learning techniques that significantly enhance accurate diagnosis and effective treatment planning. The integration of AI applications has revolutionized medical outcomes and patient care by leveraging sophisticated technologies such as natural language processing (NLP) and image recognition. In this chapter, we delve into the diverse range of AI applications that have propelled medical advancements to new heights. One of the key breakthroughs facilitated by AI is the capability to analyse medical images with remarkable precision.

Image recognition algorithms like scale invariant feature transform (SIFT) [6, 7], speeded up robust features (SURF) [8], principal component analysis (PCA) [9, 10] and linear discriminate analysis (LDA) [2, 3] enable the detection of anomalies, tumours, and other critical indicators, empowering radiologists and clinicians to make accurate diagnoses and treatment decisions. Identifying a given pattern in order to identify a disease is an important task in process of identification and diagnosis. Additionally, natural language processing (NLP) [11] techniques enable the extraction of relevant information from vast amounts of unstructured clinical data, improving the efficiency of data analysis and facilitating evidence-based decision-making.

The advent of big data analytics has further revolutionized healthcare management by enabling comprehensive data collection, storage, and data analysis. The integration of large-scale datasets has the potential to transform clinical decision-making by providing healthcare professionals with valuable insights and patterns that were previously inaccessible. By leveraging big data patterns, healthcare systems can identify trends, predict disease outbreaks, and optimize treatment strategies to deliver better patient outcomes. While the benefits of leveraging data for healthcare are immense, it is essential to address crucial issues like data privacy and security. Healthcare information is highly sensitive and subject to strict privacy regulations.

The proliferation of wearable medical devices has empowered one to monitor their health in real time and actively participate in their well-being. These devices, ranging from smartwatches and fitness trackers to biosensors, collect valuable patient data and facilitate remote monitoring. The analysis of this data allows for early detection of health issues, enabling timely intervention and personalized feedback to improve self-management. Wearable devices hold immense potential in transforming healthcare from reactive to proactive, shifting the focus from treating diseases to preventing them altogether. In addition to wearable devices, bio-signals and telemedicine have emerged as key components of modern healthcare delivery. Bio-signals, such as electrocardiograms and brain activity measurements, provide vital diagnostic information that aid in the identification and monitoring of various health conditions. Furthermore, telemedicine has bridged the gap between patients and healthcare professionals, enabling remote consultations and continuous monitoring. This capability is particularly crucial in remote areas or during emergencies, ensuring that individuals receive timely and quality care.

The extensive use of AI techniques has opened up various dimensions for medical diagnosis; e.g. telemedicine is among the prevailing technologies today. In telemedicine, medicine is prescribed to the remote patient by applying various technologies like IoT, wearable devices, remote monitoring etc. Now it is no longer needed to be present physically for medical diagnosis and treatment.

The integration of AI, big data analytics, wearable devices, bio-signals, and telemedicine has the capacity to revolutionize different aspects of healthcare. From treatment and diagnostic personalization to efficient management and improved patient experiences, these innovative solutions hold the promise of enhancing medical practices and delivering better healthcare outcomes. By leveraging advanced technological solutions, we can navigate the complexities of modern healthcare, improve patient care, and ultimately shape a healthier future. In the subsequent sections of this chapter, we will delve into the particular uses and consequences of artificial intelligence, big data analytics, wearable devices, bio-signals, and telemedicine in transforming healthcare. Through in-depth analysis and examination of case studies, our goal is to offer perspectives on the possible advantages and difficulties linked with these advancements. Ultimately, our goal is to foster a comprehensive understanding of how advanced technological solutions can shape the future of healthcare, optimize clinical decision-making, and improve patient outcomes.

This chapter emphasizes the importance of utilizing AI for medical diagnosis and implementing robust data protection measures to guarantee the confidentiality, integrity, and accessibility of healthcare data. By maintaining strict data privacy and security protocols, healthcare organizations can build trust and foster a secure environment for the utilization of advanced technologies for better treatments.

2.2 ROLE OF AI IN HEALTH DIAGNOSIS AND TREATMENT

This section will explore the role of artificial intelligence in health diagnosis and treatment. The section is further divided into various sub-sections that discuss the impact of AI in health diagnosis using some of the recent related works.

2.2.1 MEDICAL IMAGING AND ITS IMPACT ON DIAGNOSTICS

There are many medical imaging techniques available, such as image recognition, image scanning, computed tomography, nuclear medicine etc. One of the key AI applications in healthcare is image recognition, which has had a profound impact on diagnostics. AI algorithms such as deep learning models like convolutional neural networks (CNNs) [12–21] have demonstrated exceptional capabilities in analysing medical images with remarkable accuracy and efficiency. Image recognition algorithms enable the detection of abnormalities, such as tumours, lesions, and fractures, aiding in early detection and precise diagnosis.

The integration of AI in medical imaging has significantly improved diagnostic accuracy, resulting in better patient outcomes. Bastani et al. [22] provide insights and considerations for medical practitioners regarding the development and utilization of AI-powered medical image recognition using smartphone-based applications. The chapter underscores the potential benefits of these applications in enhancing diagnostic capabilities and improving patient care. It emphasizes the need for careful consideration of limitations, validation, regulatory compliance, and ethical implications when implementing AI in healthcare. AI-powered [23] medical imaging has significantly improved diagnostic accuracy across various specialities.

Deep learning models can analyse large volumes of medical images and learn complex patterns, aiding in the identification of diseases at an early stage. These models have demonstrated high sensitivity and specificity in diagnosing conditions like cancer, cardiovascular diseases, and neurological disorders. Collaboration between medical practitioners and AI developers is essential to ensure the successful integration and effective utilization of AI technologies in medical practice.

Further research and development in this field will continue to shape the future of AI-powered medical image recognition smartphone applications and their impact on healthcare. The critical review done by Susanto et al. [23] provides valuable insights into the current state and prospects of smartphone-based imaging systems for medical applications. Smartphone technology has the potential to democratize access to medical imaging and transform healthcare delivery.

By addressing the limitations and challenges outlined in this review, smartphone-based imaging systems can enhance diagnostic capabilities, improve patient outcomes, and expand access to quality healthcare, particularly in resource-limited settings. Continued innovation and collaboration will play a crucial role in harnessing the full potential of smartphones in medical imaging.

2.2.2 Natural Language Processing for Efficient Data Analysis

Hunt et al. [24] provide an insightful overview of NLP applications in smart healthcare. By leveraging NLP techniques, healthcare professionals can extract valuable insights from unstructured clinical data, improve information retrieval, enhance clinical decision-making, and facilitate personalized healthcare. While challenges exist, the chapter highlights the potential for continued advancement and interdisciplinary collaboration to overcome these obstacles and fully realize the benefits of NLP in smart healthcare environments.

Natural language processing (NLP) [11, 17] techniques have played a vital role in healthcare by enabling efficient analysis of unstructured clinical data. NLP algorithms can extract expressive information from clinical texts, such as electronic health records (EHR), research articles, and patient reports. This enables healthcare professionals to process huge volumes of textual data, identify relevant patterns, and extract valuable insights for decision-making. NLP facilitates data-driven approaches to healthcare management and research, improving efficiency and accuracy.

Zhou et al. [25] begin by highlighting the increasing availability of EHR and other textual data in primary healthcare. They discuss how NLP techniques can be applied to extract meaningful facts from unstructured clinical narratives, facilitating efficient information retrieval and analysis. The chapter explores various NLP applications in primary healthcare, including named entity recognition, information extraction, clinical decision support, and patient monitoring.

Uddin et al. [26] emphasize the application of NLP to extract valuable data from unstructured clinical narratives, facilitating efficient information retrieval and analysis. The chapter explores various NLP applications in primary healthcare, such as named entity recognition, information extraction, clinical decision support, and patient monitoring. Moreover, the chapter highlights the transformative potential of integrating big data analytics into digital health services. By utilizing advanced analytics techniques, healthcare providers can derive actionable insights from extensive digital health data, resulting in improved decision-making, personalized care, and better patient outcomes.

The chapter emphasizes the importance of ongoing research, technological advancements, and collaboration among researchers, healthcare providers, policymakers, and data scientists to overcome challenges and fully leverage the benefits of big data analytics in enhancing health services. Figure 2.1 shows the role of NLP in medical diagnosis.

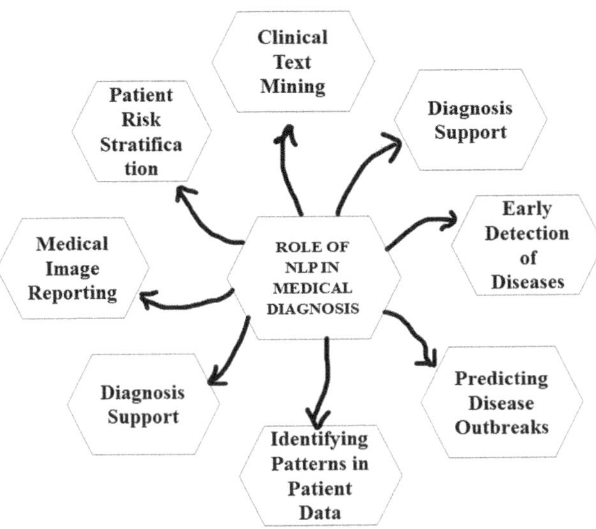

FIGURE 2.1 Role of NLP in medical diagnosis.

2.2.3 AI-Driven Decision Support Systems

AI-driven decision support systems [18, 19] leverage machine learning algorithms to provide healthcare professionals with valuable insights and recommendations for clinical decision-making. These systems analyse patient data, medical records, and relevant research to generate personalized treatment options, predict outcomes, and offer evidence-based guidance. AI-driven decision support systems have the prospective to advance the accuracy, efficiency, and consistency of clinical decisions, leading to enhanced patient care and better healthcare outcomes.

Berros et al. [27] indicate that the available evidence regarding the efficacy of AI in result-making in health and social care surroundings is scarce and conflicting. This inconsistency in findings may stem from the diverse contexts in which these technologies are implemented. The analysis pinpointed a limited selection of pertinent studies marked by considerable differences in technologies, quality, settings, and outcome. Notably none of the studies focused on social care settings, and there was a lack of investigation into the facilitators and barriers surrounding the use of data-driven AI for decision support.

While the methodology used for the review might be considered novel in a field where robust empirical evidence is still evolving, it has offered valuable perspectives on how the current evidence should be understood in this crucial yet evolving area. Consequently, further research is required to evaluate the efficacy of data-driven AI-based clinical decision support, expanding upon the discoveries made in this review.

The systematic review conducted by Cresswell et al. [28] includes a comprehensive analysis of various studies that have explored the use of AI in cardiovascular

ICUs. The review encompasses studies on arrhythmia detection, hemodynamic monitoring, predicting adverse events, and risk stratification. The authors evaluate the methodologies, outcomes, and limitations to assess the effectiveness and potential of AI in clinical decision support for cardiovascular ICU patients. The findings of the systematic review indicate that AI-based approaches have shown promising results in several areas of cardiovascular ICU patient monitoring. These include early detection of arrhythmias, predicting cardiac events, and providing personalized treatment recommendations. However, the authors note the need for further validation and standardization of AI models, as well as addressing challenges related to data quality, interpretability, and integration with existing clinical workflows.

2.2.4 AI-ASSISTED ROBOTIC SURGERY

AI has revolutionized [20, 21] the field of surgery by assisting in robotic surgical procedures. AI algorithms analyse preoperative images, surgical plans, and real-time feedback to guide the robotic surgical systems. By enhancing precision, reducing invasiveness, and providing real-time assistance, AI-assisted robotic surgery offers improved surgical outcomes, reduced complications, and enhanced patient recovery. AI algorithms can also learn from vast surgical datasets to refine surgical techniques and optimize patient-specific procedures.

The narrative review conducted by Moazemi et al. [29] encompasses a wide range of surgical specialities where robotic surgery has been utilized. These include urology, gynaecology, cardiothoracic surgery, and gastrointestinal surgery, among others. The authors discuss the specific procedures and techniques performed using robotic systems, highlighting the advantages they offer, such as reduced invasiveness, shorter recovery times, and improved patient outcomes. Furthermore, this study addresses the limitations and challenges associated with robotic surgery.

The authors discuss factors like great costs, complexity, the inadequate availability of robotic systems, and the need for specialized training for surgeons. They also examine the ethical considerations and potential risks involved in the use of robotic surgical systems. The work done by Bramhe et al. [30] focuses on the utilization of AI technologies in conjunction with robotic surgical systems to enhance surgical outcomes, efficiency, and safety. It aims to provide a broad understanding of how AI is being integrated into the domain of robot-assisted surgery and the impact it has on patient care and surgical procedures.

The authors employ a rigorous methodology to identify and analyse relevant studies and reports on AI in robot-assisted surgery. They explore different AI applications, such as image recognition, predictive modelling, decision support systems, and autonomous robots, and assess their effectiveness and limitations.

Moglia et al. [31] proposed an innovative approach to address the challenges of predicting diabetes data, encompassing both real and synthetic data. The article introduces the Generative-Adversarial-Network-Long-Short-Term Memory (GLSTM) model, which leverages the power of Generative-Adversarial-Network (GANs) to generate synthetic diabetes data while preserving its statistical characteristics. By combining this synthetic data with real-world diabetes data, the Long-Short-Term

Memory (LSTM) classification model is trained to accurately predict diabetes-related outcomes.

The review delves into the technical aspects of the GLSTM model, elaborating on how GANs generate realistic synthetic data and how the LSTM classifier is utilized to make predictions based on the combined dataset. The authors discuss the advantages of this hybrid approach, which allows for better utilization of limited real data and mitigates issues related to data scarcity. The article presents comprehensive experimental results and performance evaluations of the GLSTM model. By comparing its predictions with other existing methods, the authors demonstrate the usefulness and dominance of their proposed approach in handling diabetes data prediction tasks.

The work done by Jaiswal and Gupta [32] offers an extensive and authoritative examination of the current advancements and research directions in the field of robotically assisted surgical systems. It commences by emphasizing the importance of robotically assisted surgery in modern healthcare and its potential to address various challenges commonly associated with traditional surgical approaches. The technical aspects of these surgical systems, encompassing design, control mechanisms, and integration with cutting-edge technologies like artificial intelligence and advanced imaging systems, are thoroughly discussed.

The authors conduct a meticulous analysis of the latest developments in robotically assisted surgical systems and shed light on their practical applications. Real-world instances of these systems being employed across diverse medical specialities are provided, highlighting their impact on enhancing surgical outcomes, precision, and patient recovery times. Moreover, the authors offer valuable insights by identifying ongoing challenges and areas that necessitate further exploration, guiding researchers and practitioners in contributing to the advancement of robotically assisted surgical systems.

2.2.5 Virtual Assistants for Patient Care

Virtual assistants powered by AI technologies have emerged as valuable tools for patient care [17]. These conversational agents can provide personalized health information, answer patient queries, and offer guidance on managing chronic conditions. Virtual assistants can be integrated into telemedicine platforms, mobile applications, and smart devices, providing convenient access to healthcare information and support. By empowering patients with self-care tools and continuous monitoring, virtual assistants contribute to improved patient engagement, self-management, and overall healthcare outcomes.

The study done by Klodmann et al. [33] employs the combined qualitative and quantitative data, to comprehensively analyse cancer patients' attitudes and preferences towards virtual assistants. The authors delve into the determinants that play a crucial role in patients' willingness to accept and interact with these digital assistants as part of their healthcare journey.

Throughout the review, the researchers present a range of use cases for virtual assistants in the context of cancer care. They examine how these AI-based tools can support patients in managing their symptoms, providing essential information, and offering emotional support throughout their treatment and recovery process. The findings from both qualitative and quantitative aspects of the study contribute to a deeper understanding of patients' perceptions and the potential benefits of implementing virtual assistants in cancer care settings.

The work done by Bussel et al. [34] outlines the development and features of MEDIC, which is an AI-powered healthcare assistant designed to enhance patient care and streamline healthcare processes. The authors describe how MEDIC utilizes artificial intelligence and smart data intelligence techniques to analyse and process vast amounts of medical data efficiently. The review provides insights into the functionalities of the MEDIC AI Assistant, including its ability to offer personalized medical recommendations, facilitate remote patient monitoring, and optimize healthcare workflows. The authors present case studies and real-world applications to demonstrate the practicality and effectiveness of the MEDIC system in various healthcare scenarios. The MEDIC AI Assistant aims to give healthcare professionals useful insights and support in decision-making by utilizing cutting-edge technologies like traditional model, natural language processing, deep learning, and data analytics. This will improve patient outcomes and boost overall healthcare productivity.

2.2.6 BIO-SIGNALS: VITAL DIAGNOSTIC INFORMATION

In recent years, AI in healthcare research has seen significant advancements in the analysis of various bio-signals, offering promising diagnostic and therapeutic potential. Electrocardiograms (ECGs) have been a prominent area of focus, with their diagnostic value in cardiovascular diseases [35]. Moreover, brain activity measurements, such as electroencephalograms (EEGs), have shown promise in detecting and monitoring neurological disorders like epilepsy and Alzheimer's disease [36]. As the field continues to evolve, emerging bio-signal technologies are also gaining traction in healthcare applications, providing novel opportunities for early disease detection and personalized treatment plans [37].

The integration of AI algorithms, including ML and DL techniques, has demonstrated their efficacy in analysing and interpreting complex bio-signals, unlocking valuable insights that may not be readily discernible through traditional methods. These developments present exciting prospects for improving patient outcomes and enhancing healthcare practices through the synergy of AI and bio-signal analysis.

Patil et al. [38] have conducted a thorough examination of various AI methods employed in the analysis of bio-signals, encompassing physiological data like electrocardiograms (ECGs), electroencephalograms (EEGs), and other pertinent biometric data. They explore how AI-driven approaches have the capability to identify intricate patterns, correlations, and anomalies within these bio-signals, that may not be discernible through conventional analysis methods.

The work done by Yoon et al. [39] offers a comprehensive assessment of how bio-signals are utilized in medical applications and investigates the challenges and opportunities associated with the integration of AI in this field. The authors thoroughly explore the significance of bio-signals, encompassing diverse physiological data like electrocardiograms (ECGs), electroencephalograms (EEGs), and other relevant biometric information. They emphasize the crucial role of AI-driven approaches in analysing and interpreting these bio-signals to reveal valuable insights that may not be evident through conventional methods.

The paper delves into the technical aspects of AI algorithms applied to bio-signal processing, encompassing machine learning and deep learning techniques. Real-world examples are provided to demonstrate the successful implementation of AI models in detecting and predicting medical conditions, monitoring patient health, and improving disease management in real time. The study delves into the technical aspects of AI algorithms utilized for bio-signal processing, incorporating machine and deep learning techniques. The authors present real-world examples of how AI models have been effectively applied for the prediction and detection of medical conditions, evaluating disease progression, and providing real-time monitoring of patient health.

2.3 WEARABLE DEVICES

The term "wearable" pertains to Internet of Things (IoT) solutions that integrate hardware, software, and app development to create a platform for gathering, analysing, and overseeing health data [40]. These wearable devices, often known as smart gadgets such as wristbands, are utilized to monitor various health parameters of users, encompassing breathing rate, blood oxygen levels, calories expended, sleep quality, sleep patterns, and body temperature. They are also utilized for monitoring the condition of post-surgery patients.

These gadgets are equipped with intelligent sensors that enable the gathering and monitoring of a patient's physical readings like heart rate, blood pressure, or body temperature [41]. Wearable devices prove valuable in acquiring patients' medical data for diagnostic purposes. They rely on biosensors to gather diverse patient data, offering numerous possibilities for their application in healthcare. These devices play a crucial role in collecting patients' medical information, simplifying and enhancing the diagnostic process. The smart wearable device market reached a value of $13.8 billion in 2020 and is forecasted to hit $37.4 billion by 2028, signalling substantial growth [42].

2.3.1 TYPES OF WEARABLE DEVICES

A wearable device ranges from simple devices to more complex devices and is broadly classified into the head-mounted displays and body sensors. A study shows that there are 11 head-mounted display devices and 13 body sensor devices that are used for different monitoring [43]. Head-mounted display devices are hand-free devices mounted on the head and are used to provide medical data to the doctors while conserving infertility during operative procedures and they are reported to improve patient satisfaction during operative procedures. Devices with body sensors have been discovered to operate quite well in improving patient postures and rehabilitation. Body sensors may record any physiological function in the body and

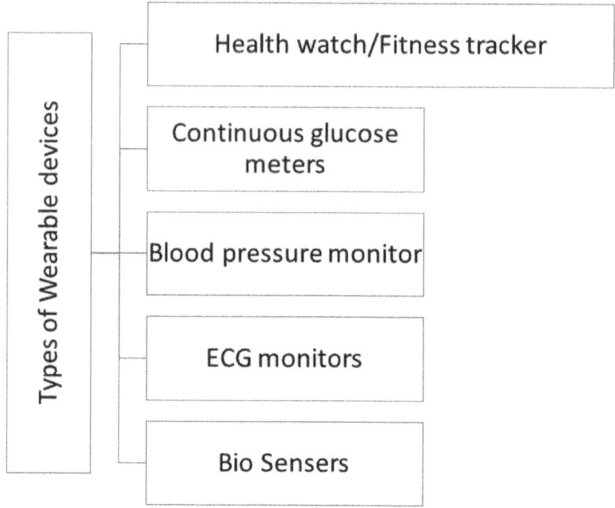

FIGURE 2.2 Types of wearable devices.

they can be further categorized into wearable and portable gadgets. Various types of wearable devices are as depicted in Figure 2.2.

2.3.1.1 Wearable Health Watch/Fitness Trackers

Wearable fitness trackers and health watches are some of the newest inventions in the healthcare sector. It is designed to monitor significant signals, including heart rate, blood pressure, and steps taken to burn calories. These gadgets can also help with fall detection, meditation, and sleep quality archiving. It is one of the most popular wearable technologies for a variety of purposes, including goal setting, sleep pattern identification, exercise tracking, calorie tracking, heart monitoring, and step counting. These straightforward and creative gadgets connect to smartphones via apps to easily track data and provide a thorough understanding of our daily lives.

2.3.1.2 Wearable Blood Pressure Monitors

These types of devices are used for monitoring blood pressure at home, and sometimes the pressure of blood, cuffs may be uneasy for old people and may lead to wrong measures due to the wrong fitting of cuffs and the wrong positioning of arms. A wearable blood pressure monitor can help alleviate this load by automating blood pressure collection and delivering data to connected apps.

2.3.1.3 Continuous Glucose Meters (CGM)

A continuous glucose monitor (CGM) is a compact device aiding people in managing diabetes by tracking their blood sugar levels. It consists of a transmitter that continuously sends data to a display, like a smartphone, and a sensor typically placed on the upper arm. Every 5 minutes, the sensor measures glucose levels in the fluid around cells and sends this information to the receiver. The transmitter promptly provides current data to the screen, presenting immediate glucose readings, patterns, and alerts. This enables users to make informed decisions based on the real-time information provided. For example, if it indicates that the patient's glucose level is rising, additional insulin can be administered.

2.3.1.4   Wearable ECG Monitors

This electronic device captures the heart's electrical patterns and aids in diagnosing conditions like arrhythmia and heart failure. Resembling a wristwatch, this wearable gadget notifies users of potential heart issues and helps doctors diagnose heart-related conditions or cardiac events.

2.3.1.5   Wearable Biosensors

There is a high need for wearable devices incorporating biosensors for healthcare applications that work differently than wrist trackers and smartwatches. One example of this form of biosensor is a self-adhesive biosensor, which can track all of a person's activity when he is moving or in motion. Flexible biosensors can provide more accurate health and data analysis than conventional wearable devices. Table 2.1 provides an overview of head-mounted devices.

Table 2.1 shows that there are a number of head-mounted device ranging from simple to complex and each device has some advantages and disadvantages. The table shows that the AI-based technology is very supportive of medical diagnosis and affects medical treatment very positively. The AI-based head-mounted devices are continuously being upgraded as per the need. Table 2.2 shows the overview of various body sensors.

Table 2.2 shows that there are a number of wearable biosensor devices ranging from high functionality to low functionality and the functions are continuously updating and it shows that it can ease the day-to-day life of a person and can help to keep track on their health.

2.4   ROLE OF NLP TO PROCESS BIG DATA FOR MEDICAL DIAGNOSIS

NLP stands as an AI-driven technology crucial for enhanced medical diagnosis, streamlining the process significantly. The abundance of medical data generated daily emphasizes the importance of big data in ensuring high-quality medical information. Integrating big data into healthcare holds the potential to transform how clinical decisions are made, identifying patterns in patient data and forecasting disease outbreaks. Through the analysis of extensive structured and unstructured data like electronic health records (EHRs), genomic information, medical imaging, and social media streams, healthcare practitioners and researchers gain invaluable insights that can ultimately enhance patient outcomes and refine public health strategies. Notably, natural language processing (NLP) exhibits significant promise in aiding medical diagnosis by extracting pertinent details from unstructured medical texts, including clinical notes, research papers, patient records, and social media updates. These

TABLE 2.1

Overview of Available Head-Mounted Devices

Literature	Device/Sensor	Device Utilization	Merits	Demerits
Lastra et al. [44], Palumbo et al. [45]	Microsoft HoloLens 2	Medical surgery, monitoring, virtual reality	• easy to use • comfortable to wear • very elegant • high quality • excellent position tracking	• battery life • less suitable for industry
Jiang et al. [46], Scherl et al. [47]	Microsoft HoloLens 1	Perforator flap transfer, surgery of the parotid gland	• comfortable • easy to use • support for MS platform	• small view • difficult to read text
Zorzal et al. [48]	Meta-vision Meta 2	Laparoscopic procedures	• improvable experience • more accurate • better connectivity	• higher cost • security issue
Mendes et al. [49]	Arzyon headset	Central venous catheterization	• good connectivity • accurate • compact	• battery life
Liounakos et al. [50]	Epson Moverio BT-300	Percutaneous endoscopic lumbar discectomy	• improved camera • lightweight • more resistant	• no zoom • no autofocus
Zhou et al. [51]	Magic Leap One	Tooth decay management	• advance technology • standalone device • lighweight and convenient • individual optics	• high cost • not impressive graphics
Boillat et al. [52]	Google Glass	Surgical time-out checklist execution	• user can easily send a mail • good connectivity • voice command and hand gesture	• user friendliness • eye problem • cannot be used while driving

(Continued)

TABLE 2.1
(Continued)

Literature	Device/Sensor	Device Utilization	Merits	Demerits
Hiranaka et al. [53]	PicoLinker glasses	Single-segment posterior lumbar interbody fusion	• simple structure • lighweight • no image delays • commercial availability	• connectivity • battery life
Inoue et al. [54]	HMZ-T2 & Wrap1200	Sonography for patient education	• comfortable • enhanced comprehension of the patient's illness • images of superior quality. • lag time	• battery issue
Yoshida et al. [55]	HMM-3000MT	Vision-based index finger tracking	• Ensure sterility while instructing • user- friendly • comfortable to wear • low cost	• delay between endoscopic image and pointer device
Schneider et al. [56]	Sony Glasstron	Personal medical imaging	• image quality • good 3D effect • excellent immersion • lens glare	• limited connectivity • difficult to adjust right

TABLE 2.2

Overview of Available Body Sensors

Literature	Device/Sensor	Device Utilization/Location to Wear	Merits	Demerits
Lui et al. [57]	Apple Watch Series 6	Heart rate monitoring, SpO2 monitoring, ECG, sleep tracking, activity tracking/wrist	• comprehensive health monitoring features • user-friendly interface • premium build and design	• costly • limited connectivity with android
Nissen et al. [58]	Fitbit Charge 4	Heart rate monitoring, sleep tracking, activity tracking, built-in GPS/wrist	• accurate heart rate tracking • built-in GPS for tracking • affordable	• limited features • limited app support
Masri et al. [59]	Samsung Galaxy Fit 2	Heart rate monitoring, sleep tracking, activity tracking, stress tracking/wrist	• slim and lightweight design • bright AMOLED display • long battery life • water-resistant • affordable	• limited function • limited third-party support
Miller et al. [60]	Whoop Strap 3.0	Heart rate monitoring, sleep tracking, strain tracking, recovery tracking/wrist	• focused on recovery and performance optimization • provides detailed insights for athletes • long battery life • water-resistant	• expensive subscription • limited smartwatch features
Welch et al. [61]	ViSi Mobile System	Vital signs monitoring/chest, shoulder, wrist, abdomen	• maximum measurement • cost-effective	• result is bounded
Donnelly et al. [62]	Aingeal	Vital signs monitoring including arrhythmia detection/upper abdomen	• portable and preferable • low false-positive rate • automation	• result is limited
Banos et al. [63]	PhysioDroid	Vital signs/chest	• operating device is easy • several parameters recorded	• need smartphone

(Continued)

TABLE 2.2
(Continued)

Literature	Device/Sensor	Device Utilization/Location to Wear	Merits	Demerits
Hollier et al. [64]	Life Vest/ Life Shirt	Ambulatory inductive plethsysmography, pulse oximeter, ECG monitoring/chest	• good results • not patient-friendly • complicated	• need smartphone
Aziz et al. [65]	Micro-stain	Posture and gait, rehabilitation/ankle, sternum	• posture guidance • more focused physiotherapy	• result is bounded
Cancela et al. [66]	Perform	Posture monitoring for Parkinson's disease/wrist, ankle	• excellent • very accurate	• few studies available

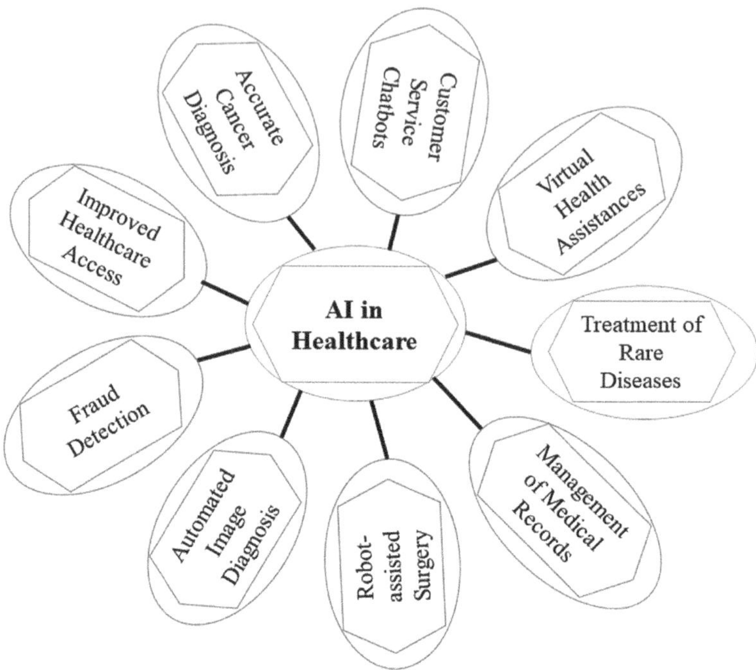

FIGURE 2.3 Contribution of AI in healthcare.

capabilities illustrate how NLP contributes to medical diagnosis within the context of processing vast amounts of data. Figure 2.3 illustrates the pivotal role of AI in healthcare.

1. **Clinical Text Mining**: NLP algorithms can analyse EHRs and clinical notes to extract critical information related to symptoms, medical history, laboratory results, and treatment plans. It enables efficient data mining and supports clinical decision-making.
2. **Diagnosis Support**: NLP models can be trained on vast amounts of medical literature and data to help physicians diagnose various medical conditions accurately and quickly. By analysing symptoms and comparing them to existing knowledge, NLP aids in identifying potential diagnoses.
3. **Early Detection of Diseases**: NLP techniques can be employed to screen large volumes of patient data and detect patterns or trends that might indicate the early stages of certain diseases, facilitating timely interventions.
4. **Medical Image Reporting**: NLP can automatically generate radiology reports by extracting information from medical images, providing more structured and standardized reports for medical professionals.

5. **Patient Risk Stratification**: NLP can assist in identifying high-risk patients based on history, lifestyle, and other factors, which can aid in targeted interventions and preventive measures.

6. **Enhancing Clinical Decision-Making**: An article published in the *Journal of the American Medical Association* established how big data analytics can be used to identify high-risk patients for early intervention. By analysing patient data from EHRs the researchers developed a predictive model that could accurately identify patients at risk of readmission within 30 days of the discharge. This model allowed clinicians to proactively address the needs of high-risk patients, reducing readmission rates and improving patient care.

7. **Identifying Patterns in Patient Data**: Big data analytics has been used to identify patterns in patient data that can lead to the quick discovery of diseases. For instance, a study published in *Nature Medicine* demonstrated how ML algorithms can analyse electronic health records and identify subtle patterns in patients' physiological data, which could predict the onset of conditions like sepsis hours before clinical symptoms become evident. Early detection allowed for timely intervention, potentially saving lives, and improving patient outcomes.

8. **Predicting Disease Outbreaks**: The potential of big data in predicting disease outbreaks was demonstrated during the Ebola outbreak in West Africa. Researchers used real-time data from various sources, including social media feeds, mobile phone data, and satellite imagery, to track the spread of the disease and predict its potential impact on different regions. This information helped public health officials allocate resources and implement preventive measures to control the outbreak.

Overall, these studies highlight the immense potential of leveraging big data in healthcare to enhance clinical decision-making, identify patterns in patient data, and predict disease outbreaks. By harnessing the power of big data analytics, healthcare providers and public health officials can make more informed decisions, improve patient care, and better respond to public health challenges.

2.5 ETHICAL CHALLENGES

There are various ethical challenges pertaining to integration of AI for healthcare diagnosis. Data security and privacy are among the most important challenges when it comes to managing sensitive healthcare information in the context of NLP and big data management. While leveraging these technologies can carry significant benefits to the medical diagnosis system, it also raises concerns about protecting patients' privacy and ensuring the confidentiality of their data [67–71]. Here's how data privacy and security are essential in this domain:

1. **Patient Confidentiality**: Healthcare data often contain highly sensitive information, including medical history, diagnoses, genetic data, and other personally identifiable information (PII). Maintaining patient confidentiality is crucial to building and maintaining trust between patients and healthcare providers.
2. **Compliance with Regulations**: Many countries have strict regulations governing the collection, storage, and use of healthcare data, such as the Health Insurance Portability and Accountability Act (HIPAA) in the United States and the General Data Protection Regulation (GDPR) in the European Union. Healthcare organizations must ensure they comply with these regulations to protect patient privacy.
3. **Data Breach Prevention**: NLP and big data management involve the storage and processing of massive amounts of healthcare data. Implementing robust security measures is essential to prevent unauthorized access, data breaches, and cyberattacks that could compromise patient information.
4. **Anonymization and De-identification**: To protect patient privacy, data should be anonymized or de-identified whenever possible, so that individual patients cannot be identified from the data. This helps strike a balance between using valuable data for analysis and preserving patient confidentiality.
5. **Access Control and Encryption**: Implementing access controls and encryption techniques ensures that only authorized personnel can access sensitive healthcare data. Encryption helps safeguard data while it is in transit and at rest.
6. **Secure Data Sharing and Collaboration**: In the context of multi-institutional research and collaborations, secure data-sharing protocols must be established to protect patient privacy when sharing data among different healthcare organizations.
7. **Users Training**: In order to integrate AI with healthcare, lots of training of users is required to be done for assuring full utilization of AI.
8. **Financial Barriers**: As we know implementing AI with healthcare data requires lots of money for integrating AI functionality with the healthcare infrastructures.

By prioritizing data privacy and security, healthcare providers and organizations can harness the benefits of NLP and big data management while maintaining patient trust and compliance with regulatory requirements. Safeguarding patient data is an ongoing process that requires a proactive and vigilant approach in the face of evolving cybersecurity challenges.

2.6 CONCLUSION

In summary, this chapter extensively explores the profound impact of AI on revolutionizing smart health treatments. The fusion of intelligent algorithms and machine learning techniques has significantly reshaped medicine, enabling precise diagnoses and effective treatment strategies. AI applications, such as image recognition and natural language processing, have notably improved medical outcomes and patient care. Moreover, integrating big data analytics has shifted healthcare management by enabling comprehensive data collection, storage, and analysis. Utilizing big data holds significant potential for refining clinical decision-making, recognizing patterns, and predicting disease outbreaks, ultimately leading to more efficient healthcare practices. The chapter emphasizes the critical need to prioritize data privacy and security to protect sensitive healthcare information. Wearable medical devices like smartwatches, fitness trackers, and biosensors empower individuals to monitor their health in real time, facilitating early detection of health issues and personalized feedback for better self-care. Additionally, the emergence of bio-signals and telemedicine in modern healthcare delivery offers innovative solutions to enhance medical practices and achieve improved healthcare outcomes. As AI and technology advance, the healthcare sector must responsibly embrace these advancements, addressing ethical concerns and ensuring patient privacy and data security. Balancing innovation with responsible implementation will unleash AI's full potential for smart health diagnosis and treatment, ushering in a new era of more efficient, accessible, and patient-focused healthcare systems.

REFERENCES

1. Cortes, C., & Vapnik, V. (1995). Support-vector networks. 20(3), 273–297. https://doi.org/10.1007/BF00994018
2. Martinez, A.M., & Kak, A.C. (2001). PCA versus LDA. *IEEE Transactions on Pattern Analysis and Machine Intelligence.* 23(2), 228–233. https://doi: 10.1109/34.908974
3. Jaiswal, S., & Pandey, M.K. (2023). Linear discriminate analysis based robust watermarking in DWT and LWT domain with PCA based statistical feature reduction. *International Journal of Image, Graphics and Signal Processing (IJIGSP).* 15(2), 73–88, https://doi.org/10.5815/ijigsp.2023.02.07
4. Simon, H.S. (1999). *Neural Networks: A Comprehensive Foundation.* Prentice Hall. OCLC 38908586
5. Raina, R.M., & Andrew, Ng. (2009). Large-scale deep unsupervised learning using graphics processors. *ICML*, 873–880. https//doi:10.1145/1553374.1553486
6. Kher, H.R., & Thakar, V.K. (2014). Scale invariant feature transform based image matching and registration. Fifth International Conference *on* Signal *and* Image Processing, Bangalore, India, 50–55. https//doi:10.1109/ICSIP.2014.12
7. Nguyen, T., Park, E.A., Han, J., Park, D.C., & Min, S.Y. (2014). Object detection using scale invariant feature transform. In Pan, J.S., Krömer, P., & Snášel, V. (eds.) *Genetic and Evolutionary Computing. Advances in Intelligent Systems and Computing.* Springer, 238. https://doi.org/10.1007/978-3-319-01796-9_7
8. Bay, H., Tuytelaars, T., & Van Gool, L. (2006). SURF: speeded up robust features. In Leonardis, A., Bischof, H., Pinz, A. (eds.) *Computer Vision – ECCV. Lecture Notes in Computer Science*, 3951. https://doi.org/10.1007/11744023_32
9. Labrín, C., & Urdinez, F. (2020). Principal component analysis. In Francisco Urdinez, Andres Cruz (eds.) *R for Political Data Science.* Chapman and Hall/CRC, 375–393
10. Jaiswal, S., & Pandey, M.K. (2022). Robust digital image watermarking using LWT and Random-Subspace-1DLDA with PCA based statistical feature reduction. In Francisco Urdinez, Andres Cruz (eds.) Second International Conference *on* Computer Science, *Engineering and* Applications *(ICCSEA).* Gunupur, India, 1–6. https//doi:10.1109/ICCSEA54677.2022.9936355

11. Nadkarni, P.M., Machado, L.O., & Chapman, W.W. (2011). Natural language processing: An introduction. *Journal of the American Medical Informatics Association JAMIA*. 18(5), 544–551. https://doi.org/10.1136/amiajnl-2011-000464

12. Gulshan, V., Peng, L., Coram, M., Stumpe, M.C., Wu, D., Narayanaswamy, A., Venugopalan, S., Widner, K., Madams, T., Cuadros, J., Kim, R., Raman, R., Nelson, P.C., Mega, J.L., & Webster, D.R. (2016). Development and validation of a deep learning algorithm for detection of diabetic retinopathy in retinal fundus photographs. *JAMA*. 316(22), 2402–2410. htpps://doi:10.1001/jama.2016.17216

13. Esteva, A., Kuprel, B., Novoa, R.A., Ko, J., Swetter, S.M., Blau, H.M., & Thrun, S. (2017). Dermatologist-level classification of skin cancer with deep neural networks. *Nature*. 542(7639), 115–118. https//doi:10.1038/nature21056

14. Litjens, G., Kooi, T., Bejnordi, B.E., Setio, A.A.A., Ciompi, F., Ghafoorian, M., van der Laak, J.A.W.M., van Ginneken, B., & Sánchez, C.I. (2017). A survey on deep learning in medical image analysis. *Medical Image Analysis*. 42, 60–88. https//doi:10.1016/j.media.2017.07.005

15. Shen, D., Wu, G., & Suk, H.I. (2017). Deep learning in medical image analysis. *Annual Review of Biomedical Engineering*. 19, 221–248

16. Rajkomar, A., Oren, E., Chen, K., Dai, A.M., Hajaj, N., Hardt, M., & Esteva, A. (2018). Scalable and accurate deep learning with electronic health records. *NPJ Digital Medicine*. 1(1), 1–10

17. Liao, K.P., & Cai, T. (2020). Natural language processing in rheumatic diseases: using text mining to build knowledge and discover novel patterns. *Rheumatic Disease Clinics*. 46(1), 1–20

18. Kudyba, S., & Porter, P. (2019). The emerging role of artificial intelligence in health care: Will medical professionals be replaced? *Health Policy and Technology*. 8(2), 198–206

19. Golden, S.H., & Robinson, K.A. (2017). Using machine learning to improve clinical decision making: Pitfalls and opportunities. *Current Diabetes Reports*. 17(12), 1–9

20. Elmi-Terander, A., Skulason, H., Sánchez, I., Han, S., & Darzi, A. (2019). Surgical robotics beyond enhanced dexterity instrumentation: A survey of machine learning techniques and their role in intelligent and autonomous surgical actions. *International Journal of Robotics Research*. 38(9), 987–1003

21. Wagner, C.R., Stylopoulos, N., & Jackson, P.G. (2018). Surgical robotics: Systems applications and visions. *International Journal of Medical Robotics and Computer Assisted Surgery*. 14(1), 1–18

22. Bastani, H., Ghasemzadeh, H., & Dutt, N. (2018). Machine learning for mental health: A review. Proceedings of the 24th ACM SIGKDD International Conference on Knowledge Discovery & Data Mining, 2297–2306

23. Susanto, A.P., Winarto, H., Fahira, A., Abdurrohman, H., Muharram, A.P., Widitha, R.U., Efirianti, G.E.W., George, Y.A.E., & Tjoa, K. (2022). Building an artificial intelligence-powered medical image recognition smartphone application: What medical practitioners need to know. *Informatics in Medicine Unlocked*. 32, 101017, ISSN 2352-9148. https://doi.org/10.1016/j.imu.2022.101017

24. Hunt, B., Ruiz, A., & Pogue, B. (2021). Smartphone-based imaging systems for medical applications: A critical review. *Journal of Biomedical Optics*. 26(4), 040902. https://doi: 10.1117/1.JBO.26.4.040902

25. Zhou, B., Yang, G., Shi, Z., & Ma, S. (2022). *Natural Language Processing for Smart Healthcare, IEEE Reviews in Biomedical*. Engineering Institute of Electrical and Electronics Engineers (IEEE), 1–17. https://doi 10.1109/rbme.2022.3210270

26. Uddin, Y., Nair, A., Shariq, S., & Hannan, S.H. (2023). Transforming primary healthcare through natural language processing and big data analytics. *BMJ*, 381–948. https://doi: 10.1136/bmj.p948

27. Berros N., El, Mendili, F., Filaly Y., El, & Bouzekri El, I.Y. (2023). Enhancing digital health services with big data analytics. *Big Data and Cognitive Computing.* 7(2). https://doi.org/10.3390/bdcc7020064

28. Cresswell, K., Callaghan, M., Khan, S., Sheikh, Z., Mozaffar, H., & Sheikh, A. (2020 September). Investigating the use of data-driven artificial intelligence in computerised decision support systems for health and social care: A systematic review. *Health Informatics Journal.* 26(3), 2138–2147. https://doi.org/10.1177/1460458219900452

29. Moazemi, S., Vahdati, S., Li, J., Kalkhoff, S., Castano, L.J.V., Dewitz, B., Bibo, R., Sabouniaghdam, P., Tootooni, M.S., Bundschuh, R.A., Lichtenberg, A., Aubin, H., & Schmid, F. (2023). Artificial intelligence for clinical decision support for monitoring patients in cardiovascular ICUs: A systematic review. *Frontiers of Medicine (Lausanne).* 10, 1109411. https://doi: 10.3389/fmed.2023.1109411

30. Bramhe, S., & Pathak, S.S. (2022). Robotic surgery: A narrative review. *Cureus.* 14(9), e29179. https://doi:10.7759/cureus.29179

31. Moglia, A., Georgiou, K., Georgiou, E., Satava, R.M., & Cuschieri, A. (2021). A systematic review on artificial intelligence in robot-assisted surgery. *International Journal of Surgery.* 95, 106151. ISSN 1743-9191. https://doi.org/10.1016/j.ijsu.2021.106151

32. Jaiswal, S., & Gupta, P. (2023). GLSTM: A novel approach for prediction of real & synthetic PID diabetes data using GANs and LSTM classification model. *International Journal of Experimental Research and Review.* 30, 32–45. https://doi.org/10.52756/ijerr.2023.v30.004

33. Klodmann, J., Schlenk, C., Hellings-Kuß, A. et al. (2021). An introduction to robotically assisted surgical systems: Current developments and focus areas of research. *Current Robotics Reports.* 2, 321–332. https://doi.org/10.1007/s43154-021-00064-3

34. Bussel, M.J.P., Schröder, O.G.J., Ou, C. et al. (2022). Analyzing the determinants to accept a virtual assistant and use cases among cancer patients: A mixed methods study. *BMC Health Services Research.* 22(1), 890. https://doi.org/10.1186/s12913-022-08189-7

35. Swapna, M., Viswanadhula, U.M., Aluvalu, R., Vardharajan, V., & Kotecha, K. (2022). Bio-signals in medical applications and challenges using artificial intelligence. *Journal of Sensor and Actuator Networks.* 11(1), 17. https://doi.org/10.3390/jsan11010017

36. Tang, Z., Hu, H., Xu, C., & Zhao, K. (2021). Exploring an efficient remote biomedical signal monitoring framework for personal health in the COVID-19 pandemic. *International Journal of Environmental Research and Public Health.* 18(17), 9037. https//doi:10.3390/ijerph18179037

37. Dey, N., & Rajinikanth, V. (2022). Abnormality detection in heart MRI with spotted hyena algorithm-supported Kapur/Otsu Thresholding and level set segmentation. In *Primers in Biomedical Imaging Devices and Systems, Magnetic Resonance Imaging.* Academic Press, 105–126. https://doi.org/10.1016/B978-0-12-823401-3.00006-7

38. Patil, S., Darji, J., Hingu, S., & Thakkar, A. (2021, May 24). Medic: Smart healthcare AI assistant. Proceedings of the International Conference on Smart Data Intelligence (ICSMDI 2021). https://ssrn.com/abstract=3852150 or http://dx.doi.org/10.2139/ssrn.3852150

39. Yoon, D., Jang, J.H., Choi, B.J., Kim, T.Y., & Han, C.H. (2020). Discovering hidden information in biosignals from patients using artificial intelligence. *Korean Journal of Anesthesiology.* 73(4), 275–284. https//doi:10.4097/kja.19475

40. Aileni, R.M., Valderrama, A.C., & Strungaru, R. (2017). *Wearable Electronics for Elderly Health Monitoring and Active Living, Ambient Assisted Living and Enhanced Living Environments.* Butterworth-Heinemann, 247–269. https://doi.org/10.1016/B978-0-12-805195-5.00010-7

41. Web. https://www.velvetech.com/blog/wearable-technology-in-healthcare. Accessed on July 12, 2023

42. Web.   https://builtin.com/healthcare-technology/wearable-technology-in-healthcare Accessed on July 12, 2023

43. Iqbal, M.H., Aydin, A., Brunckhorst, O., Dasgupta, P., & Ahmed, K. (2016). A review of wearable technology in medicine. *Journal of the Royal Society of Medicine.* 109(10), 372–380. https//doi: 10.1177/0141076816663560

44. Lastra, A., Ungi, T., Morton, D. et al. (2023). Real-time integration between Microsoft HoloLens 2 and 3D Slicer with demonstration in pedicle screw placement planning. *International Journal of Cars.* https://doi.org/10.1007/s11548-023-02977-0

45. Palumbo, A. (2022). Microsoft HoloLens 2 in medical and healthcare context: State of the art and future prospects. *Sensors (Basel).* 22(20), 7709. https//doi: 10.3390/s22207709

46. Jiang, T., Yu, D., Wang, Y., Zan, T., Wang, S., & Li, Q. (2020). HoloLens-based vascular localization system: Precision evaluation study with a three-dimensional printed model. *Journal of Medical Internet Research.* 22(4), e16852

47. Scherl, C., Stratemeier, J., Karle, C., Rotter, N., Hesser, J., Huber, L., Dias, A., Hoffmann, O., Riffel, P., Schoenberg, S.O., et al. (2021). Augmented reality with hololens in parotid surgery: How to assess and to improve accuracy. *European Archives of Otorhinolaryngol,* 278, 2473–2483. https://doi.org/10.1007/s00405-020-06351-7

48. Zorzal, E.R., Gomes, J.M.C., Sousa, M., Belchior, P., DaSilva, P.G., Figueiredo, N., Lopes, D.S., & Jorge, J. (2020). Laparoscopy with augmented reality adaptations. *Journal of Biomedical Informatics.* 107, 103463

49. Mendes, H.C.M., Costa, C.I.A.B., DaSilva, N.A., Leite, F.P., Esteves, A., & Lopes, D.S. (2020). PIÑATA: Pinpoint insertion of intravenous needles via augmented reality training assistance. *Computer Med. Imaging Graph.* 82, 101731

50. Liounakos, J.I., Urakov, T., & Wang, M.Y. (2020). Head-up display assisted endoscopic lumbar discectomy–a technical note. *International Journal of Medical Robotics and Computer Assisted Surgery.* 16(3), e2089

51. Zhou, Y., Yoo, P., Feng, Y., Sankar, A., Sadr, A., & Seibel, E.J. (2019). Towards ar-assisted visualisation and guidance for imaging of dental decay. *Healthcare Technology Letters.* 6(6), 243–248

52. Boillat, T., Grantcharov, P., & Rivas, H. (2019). Increasing completion rate and benefits of checklists: Prospective evaluation of surgical safety checklists with smart glasses. *JMIR mHealth and uHealth.* 7(4), e13447

53. Hiranaka, T., Fujishiro, T., Hida, Y., Shibata, Y., Tsubosaka, M., Nakanishi, Y., Okimura, K., & Uemoto, H. (2017). Augmented reality: The use of the PicoLinker smart glasses improves wire insertion under fluoroscopy. *World Journal of Orthopedics.* 8(12), 891–894. https//doi:10.5312/wjo.v8.i12.891

54. Inoue, M., Kihara, K., Yoshida, S., Ito, M., Takeshita, H., Ishioka, J., et al. (2015). A novel approach to patient self-monitoring of sonographic examinations using a head-mounted display. *Journal of Ultrasound in Medicine.* 34(1), 29–35

55. Yoshida, S., Kihara, K., Takeshita, H., & Fujii, Y. (2014). Instructive head-mounted display system: Pointing device using a vision-based finger tracking technique applied to surgical education. *Videosurgery Other Miniinvasive Technique.* 9(3), 449–452

56. Schneider, S.M., Ellis, M., Coombs, W.T., Shonkwiler, E.L., & Folsom, L.C. (2003). Virtual reality intervention for older women with breast cancer. *Cyber Psychology and Behavior.* 6(3), 301–307. https//doi:10.1089/109493103322011605

57. Lui, G.Y., Loughnane, D., Polley, C., Jayarathna, T., & Breen, P.P. (2022). The apple watch for monitoring mental health-related physiological symptoms: Literature review. *JMIR Mental Health.* 9(9), e37354. https//doi:10.2196/37354

58. Nissen, M., Slim, S., Jäger, K., Flaucher, M., Huebner, H., Danzberger, N., Fasching, P.A., Beckmann, M.W., Gradl, S., & Eskofier, B.M. (2022). Heart rate measurement accuracy of Fitbit Charge 4 and Samsung galaxy watch Active2: Device evaluation study. *JMIR Formative Research.* 6(3), e33635. https//doi:10.2196/33635

59. El-Masri, M., Al-Yafi, K., & Kamal, M.M. (2023). A task-technology-identity fit model of Smartwatch utilisation and user satisfaction: A hybrid SEM-neural network approach. *Information Systems Frontiers*. 25(2), 835–852, https://doi.org/10.1007/s10796-022-10256-7

60. Miller, D.J., Sargent, C., & Roach, G.D. (2022). A validation of six wearable devices for estimating sleep, heart rate and heart rate variability in healthy adults. *Sensors (Basel)*. 16(16), 6317. https//doi:10.3390/s22166317

61. Welch, J., Kanter, B., Skora, B., McCombie, S., Henry, I., McCombie, D., et al. (2016). Multi-parameter vital sign database to assist in alarm optimization for general care units. *Journal of Clinical Monitoring and Computing*, 30, 895–900.

62. Donnelly, N., Hunniford, T., Harper, R., Flynn, A., Kennedy, A., Branagh, D., et al. (2013). Demonstrating the accuracy of an in-hospital ambulatory patient monitoring solution in measuring respiratory rate. *Conference Proceedings – IEEE Engineering in Medicine and Biology Society*, 6711–6715

63. Banos, O., Villalonga, C., Damas, M., Gloesekoetter, P., Pomares, H., & Rojas, I. (2014). PhysioDroid: Combining wearable health sensors and mobile devices for a ubiquitous, continuous, and personal monitoring. *Scientific World Journal*, 490824

64. Hollier, C.A., Harmer, A.R., Maxwell, L.J., Menadue, C., Willson, G.N., Black, D.A., et al. (2014). Validation of respiratory inductive plethysmography (LifeShirt) in obesity hypoventilation syndrome. *Respiratory Physiology and Neurobiology*. 194, 15–22

65. Aziz, O., Park, E.J., Mori, G., & Robinovitch, S.N. (2014). Distinguishing the causes of falls in humans using an array of wearable tri-axial accelerometers. *Gait and Posture*. 39(1), 506–512

66. Cancela, J., Pastorino, M., Tzallas, A.T., Tsipouras, M.G., Rigas, G., Arredondo, MT., et al. (2014). Wearability assessment of a wearable system for Parkinson's disease remote monitoring based on a body area network of sensors. *Sensors (Basel)*. 14(9), 17235–17255

67. Treviso, M., Lee, J.U., Ji, T., Aken, V.B., Cao, Q., Ciosici, M.R., Hassid, M., Heafield, K., Hooker, S., Raffel, C., Martin, P.H., Martins, A.F.T., Forde, J.Z., Milder, P., Simpson, E., Slonim, N., Dodge, J., Strubell, E., Balasubramanian, N., Derczynski, L., Gurevych, I., & Schwartz, R. (2023). Efficient methods for natural language processing: A survey. *Transactions of the Association for Computational Linguistics*. 11, 826–860. https//doi:10.1162/tacl_a_00577

68. Abouelmehdi, K., & Beni- hessane, A.H. (2018). Big healthcare data: preserving security and privacy. *Journal of Big Data*. 5(1), 1. https://doi.org/10.1186/s40537-017-0110-7

69. Xiang, D., & Cai, W. (2021). Privacy protection and secondary use of health data: Strategies and methods. *BioMed Research International*, 6967166. https://doi:10.1155/2021/6967166

70. Keshta, I., & Odeh, A. (2021). Security and privacy of electronic health records: Concerns and challenges. *Egyptian Informatics Journal*, 22(2), 177–183. https://doi.org/10.1016/j.eij.2020.07.003

71. Paul, M., Maglaras, L., Ferrag, M.A., & Almomani, I. (2023). Digitization of healthcare sector: *A study on privacy and security concerns. ICT Express*, 2405–9595. https://doi.org/10.1016/j.icte.2023.02.007

3

Different Smart Diagnosis Processes of Alzheimer's Brain Disease Using AI Techniques

Nivedita Manohar Mathkunti
and Shanta Rangaswamy

3.1 INTRODUCTION

In the human body, the complex organ is the brain which regulates the neurological system and its central portion of the brain. All the functions of the human body are regulated and coordinated under the responsibilities of the brain. The main functions of the brain include controlling the movement of other organs, processing sensory information, and most importantly higher cognitive activities such as memory, emotions, and thinking. The regions of the brain play a unique role in processing information and regulating bodily functions. Neurons are the building blocks of the brain and are responsible for transmitting electrical and chemical signals. The complex network formed by these neurons is used to communicate with each other at Synapses. Synapses are notable junctions between neurons in the brain and the nervous system. These components play a significant role. Synaptic connectivity determines the flow of information within neural circuits. It also offers the overall functions and processing capabilities of the brain. During aging, iron accumulates in the brain which causes neuronal impairment due to radical formation and it is a pathogenic factor. There are many brain diseases caused by neurological disorders such as Pick's Disease (PiD), Argyrophilic Grain Disease (AGD), Cortico Basal Degeneration (CBD), Progressive Supranuclear Palsy (PSP), as well as Alzheimer's Disease (AD) based on Tauopathies. Fronto Temporal Lobular Dementia (FTLD), Multiple System Atrophy (MSA) Parkinson's Disease (PD), Dementia with Lewy Bodies (DLB), based on α-Synucleinopathies, and based on TDP-43 Proteinopathies Amyotrophic Lateral Sclerosis (ALS) Proteinopathies in the brain [1].

The present study has identified that 1/9th of the population is suffering from neurodegenerative diseases such as AD and expects that by 2050 it may reach 1/3rd of

DOI: 10.1201/9781003464884-5

the population [2]. It is essential to diagnose the degenerative condition of the brain with technology to prevent the expected.

AD, a brain disease, is caused by a disorder of the neurological functions and is progressive with cognitive disturbance, loss of memory, and altered perception. In the cortex and hippocampus sections of the brain, the presence of amyloid plaques and neurofibrillary tangles are identified. These are also some of the sources of AD which left uncured places a significant burden on the caretaker and society as patients must be reliant on caretakers [3, 4]. The main cause of this disease is still unclear. After studying the stress and its contribution, it is identified that it leads to AD as it promotes production of oxidative to neuronal degeneration. Iron transition metal accelerates oxidative radical production. It is an escalating effect of AD. The accumulation of iron on the regional part of the brain increases with age, driven by changes in protein determines the exact density and severity of the disease.

In order that the AD patients get relief it is necessary to address the excessive iron in the brain. Deferoxamine (DFO) and Deferiprone (DFP) which are metal chelators have been found promising in clinical trials to slow AD progression. However, limitations rooted in their biochemistry hinder AD effectiveness. The DFO binds the iron but then again DFP adversely affects blood count.

The development of an urgent need for a safe, nontoxic iron chelator to mitigate brain iron deposits holds promising improvement in AD's impact [3, 4].

As mentioned here, the chapter reveals many factors for brain diseases and some of the diagnosing methods with Artificial Intelligence (AI) techniques and its tributaries such as Deep Learning [DL] algorithms and Machine Learning (ML) algorithms.

3.2 DEMENTIA TYPES

The term "cognition" refers to a broad variety of mental functions, including problem-solving, memory, comprehension, and knowledge acquisition. These cognitive skills, which are necessary for doing daily tasks, rely on higher-order brain functions that control memory, learning, and reasoning rather than merely on information. Memory skills are greatly influenced by neural networks, particularly those in the frontal and temporal lobes, two specialized brain regions. Acetylcholine, dopamine, serotonin, and glutamate are just a few examples of the neurotransmitters that neurons use to interact with one another and affect brain function via stimulating or depressing receptors and neurotransmission. The neurotransmitters' ability to bind and fit into receptors is influenced by the type and quantity of these molecules, which have an impact on the functions of the brain, particularly on cognitive activity. Such a process is influenced by following a nutritious diet, an active lifestyle, maintaining dehydration, nutrition, and balancing of hormones [5, 6]. The processing of neurotransmitters can be impacted by insufficient nutrition, whereas hypoperfusion impacts the nutrient status of the brain and cognitive functions, potentially resulting in cognitive decline. The phrase "hormonal misconnection syndrome," which is characterized by altered thinking, speech, attention, memory, behavior, and spatial skills describes how long-term imbalances, particularly hormonal ones, can adversely disrupt brain function [7–10].

A group of cognitive impairments that cumulatively impair a person's capacity to perform daily chores is referred to as dementia. With a more severe decrease in cognitive function than is typical with aging, it is more of a syndrome than a specific disease. Memory, thinking, reasoning, language, as well as behavior are all capable of being impacted by dementia. It commonly advances over time and can significantly affect a person's quality of life and capacity for independent living.

Given its complexity and difficulty, dementia calls for both extensive medical care and social support. Work is being done to expand the care and excellence of the lifestyle for those with dementia as well as their caregivers, as knowledge of the underlying causes and treatments grows via research. Dementia-related key points include dementia types, symptoms, risk factors, underlying causes, diagnosis, caregiver impact, and prevention.

The decline in brain activity may be due to Vascular Dementia (VD), Mild Cognitive Impairment (MCI), Front Temporal Dementia (FTD), Behavioral FTD (bvFTD), Parkinson's, Lewy Body Dementia (LBD), mixed dementia, Huntington's Disease etc. A few dementias are discussed in this chapter. The techniques used to diagnose brain disease AD are also discussed.

Numerous cognitive impairments that afflict the elderly, including conditions like AD and Vascular Dementia (VD), frequently overlap. This makes it challenging to definitively attribute cognitive decline solely to vascular problems or to underlying brain pathologies like AD. The distinction is frequently difficult to ascertain. Several factors contribute to Vascular Dementia risk, such as advancing age and genetic predisposition, many of which are beyond control. Nevertheless, modifiable lifestyle elements (e.g., diet, exercise, obesity, alcohol, smoking) and physiological conditions (hypertension, diabetes, hypercholesterolemia) can be managed through appropriate medical interventions [11].

VD is caused due to slow blood flow to all the organs of the body especially the brain. Based on different portions of the brain its effect varies. But in general, these patients exhibit problems in reasoning, thinking, as well and memory. As shown in Figure 3.1 VD witnesses the symptoms of AD as well as sometimes it is difficult to judge the difference between VD and other dementia.

VD risk factors are many such as aging and genetic factors, which cannot be modified. The factors that depend upon our lifestyle which include diet, physical activity, obesity, alcohol consumption, tobacco consumption, hypertension, diabetes, etc., can be treated by proper medical observation [11].

MCI is a phrase used to describe the stage of cognitive function that exists between healthy cognitive functioning and nonhealthy cognitive functioning i.e. dementia. The frequency of MCI in the aged population ranges from 3% to 19%, with an annual occurrence of 58 occurrences per 1,000 people. The idea of Moderate Cognitive Impairment (MCI) is a cognitive condition in between dementia and normal brain function.

MCI is defined by observable cognitive deterioration that is more noticed than would be predicted for a patient's age and level of education, but not to the extent that it significantly affects everyday activities. There are various factors related to MCI,

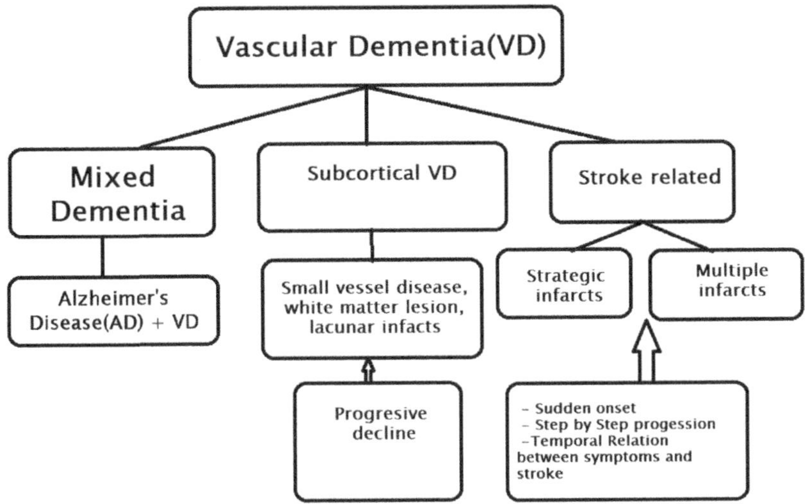

FIGURE 3.1 Versatility of vascular dementia.

its progression, and the potential for reversion to normal cognition or advancement to dementia. Apart from this 11% to 33% population of MCI progresses into dementia within a span of 2 years. Continuous medical treatment is aimed to alter and slow down the natural course of disease progression. This imparts the considerable attention in identifying an early diagnosis [12–15].

The LBD exists as a disease due to a neurological disorder distinguished by the expansion of aberrant alpha-synuclein protein deposits in the brain. Lewy bodies are the name for these deposits, which cause a variety of motor, behavioral, cognitive, and temper-connected problems [16].

3.2.1 Parkinson's Disease (PD)

Parkinson's Disease (PD) is a progressive neurological disorder that causes a range of movement and non-motor symptoms. Over time, PD decreases functionality. This review emphasizes the unique clinical characteristics of PD that set it apart from other Parkinson's Diseases. PD's hallmark is its worsening nature, encompassing a variety of symptoms affecting both motor and non-motor functions [15–17]. There are around 0.01 billion cases of PD globally. It is mostly a neurological disorder that progresses and predominantly affects emotional and motor imbalance. The four main symptoms are slowness of movement, tremor development, stiffness and rigidity, and dysphonia. Melancholy, anxiety, pain, weariness, constipation, and other symptoms of Parkinson's Disease (PD) can all have a major impact on a person's daily activities. When a person is born, their brain has an optimal number of neurons, but as they grow older, those neurons die and stop functioning interchangeably because a specific group of brain cells necessary for producing neurotransmitters like dopamine has died. PD most commonly affects older persons over the age of 50 [18].

3.2.2 WHITE MATTER

Myelin, a fatty material that insulates and speeds up the passage of electrical signals between various parts of the brain, is a tissue found in the central part of the nervous system and is identified as "white matter." Gray matter, which houses the cell bodies of neurons, is connected to other regions of the brain by white matter, which also makes communication and coordination across other brain regions easier.

The myelin sheaths that cover the nerve fibers give white matter its white appearance. It is essential for information transmission throughout the brain, letting diverse brain regions cooperate and facilitate varied cognitive activities.

White Matter Hyperintensities (WMH) are regions of increased signal intensity seen on Magnetic Resonance Imaging (MRI) images of the brain. These hyperintensities show regions of harmed or diseased white matter, frequently brought on by conditions like small artery disease, persistent hypertension, or other vascular problems. WMH can affect how the brain functions cognitively because it can disrupt the connections between various brain regions, which could result in cognitive decline or other neurological symptoms.

In this way, many dementia types exhibit changes in the beginning and some of them do not exhibit any changes in the beginning. In the next section, the different methods for identification are discussed [19].

3.2.3 ALZHEIMER'S DISEASE

One common neurodegenerative disease that mostly affects the elderly is Alzheimer's Disease, though it is also increasingly seen in younger persons. It is characterized by amyloid-β plaques, neurofibrillary tangles, inflammation, impaired synaptic function, and neuronal death, and it causes gradual cognitive deterioration. Its incidence and progression are influenced by various risk factors, including oxidative stress, lifestyle, genetics, and environment. Misfolded protein aggregates in the brain plays a crucial role in the etiology (cause) of AD. For this disease, extracellular amyloid-β plaques, inflammation synaptic dysfunction, intracellular neurofibrillary tangles, and neuronal death are important markers of neuropathology [20].

AD symptoms include the following: Daily living is disrupted by memory loss, difficulties with organizing or solving problems, trouble doing routine activities, uncertainty about location or time, difficulty making sense of spatial relationships and visual representations, fresh issues while using words when writing or speaking, losing track of where you put items and your capacity to go back, reduced or subpar judgment, retreating from social or professional activity, alterations in personality or mood.

3.2.4 FRONTO TEMPORAL DEMENTIA

Fronto Temporal Dementia (FTD), an infrequent manifestation of dementia, is characterized by unconventional symptoms. In this chapter, the authors examine the process of diagnosing and treating this condition, as well as the genetic and clinical indications. This chapter presents a thorough overview of Fronto Temporal Dementias (FTD), including differential diagnosis, clinical manifestations, underlying neuropathological and genetic variables, current therapy choices, and diagnostic procedures. FTD, in contrast to Alzheimer's Disease, frequently manifests as unusual symptoms that might not be detected right away. The chapter explores Fronto Temporal Dementias' clinical signs, brain pathology, hereditary factors, diagnostic techniques, and possible therapies. The fluctuation in symptomatology is the reason for the illness's delayed diagnosis. This study does a systematic comparison between the signs and symptoms of FTD and Alzheimer's Disease. It provides a comprehensive analysis of the diagnostic techniques, treatments that are now accessible, genetic and neuropathological underpinnings, diagnosis possibilities, and clinical symptoms of FTD [21].

3.2.5 DEMENTIA TESTS FOR DIAGNOSIS

Dementia diagnosis is a comprehensive procedure carried out using many methods. This involves a neurological evaluation, in which a physician evaluates the functions of the patient's nervous system. The goal of a psychiatric evaluation is to comprehend mental and emotional health. Behavior and cognitive functions are assessed with the use of cognitive and neuropsychological testing. Brain anatomy can be understood using brain imaging techniques like CT or MRI scans. Blood tests could be performed to rule out further possible reasons. Functional assessment evaluates a person's capacity to carry out daily duties. Family and caregiver involvement is also very important as they provide insightful viewpoints on the patient's behavior and how it develops over time. A thorough medical history and physical examination are frequently the first steps in the process of gathering data on the development, course, and severity of the symptoms. They also perform a physical check in order to regulate any deeper health issues that might be the cause of the symptoms. In neurological evaluation, reflexes, motor skills, and other neurological functions can all be assessed via a neurological examination. It can also provide cues as to the presence of specific types of dementia, such as Fronto Temporal Dementia.

Evaluation by a psychiatrist: Some mental illnesses, such as depression, might resemble dementia symptoms. If a psychiatric disease is the primary cause of the symptoms, a psychiatric evaluation can help identify this.

Tests for memory, attention, language, problem-solving, and other cognitive abilities are part of the cognitive and neuropsychological evaluation process. These tests can assist in distinguishing between different types of dementia and can help determine the degree of cognitive impairment.

A series of assessments intended to evaluate cognitive abilities such as memory, attention, language, problem-solving, and other areas. These assessments can help distinguish between various forms of dementia and determine the degree of cognitive impairment. This test is referred to as Cognitive and Neurological Testing.

Precision images of the brain can be obtained from MRI and Computed Tomography (CT) scans of the brain. These types of brain scans can assist in identifying anatomical alterations in the brain that may be indicative of various forms of dementia.

The Mini-Mental State Examination (MMSE), a well-liked cognitive screening examination, evaluates a variety of cognitive processes, such as direction, focus, recall, communication, and visuospatial skills. It is frequently used by medical professionals to quickly evaluate a patient's cognitive health and check for any potential cognitive impairment, such as that seen in AD and other types of dementia. Healthcare professionals can take this test. The Mini-Mental State Examination, also known as the MMSE comprises tasks related to orientation, registration, attention, and computation, as well as language assessments and design copy [19].

These tests produce data types such as images, demographics, multi-omics, electronic health records, biological data, and neurological test results, which can be referred to for further study or research.

3.3   STUDY ON ALZHEIMER'S DISEASE AND AI

According to the study, Artificial Intelligence (AI) offers capabilities for complex, large-scale data analysis in AD research, such as risk assessment and patient categorization for tailored care and diagnosis. Additionally, it was determined that AI offers methods for the processing of large and complex data in AD research. AI can assist in diagnosing AD and creating customized treatment programs. AI offers methods for procedures. The knowledge and research on Alzheimer's Disease is lacking. Initiatives for open data sharing offer a wealth of knowledge about the illness.

AI-assisted clinical practice supported for patient classification for evaluating vast and complicated datasets with possible application of AI for the detection and management of AD. Combining being data from multiple-omics research studies that collect biological, clinical, and lifestyle data from AD patients is the contribution. AI can enhance AD prediction and diagnosis. One way to list the practical consequences is that AI can provide personalized treatment approaches for AD. There are some limits. For diagnosis of AD, this work suggests using data types such as biological images, demographics, neuropsychological test results, Electronics Health Record, and multi-omics data. These data can be processed with algorithms such as classification, regression, and clustering to get outcomes.

Figure 3.2 shows how AI can be used in Health Science to diagnose a disease in the early stage, check disease progression, and conversion predictions in the monitoring of symptoms, and categorize the patients [21].

This groundbreaking study has paved the way for the development of highly precise blood-based diagnosis biosignatures for AD using advanced automated Machine Learning algorithms. By carefully examining transcriptome and proteome data, the team has discovered three unique biosignatures, which constitute a main development in our understanding of Alzheimer's Disease. These complex molecular indicators not only help us understand the disease better, but they may also revolutionize early diagnosis and expedite the creation of specialized treatments for this challenging neurodegenerative disease.

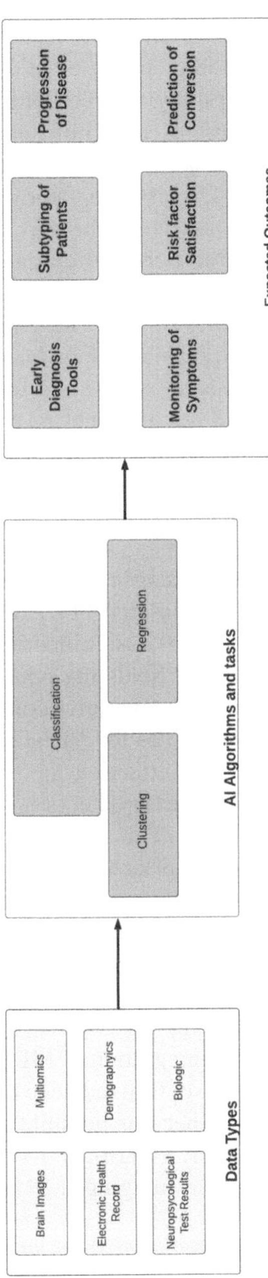

FIGURE 3.2 AI in diagnosing the diseases.

The work uses state-of-the-art techniques such as Support Vector Machines with miRNA (Micro Ribonucleic Acid) predictors and Classification Random Forests with mRNA (Messenger Ribonucleic Acid) predictors. This groundbreaking study explores blood-based biosignatures in an effort to clarify the intricate molecular processes linked to AD. By employing cutting-edge automated Machine Learning techniques, scientists may carefully study complex patterns and signs found in blood samples. This novel method represents a significant advance in neurodegenerative disease research as well as clinical practice by offering an improved and more accurate diagnosis of Alzheimer's Disease. The study's conclusions highlight how technology may change medicine and point the way for earlier and more precise diagnoses. Scientists have successfully created diagnostic biomarkers by utilizing automated Machine Learning techniques. These biomarkers provide complicated insights into the underlying intricacies of AD. These findings not only improve our ability to diagnose patients but also open the door for more advances in treatments and interventions. Ultimately, this study shows the remarkable impact of cutting-edge technology on patient care and research into AD, marking a significant breakthrough in both improved scientific knowledge and medical procedures [22].

In this study, researchers explore AD diagnosis using advanced MRI scans and cutting-edge feature extraction methods coupled with Machine Learning algorithms. Their goal is to enhance Alzheimer's diagnosis precision by employing deep learning to thoroughly analyze brain images. The research, backed by meticulous examination and validation, offers crucial insights, paving the way for reliable diagnostic tools. This breakthrough signifies a significant stride in rapid and accurate Alzheimer's diagnosis through MRI. It holds the potential to enhance patient outcomes and deepen knowledge of neurodegenerative conditions. The study delves into the realm of Machine Learning techniques for Alzheimer's diagnosis, emphasizing early detection and advanced feature extraction methods. This study underscores the utilization of AI for early-stage disease detection, emphasizing the crucial role of accurate feature extraction methods. The research highlights the importance of prompt intervention by placing a high priority on early detection. It also provides insightful information regarding the advancement of effective diagnostic methods for Alzheimer's Disease. The study's conclusions provide a thorough investigation of Machine Learning techniques for MRI image-based AD diagnosis. It delves into various methods of feature amalgamation and extraction, shedding light on the methodologies employed by scientists [23].

The study in [24] investigates the integration of MRI and PET scans intended for the categorization of AD using Pareto-optimized deep learning models. The purpose of this article was to investigate whether it is possible to use pre-existing models—the Visual Geometry Group (VGG) 11, VGG16, and VGG19 architectures—to integrate images from Magnetic Resource Imaging (MRI) and Pareto-optimized deep learning methodologies (PET).

In image fusion, VGG19 performs better than VGG16 and VGG11. There are documented Structural Similarity Index Method (SSIM) values for the Cognitively Normal (CN), AD, and MCI stages. The viability of classifying Alzheimer's illness by image fusion using Pareto-optimized deep learning is discussed in the references

[25]. When it comes to extracting meaningful features from MRI and PET data, VGG19 performs better than VGG16 and VGG11. In image fusion, VGG19 performs better than VGG16 and VGG11. Mean SSIM ratings for the CN, AD, and MCI phases are considered. In [24], the deep learning is used to investigate AD. Here it makes use of Pareto-optimized techniques to fuse images. Image fusion using a transposed convolution layer is used as a method for deep learning with Pareto-optimization.

The study [25], obtains great classification accuracy by predicting AD using brain MRI scans and AI algorithms. In this work, the authors classified AD from brain MRI scans using three distinct deep CNN models such as VGG-16, Inception-V3, and Xception. High classification accuracy was attained by three deep CNN models. The different types of AD are classified into several methods is also studied. Detecting AD with deep learning methods with CNN models, high classification accuracy was attained. From the experiment VGG-16 model's accuracy was 75%. The algorithm Xception results in accuracy and Inception V3 models were 70%. The VGG-16 model's accuracy was 75%. The accuracy of the Xception and Inception-V3 models was 70%. The objective of this study was to develop an AD prediction mode. In this article, it uses brain MRI scans and AI algorithms to forecast Alzheimer's Disease. AI algorithm which belongs to CNN models is VGG-16, Inception, and Inception-V3. AI algorithms have been developed to forecast Alzheimer's illness. Three distinct deep CNN models were trained and assessed. AI algorithms have been developed to forecast Alzheimer's illness [25].

The study successfully classified AD and Fronto Temporal Dementia using Machine Learning with MRI data. In the referred paper [27], the scientists used brain Magnetic Resonance Imaging (MRI) to combine unsupervised and supervised Machine Learning techniques to distinguish between FTD and AD (AD). FTD and AD are correctly classified by Machine Learning. A single characteristic is utilized for classification, and accuracy is high. FTD and ADs are classified based on Machine Learning; classification accuracy increased with longitudinal data. Classification accuracy over the long term: CTR vs AD—90.0%, CTR vs FTD—88.0%; CTR vs AD—83.3%, CTR vs FTD—82.1%. Cross-sectional and longitudinal MRI data were evaluated to classify Alzheimer's and Fronto Temporal Dementia using Machine Learning. Dimensionality reduction and support vector machine classification are two examples of unsupervised and supervised Machine Learning. Combining supervised and unsupervised Machine Learning techniques produced measurements of the cortical thickness and subcortical gray matter volume [26]. This helps to identify the content of the brain in terms of gray matter and thickness.

In order to forecast AD using clinical and neuroimaging tests—including the application of artificial intelligence techniques on MRI images—the research suggests comparing the efficacy of data mining techniques. A comparison of data mining methods' efficacy on both datasets involving clinical and imaging testing with AD indicates that the CHFS model is better in the early stages of the disease prediction when compared to the clinical medical dataset (MRI). The suggested paradigm increases the accuracy of AD diagnosis. The Composite Hybrid Feature Selection (CHFS) model performs better than conventional methods for categorization.

An analysis of comparing neuroimaging and clinical tests for AD prediction shows that the proposed model increases the precision of clinical diagnosis prediction. The clinical dataset gives 96.90% accuracy in working with the proposed model which yields 80.21% on the MRI dataset. The study focuses on predicting neurodegenerative illnesses using Artificial Intelligence methods using the Stack Hybrid Classification (SHC) model and Composite Hybrid Feature Selection (CHFS) model. A comparative analysis of neuroimaging and clinical testing of these two models are studied.1 A hybrid feature extraction approach for MRI images is proposed. Early AD diagnosis increased neuroimaging test classification accuracy with this method [27].

The study [28] suggests a deep learning architecture that is led by attention to diagnosing dementia from structural MRI (sMRI) data. Present reference shows that a hybrid network is developed to concurrently train an entirely convolutional network built to autonomously locate the prejudiced brain areas in a partially supervised manner, and merge multilevel sMRI information for the production of CAD models. The suggested approach performs better in MCI conversion prediction and AD diagnosis than cutting-edge techniques. Deep learning techniques are used with sMRI to diagnose dementia as a framework for dementia diagnosis that is directed by attention and concentration of the patient. The attention-guided framework that has been proposed performs better. When it comes to AD diagnosis and MCI conversion prediction, the recommended method outperforms state-of-the-art methods evaluated using the Alzheimer's Disease Neuroimaging Initiative (ADNI-1), ADNI-2, and Australian Imaging Biomarkers and Lifestyle Study (AIBLs) public datasets. A suggested deep learning technique for dementia detection using sMRI data is called an attention-guided Hybrid Network for CAD model development. Every subject's identified brain areas were positioned exactly the same. Training of the model involved strictly specified local areas or patches. To train and combine multilayer sMRI characteristics in the suggested attention-guided deep learning framework for dementia detection, a hybrid network was developed. CAD model building using a framework for attention-guided deep learning improved dementia identification with structural MRI data [28].

The study assesses the efficiency of neuropsychological testing in the classification of AD and pinpoints the most important characteristics for precise categorization. Previous correlation studies have shown that processing several neuropsychological tests requires a large amount of computer time. As a result, attribute selection methods are used for the test scores. The top four characteristics are important for classifying AD; 99.1% accuracy and 0.999 ROC area were attained. Neuropsychological assessments are performed to assess the course of AD. Machine Learning classifiers and attribute selection techniques are applied. Using InfoGain AttributeEval with the Bayes Net classifier, the top six attributes yielded an accuracy of 99.1% and a ROC area of 0.999. Comparable outcomes were obtained using the BayesNet classifier and OneRAttributeEval for the top seven attributes. AD is a type of dementia that cannot be reversed. Tests of neuropsychology are used to evaluate cognitive deterioration. Supervised classifiers are the attribute selection algorithms employed in this instance. Using classifiers and attribute selection algorithms, neuropsychological test evaluation is done to accurately classify cases of Alzheimer's Disease.

The top four characteristics significantly influence how AD is classified; neuropsychological scores with data availability < 50 are not included [29].

In order to distinguish between AD and AD along with Lewy Bodies Disorders (LBD), the study looked at the use of neuropsychological testing. This study looked at neuropsychological functioning differences between pathologically proven groups and the capacity of particular tests to classify patients with AD and LBD. The vasoconstriction, phonemic fluency, and processing speed of individuals with AD were superior to those with AD with Lewy Body Dementia (LBD. The pathological finding of AD and AD with LBD was predicted by processing speed and vasoconstriction. Cognitive testing helps distinguish Alzheimer's from AD associated with Lewy Body Dementia (LBD). The pathological group is predicted by vasoconstriction and the speed of the process. Compared to patients with AD with LBD, people with AD exhibited superior vasoconstriction, phonemic fluency, and processing speed. The pathological vasoconstriction is difficult to distinguish AD from AD with LBD clinically. Many examinations have to be carried out to test the same, in which cognitive differences are measured. Binary logistics regressions, one-way ANOVAs and $\chi2$ analysis are the methods used for the same. The considerable amount of time required to gather pathology specimens. Neuropsychological functional disparities in between AD and AD with LBD are evaluated. The pathological group is predicted by vasoconstriction and processing speed.

Cognitive assessments can help distinguish AD from AD in conjunction with LBD illnesses. Vasoconstriction and processing speed are predictive of pathological diagnosis [31].

The study investigated the connection between cortical shrinkage and specific cognitive impairments in the Alzheimer's continuum. Because poor performance on most neuropsychological tests is closely associated with cortex thinning in particular brain locations, an accurate examination of these assessments in clinical settings may forecast the cerebral atrophy distribution among individuals with Alzheimer's Disease. Specific brain areas that have seen cortical shrinkage are linked to neuropsychological abnormalities in the Alzheimer's continuum. A precise examination of neuropsychological assessments can forecast the pattern of brain atrophy in individuals suffering from AD. Examined the co-relation between cortical atrophy and cognitive deficiencies. Poor performance on cortical thinning test results in the Alzheimer's. In the Alzheimer's continuum, the majority of cognitive abnormalities are linked to cortical atrophy in certain brain areas these gives cortical thinning. The association between particular cognitive abnormalities in the Alzheimer's continuum and cortical atrophy was examined in this study. Since poor performance on most neurological examinations is closely associated with cortical thinning in specific brain locations in AD, a precise evaluation of neurocognitive findings would result in an estimate of the brain degeneration sequence in patients with the illness. Cortical atrophy in particular brain regions is linked to neuropsychological abnormalities in AD. Brain part atrophy patterns in patients with AD range can be predicted with precision through the examination of neuropsychological test results. The majority of cognitive impairments in the Alzheimer's spectrum are linked to cortical atrophy in particular brain areas [31].

According to the study, there is a correlation between the component Brain–Age–Score (BAS) and conventional neuropsychological screening instruments for AD. Using MRI scans, a completely automated methodology is constructed to estimate the component BAS in normal healthy controls and people with MCI or AD. The Brain-Age Score (BAS) and conventional AD screening instruments have a correlation. Measurements from anatomical MRI are also linked to BAS. The AD Brain–Age–Score (BAS) is an MRI-based indicator. BAS corresponds with both MRI measures and conventional screening techniques. Anatomical MRI data and conventional methods of AD screening are associated with the Brain–Age–Score (BAS). When it comes to clinical applications and neuropsychological screening tools, the BAS can be a dependable automated indicator.

AD's intensity is measured based on BAS as well, which can be used to diagnose the degree of brain atrophy as well as a dependable automated measure for neuropsychological screening and clinical applications which is created a completely automated system to use MRI scans to estimate the Brain-Age Score (BAS). 385 healthy controls were used to train the framework, and people with Mild/Moderate Cognitive Impairment (MCI) or AD were used to evaluate it. The Brain–Age–Score (BAS), an MRI-based marker for AD, showed a relationship between BAS and conventional screening methods as well as measurements from anatomical magnetic resonance imaging. Brain atrophy level can be diagnosed using BAS. It can also be a useful automated indicator for neuropsychological screening tools and clinical applications [32].

The research presents an up-to-the-minutes ML model for AD that guarantees early and affordable diagnosis with an astounding 90% accuracy rate. With only three tests and four clinical visits needed for diagnosis, this model is efficient and reliable, demonstrating 87% accuracy and 79% recall. The study suggests a productive Machine Learning model that may diagnose AD early and affordably, doing away with the necessity for in-depth examinations and visits. The model, which achieves over 90% accuracy and recall, also offers an efficient "lean" diagnostic technique with 87% accuracy, highlighting its efficacy in anticipating the onset of Alzheimer's Disease. Important elements are missed by the research: demographic and biomarker information is not disclosed, nor is data specifics from AIBL and ADNI trials included. Unaddressed are biases, confounding variables, and difficulties in implementing the reduced diagnostic protocol, which cast doubt on the accuracy and practicality of the approach. Important elements are missed by the research: demographic and biomarker information is not disclosed, nor are data specifics from AIBL and ADNI trials included. Unaddressed are biases, confounding variables, and difficulties in implementing the reduced diagnostic protocol, which cast doubt on the accuracy and practicality of the approach. Potential limits and biases in the suggested AD predictive model should be investigated and validated using a variety of datasets, and long-term studies should be carried out to evaluate the model's stability. Furthermore, investigating the "lean" diagnostic protocol's viability in the real world while taking patient acceptability and cost into account is essential for its effective use [33].

There is no mention of neuropsychological testing for AD in the information that is presented. The referred articles [34] explain the pathologic features of AD associated with its genesis as well as those that cannot be prevented and are of dubious importance, such as granulovacuolar degeneration and Hirano bodies. The absence of standard diagnostic instruments to detect patients sufficiently early, in their treatment regimen, and insufficient alternatives for effective treatment after the illness process is identified. A neurodegenerative condition that progresses over time is Alzheimer's Disease. Diagnosis requires the presence of neurofibrillary tangles and amyloid plaques. AD is a mixture of proteins such as tau and amyloid in a part of the brain, which is linked to other age-related conditions like Lewy Body Disease and cerebrovascular illness. Patients over the age of 80 are frequently found to have independent protein tau pathologies, namely Primary Age-Related Tauopathy (PART) and Aging-Related Tau Astrogliopathy (ARTAG). AD is a neural disorder that progresses as time passes and is typified by cognitive decline and memory problems. A neuropathologic alteration characteristic of AD can be identified by staining and microscopic inspection of several brain areas. The absence of routine diagnostic instruments for early detection is required. There is an absence of efficient treatment alternatives for diagnosed diseases. Lewy Body Dementia (DLB and PDD) is caused by PART and ARTAG. inadequate therapeutic alternatives for therapy.

3.4 DEMENTIA DIAGNOSIS WITH AI TECHNIQUE

For any disease, proper diagnosis at the right time is very important. As there are many dementia types, diagnosis method also varies from one to the other. In some cases, overlapping symptoms are exhibited in a patient which is difficult to diagnose by a physician. Typically, dementia diagnosis entails a thorough and detailed examination process that includes methods such as Medical History and Physical Examination, Cognitive and Neuropsychological Testing, Brain Imaging, Blood Tests, Neurological Evaluation, Psychiatric Evaluation, Functional Assessment, and Family and Caregiver Input.

In [35, 36] Convolutional Neural Networks (CNNs) are used for transfer learning in two ways: first, by using the output of the classification layer to transfer knowledge from components of CNN to other CNN layers, and second, by using trained CNN for the purpose of feature extraction. In many evaluation tasks, feature extraction is a common method. Transfer learning methodologies are being included in CAD systems to increase adaptability and expedite operational processes. It's important to keep in mind that one of the most prevalent forms of dementia worldwide is still AD. Nowadays, a lot of cutting-edge research and clinical settings employ ML techniques for diagnosis and classification.

This chapter presents a method for converting 2D MRI scan data into a Machine Learning classification format. The technology uses either a custom-trained Convolutional Neural Network (CNN) or a pre-trained AlexNet CNN to extract significant properties from 2D photos. Additionally, methods for reducing dimensionality like Principal Component Analysis (PCA) and t-Distributed Stochastic Neighbour Embedding (t-SNE) are used to condense the feature space.

The methodology results in two classifiers: one employs a feed-forward Artificial Neural Network (ANN), while the other employs the K-Nearest Neighbors (K-NN) method. These classifiers were created specifically to distinguish between typical and abnormal human MRI data. The analysis of these classifiers reveals that the K-Nearest Neighbors (K-NN) classifier has an even higher accuracy rate of 98% than the Feed-forward Neural Network (FP-ANN) classifier, which already has an amazing accuracy rate of 97%. When compared to recent efforts in the same subject, these amazing findings show how successful and simple the suggested approach is. The combination of the FP-ANN and K-NN classifiers shows the resilience and accuracy of the system, offering it a promising solution for the essential issue of reliably and quickly detecting anomalies in MRI scans. Convolutional Neural Networks (CNNs) using pre-trained features provide an invaluable resource for training classifiers. In comparison to building a full CNN network from scratch, these classifiers usually perform better when they are built on top of CNN features. However, the key to obtaining improved outcomes depends on the careful management of characteristics and the categorization procedure.

In the reference [37], a new Weakly Supervised Model (WSDL) is developed for training and learning on specific medical datasets without complete labels. Weakly Supervised Learning, regularization terms, attention mechanisms, the Effective Net Deep Learning Model, and Mixture data improvement techniques are all used in WSDL. First, data improvement pre-processing is applied to the two ADNI2 datasets. Our proposed WSDL model then instructs the data for different levels of missing labels. The model can distinguish between samples with verified cases of AD and Normal Controls (NC), as well as between AD patients in two distinct developmental stages and NC. It is highly validated by experimental results that the WSDL approach outperforms the other baselines for each performance metric that has been looked at. Axial and sagittal views can both be used for training. Using image data from various diseases, it is also feasible to train WSDL and make an effort to advance it in order to obtain better performance [37].

In [38] the Spontaneous Homeopathic Syndrome (SHS) diagnosis and therapy are represented by suggesting a model that has significantly improved the treatment. In order to offer a comprehensive solution, this comprehensive framework makes use of the interactions between data mining, Machine Learning, and Internet of Things (IoT) technologies. Its main objectives include strengthening real-time monitoring of SHS cases, treating patients with individualized treatment programs, and improving diagnosis accuracy.

The model can effectively filter through enormous information to find patterns and trends that may escape human observers by utilizing data mining techniques. IoT device integration enables continuous and remote patient monitoring, providing insightful data on the development of SHS and patient responses to therapies.

At the end of the day, our concept has the potential to change the diagnosis and treatment of SHS, ushering in a time of more precise diagnoses, individualized care, and better patient outcomes. Its wider implications extend to the broader medical community, as data-driven methodologies hold enormous potential for revolutionizing healthcare procedures.

As the average age of the population rises, early diagnosis of cognitive impairment in the elderly has become a critical objective for healthcare systems worldwide [39].

This chapter provides a thorough examination of the different technologies and methods used to diagnose the symptoms of Neurodegenerative Disorders (NDDs), including the analysis of locomotion sensor data and Artificial Intelligence (AI) algorithms. Dementia detection (37%), Huntington's disease (11%), and Parkinson's disease (44%), which were the main topics of 128 peer-reviewed studies that were meticulously studied for this study, were the key topics. Some publications also discussed disorders that coexisted, such as PD and HD (4%), or PD and dementia (4%). These studies' testing results repeatedly show that these new technologies have a great deal of promise to help medical professionals and carers. They improve patient management as well as the diagnostic process. This chapter offers a thorough summary of the various technologies and AI techniques used to identify NDD symptoms, mostly through the use of locomotion sensor data. In addition, it explores the difficulties currently faced and suggests prospective solutions to make NDD symptom detection more approachable and advantageous for the scientific community and clinical practice. This study contributes to the improvement of early diagnosis and better care for those dealing with NDDs by bridging the gap between technology and healthcare, aligning with the changing needs of an aging global population.

In the study [40], we thoroughly evaluated each Machine Learning model using the Receiver Operating Characteristic (ROC) curve and its matching Area Under the Curve (AUC) score. These evaluations were crucial in determining how well the models could distinguish between various classes and correctly classify the data. We chose a baseline value of 0.5, which represents random performance, as a standard for comparison in the context of AUC. The outcomes, as seen in Figure 3.3, are encouraging. Each model we examined performed much better than the arbitrary baseline of 0.5, demonstrating its suitability for the task at hand. Notably, the top-performing models were two models: neural networks and logistic regression. While neural networks demonstrated even stronger discriminatory ability with an average AUC value of 0.848, logistic regression produced a remarkable average AUC score of 0.815.

Three algorithms Support Vector Machine (SVM), K-Nearest Neighbour (KNN), and Linear Discriminant Analysis (LDA) were used in an analysis employing a dataset from the online source UCI-based Machine Learning Repository to generate accuracy, recall, and confusion matrices for disease detection. The findings demonstrated extraordinary accuracy: SVM and KNN both obtained 100% accuracy, while LDA achieved 80%. The dataset has 196 entries, each with 22 parameters, including 5 key parameters deemed important for disease diagnosis. The study was conducted in two versions: one with all 22 parameters and one with only the 5 most important ones. Each version employed a 70% training, 30% test data split. SVM regularly outperformed the other algorithms, demonstrating its diagnostic efficacy. This approach not only aids in disease diagnosis but also sheds light on the significance of key factors in real-world datasets [41].

In our investigation, the strongest association was found between the outcome variable and the SUBTL measure of linguistic richness across eight of the nine folds. The portrayal of this correlation (Figure 3.3) graphically provides compelling insight into each blog post's SUBTL scores in the referred corpus. These rankings

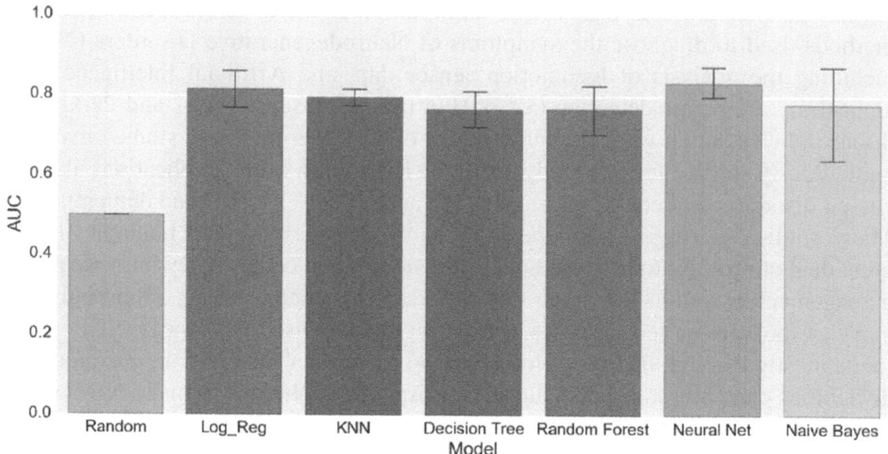

FIGURE 3.3 Comparison of model: To evaluate the efficacy of the model, evaluated the mean AUC and 90% confidence intervals using a ninefold cross-validation procedure. To avoid overlapping the training and test sets, each blog's entries were only included in one of them.

are deliberately arranged by blog, with bloggers who have dementia displayed in the front row.

Interestingly, bloggers with dementia were significantly less likely to have lower SUBTL scores, which are a sign of a broader vocabulary, demonstrating linguistic diversity in this group. It's interesting to note that our longitudinal investigation did not find any discernible deterioration in the richness of the vocabulary across the observed time frame. With this discovery, researchers can now better understand how language dynamics in dementia patients change.

As part of our ongoing research, researchers rigorously investigated additional features with high predictive power for his/her target variable. These upcoming discoveries should improve our understanding of this challenging topic. In order to further our collective knowledge and improve assistance for those dealing with dementia, we are excitedly anticipating addressing these insights and encouraging collaborative conversation during our next workshop.

All research gives a ray of hope to all mental patients and neurologists. These solutions can also be expanded with other algorithms. These research works show a lot of hope and promise in the present developments in the field of mental healthcare. The field of mental healthcare is being transformed by these methods, which cover a wide range of modalities from psychotherapy and pharmacology to cutting-edge technology like telehealth and digital treatments. Here are some important things to think about: personalized care, neuroscience and medicine, digital mental health, psychotherapy and behavioral interventions, research, and innovations are the future discoveries and therapies that could result from current research in fields like neuroplasticity, and psychedelics with artificial intelligence.

3.5 RESULT ANALYSIS OF DIFFERENT METHODS

Researchers presented DL models for the categorization of MRI images of (1) AD and sMCI participants, and (2) AD, sMCI, and CN patients. For job one, the team used a special E2EL and TL fusion method, as shown in Figure 3.4. They used fivefold stratified cross-validation to train the model from scratch in the first fold (E2EL), utilized the best epoch's final weights from fold 1 as the initial weights for fold 2 after later validating the model (TL) [42].

The ML algorithm showed a 92% accuracy rate in predicting a 2-year incidence of dementia in comparison to other neurodegeneration risk-predicting mathematical models, such as the Cardiovascular Risk Factors, Aging, and Incidence of Dementia (CAIDE) Risk Score and the Brief Dementia Screening Indicator (BDSI). Additionally, 84% of individuals were identified by the model as potentially misdiagnosed with dementia, and these patients had their diagnosis altered to either cognitively normal or Mild Cognitive Impairment (MCI). One hopeful application of AI in clinical settings is the prediction of dementia progression over a two-year period, as demonstrated by a large-scale study. Within two years of the first assessment, Machine Learning correctly identified dementia subtypes (vascular, Lewy Body, Alzheimer's, and others) in this University of Exeter study with 15,307 participants, indicating a significant clinical diagnosis. The AI has both pros and cons. The study revealed that the ML system outperformed models such as the Brief Dementia Screening Indicator (BDSI) and Cardiovascular Risk Factors, Aging, and Incidence of Dementia (CAIDE) Risk Score, demonstrating a 92% accuracy rate in predicting dementia occurrence over two years in clinical research that used AI. Remarkably, 84% of patients who were originally misdiagnosed with dementia were subsequently corrected to moderate cognitive.

Impairment of neurological function or cognitively normal status were recognized by the AI model. The growing amount of radiographic pictures in the world highlights how AI may help radiologists analyze data more efficiently and reduce their expanding workload. Radiologists prioritize using Artificial Intelligence (AI), and this is especially true in light of the difficulties caused by COVID-19. The pandemic has resulted in longer wait times for diagnostic imaging services, with CT and MRI tests in Canada averaging between 50 and 89 days. Every year, hospitals across the globe complete 3.6 billion imaging procedures and generate 50 petabytes of data. Radiologists struggle to discover effective ways to handle the massive number of data they are required to collect, read, and process promptly. Not all diseases respond well to medicine's "one-size-fits-all" approach. To prevent, diagnose, and cure diseases, precision or personalized medicine is a new branch of medicine that takes into account an individual's genetic composition, environment, and lifestyle [43].

Neurocognitive symptoms include obvious memory loss, difficulty with routine tasks, confusion, personality changes, etc. that patients present with. In a clinic, a brain scan is carried out with suitable modalities, such as CT, MRI, or PET. The image is processed by an artificial intelligence-based system to identify and categorize low, moderate, and high-priority brain scans, and it is then stored in the

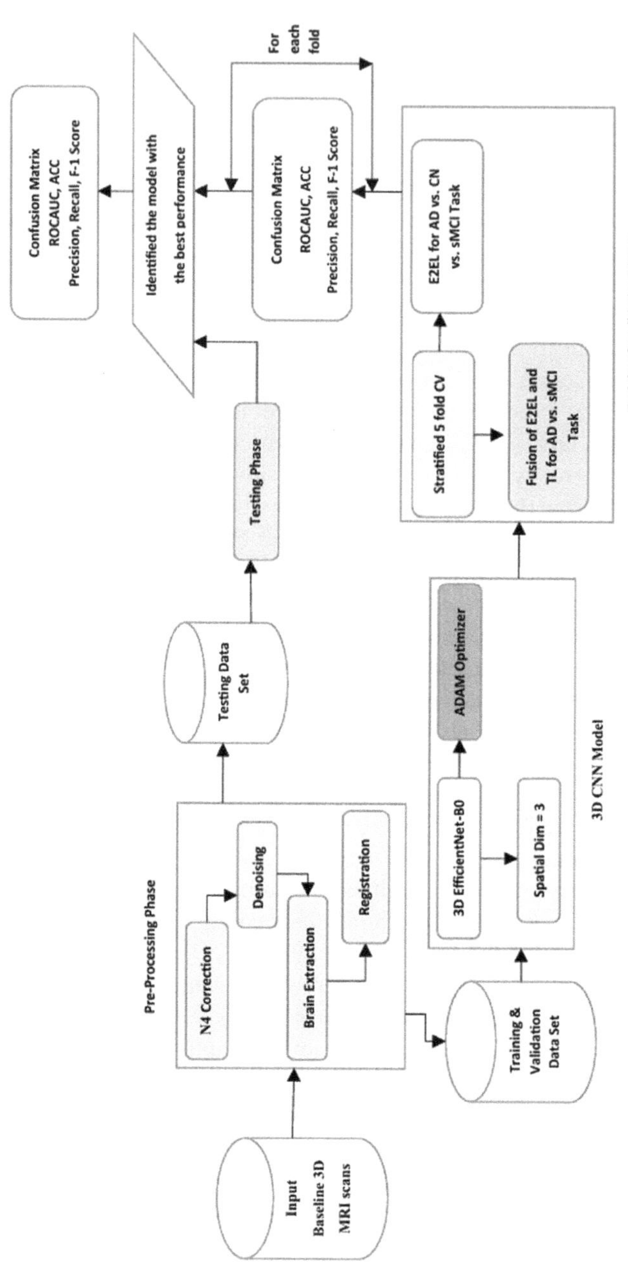

FIGURE 3.4   Model to categorize MRI images.

Picture Archiving and Communication Systems (PACS) database. The radiologists assess high-priority patients first, then moderate and low-priority cases. Following a diagnosis, the results are cross-referenced with the AI database. Before determining a diagnosis with certainty, a second opinion is required if the radiologist's judgment conflicts with the AI system. Following a diagnosis, the results are cross-referenced with the AI repository. A second opinion is required before determining a diagnosis with certainty if the radiologist's judgment conflicts with the AI system. Patients can discuss recommendations for future treatment with their practitioner after a definitive diagnosis has been made. The process is shown in Figure 3.5 [44].

As the most common type of progressive degenerative dementia with a significant socioeconomic impact in Western nations, AD is currently one of the most active study topics. A post-mortem examination of the patient's brain tissue is required for definitive confirmation of the diagnosis, which is occasionally established by ruling out other dementias. With automatic analysis carried out by non-invasive intelligent approaches, the goal of this chapter is to enhance the early detection of AD and its severity. Here, the techniques of Automatic Spontaneous Speech Analysis (ASSA) and Emotional Temperature (ET) have been chosen since they are noninvasive, inexpensive, and free of negative consequences. Figure 3.6 and Figure 3.7 show drastic changes after experiments. Experiments measuring emotional temperature include the first series of tests. The suggested measures' capacity for discrimination has been

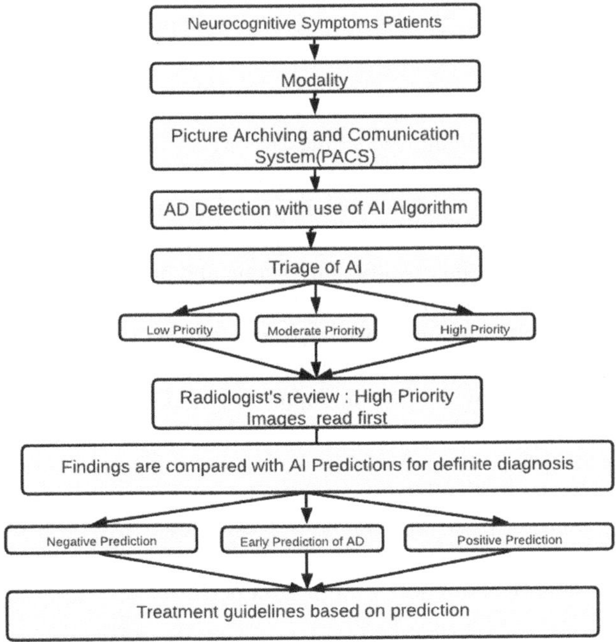

FIGURE 3.5   Model to diagnose AD.

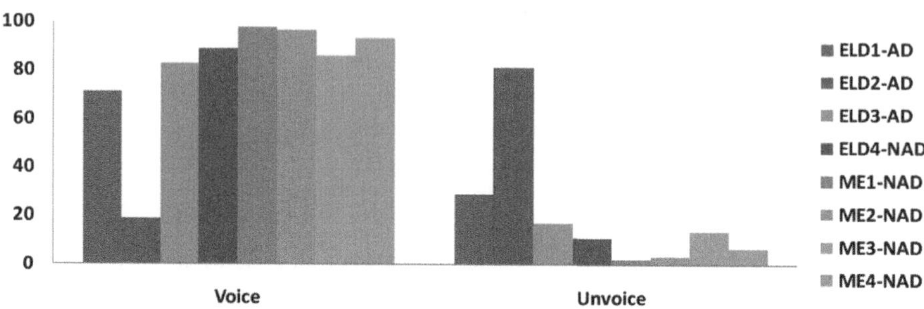

FIGURE 3.6 Percentage in the spon for voiced and unvoiced.

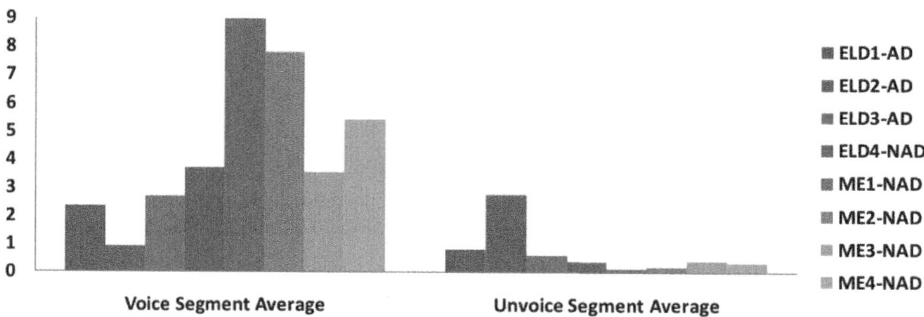

FIGURE 3.7 Percentage in the spon for voiced segment average and unvoiced segment average.

measured using Support Vector Machines (SVM). Utilizing a radial basis kernel function, we implemented our method using the publicly available LIBSVM [45].

Different brain regions change as a result of various brain problems. Cognitive problems including disorientation and memory loss are hallmarks of Alzheimer's Disease, a chronic illness that results in dementia and brain cell death. AD has been identified thanks to the combination of ML algorithms and image processing techniques. In order to differentiate between people with AD and healthy persons, this study employs brain magnetic resonance imaging. To do this, a convolutional neural network is fed 2D anatomical slices as input using a deep learning technique. This study used a 2D-based Alzheimer's network (AlzNet) to reach a 99.30% accuracy rate, in contrast to prior research that frequently used 3D convolutional neural networks. The study methodically investigated the effects of variables such as layer number, filters, and dropout rate on AlzNet using data from the OASIS website. When the data were assessed using other performance criteria, they provided fascinating new information about how well AlzNet performs in identifying Alzheimer's illness.

3.6 CONCLUSION

Overall, the study emphasizes the need for greater knowledge and comprehension of these brain diseases in order to enhance the disease's early detection and treatment. Device based on biological traits for intelligent auxiliary dementia diagnosis is required and AI is supporting in fulfilling this requirement. Integrating Large Data from Various Omics Studies with AI can enhance AD prediction and diagnosis. As per the study, AI is supporting to do research with types of data such as images, biological data, neuropsychological test data, and electronic data which are available as open source. These can be used for study and research to improve the process. It is necessary to modify diagnostic standards as brain diseases such as FTD, AD, etc., which are influenced by socioeconomic, linguistic, cultural, and educational characteristics. In some diseases such as FTD, neuroimaging serves as a pivotal biomarker. So, specialized neuroimaging methodologies are imperative for both diagnosing and monitoring the condition. As mentioned here all types of data yield proper output. But, to fortify the diagnosis methods in view of patients we can research with new technologies as well. AI has both pros and many challenges. Lack of an in vivo gold standard for diagnosis, physician prejudice, distrust in the medical community, generalization issues, and patient privacy concerns are some of the problems faced while using AI.

Other than AI, a new technology is also evolving in health science as well, which is identified as Quantum Computing. Beyond the scope of AI, there is a ray of hope with Quantum Computing. This technique is also booming in all fields. The field of Quantum Computing holds great potential for transforming healthcare, specifically in the areas of complex diseases, where it can provide improved precision and effectiveness. Because of its special computational powers, it has the potential to revolutionize illness prediction and detection.

REFERENCES

1. Fan, Y., Zhao, W., Ni, Y., Liu, Y., Tang, Y., Sun, Y., Liu, F., Yu, W., Wu, J., & Wang, J. (2023). Newly identified transmembrane protein 106B amyloid fibrils in the human brain: Pathogens or by-products? *Ageing Neur Dis*, 3(1), 4. doi: 10.20517/and.2022.30.
2. Simpson, B.N., Kim, M., Chuang, Y.F., Beason- Held, L., Kitner- Triolo, M., Kraut, M., Lirette, S.T., Windham, B.G., Griswold, M.E., Legido-Quigley, C., & Thambisetty, M. (2015, October 29). Blood metabolite markers of cognitive performance and brain function in aging. *Journal of Cerebral Blood Flow and Metabolism*, 36(7), 1212–1223.
3. Zoua, Zhenyou, et al. (2019). Linking the low-density lipoprotein receptor-binding segment enables the therapeutic 5-YHEDA peptide to cross the blood-brain barrier and scavenge excess iron and radicals in the brain of senescent mice Alzheimer's & Demntia: Translational research & clinical. *Interventions*, 5, 717–731.
4. Gonnabathula, Pavani K., & Yakubu, Momoh A. The impact of sex hormones on cognition and treatment: A review. *International Journal of Medical, Pharmacy and Drug Research(IJMPD)*. http://dx.doi.org?10.22161/ijimpd.7.3.2.
5. Johansson, M. *Cognitive Impairment and Its Consequences in Everyday Life* (Doctoral dissertation, Linköping University Electronic Press).

6. Vincent,A., & Fitzpatrick, L.A. (2000). Soy isoflavones: Are useful in menopause? *Mayo Clinic Proceedings*, 75(110), 1174–1184. https://doi.org/10/4065/75.11.1174.

7. Johansson, M. (2015). *Cognitive Impairment and Its Consequences in Everyday Life.* Linkoping University Medical dissertation No.1452. Sweden: LiU-Press, pp. 1–3.

8. Steel, N., Huppert, F.A., McWilliams, B., & Melzer, D. (2004). *Physical and Cognitive Function Institute for Fiscal Studies.* Cambridge: Department of Public Health and Primary Care.

9. Paterson, Sarah J. (2006). Sabine Heim Jennifer Thomas Friedman Naseen Choudhury and April A. Benasich development of structure and function in the infant's brain: Implications for cognition, language and social behavior. *Neuroscience and Biobehavioral Reviews*, 30(8), 1087–1105.

10. Dr Gayatri Devi, M.D. (2000). *Estrogen Memory & Menopause.* New York, NY: Alpha Sigma Books.

11. Macoir, Jo El. (2024). Language impairment in vascular dementia: A clinical review. *Journal of Geriatric Psychiatry and Neurology*, 37(2), 87–95.

12. Isordia-Martinez, J., Gongora-Rivera, F., Leal-Bailey, H., & Ortiz-Jimenez, X. (2014). Mild cognitive impairment. *Medicina Universitaria*, 16(62), 28–36.

13. Accessed in January 2014: http://www.fda.gov/Drugs/DrugSafety/PostmarkeretDrugSafetyInformationforPatientsandProviders/DrugSafetyInformationforHealthcareProfessionals/ucm085186.htm.

14. Winblad, B., Gauthier, S., Scinto, L., et al. (2008). Safety and efficacy of galantamine in subjects with mild cognitive impairment. *Neurology*, 70(22), 2024–2035.

15. Barnes, D.E., & Yaffe, K. (2005). Vitamin E and donepezil for the treatment of mild cognitive impairment. *New England Journal of Medicine*, 353(9), 951–952.

16. National Institutes of Health. (2013). Lewy Body Dementia: Information for Patients, Families, and Professionals. Retrieved from: https://www.nia.nih.gov/alzheimers/publication/lewy-body-dementia/introduction

17. Jankovic, J. (2008). Parkinson's disease: Clinical features and diagnosis. *Journal of Neurology, Neurosurgery, and Psychiatry*, 79(4), 368–376. doi: 10.1136/jnnp.2007.131045.

18. Boruah, Arpita Nath, Biswas, Saroj Kr., Bandyopadhyay, Sivaji, & Sarkar, Sunita (2020). *An Expert System for Identification of Key Factors of Parkinson's Disease: B-TDS-PD.* IEEE India Council International Subsections Conference(INDISCON).

19. Alber, Jessica, et al. (2019). Perspective white matter hyperintensities in vascular contributions to cognitive impairment and dementia(VCID): Knowledge gaps and opportunities. *Alzheimer's and Dementia: Translational Research and Clinical Interventions*, 5107–5117.

20. Vijay, K.K. (2023). Alzheimer's disease. doi: 10.1016/b978-0-323-91890-9.00020-9.

21. Janine, Diehl-Schmid (2023). Rare dementias: Frontotemporal dementia. *Fortschritte der Neurologie-Psychiatrie.* doi: 10.1055/a-2055-4496.

22. Chatzaki, E., Tsamardinos, I., Gourlia, K., & Karaglani, Makrina (2020). Accurate blood-based diagnostic biosignatures for Alzheimer's disease via automated machine learning. *Journal of Clinical Medicine*, 9(9). doi: 10.3390/jcm9093016.

23. Palak, Goyal, Rinkle, Rani, & Karamjeet, Singh (2021). State-of-the-art machine learning techniques for diagnosis of Alzheimer's disease from MR-images: A systematic review. *Archives of Computational Methods in Engineering*, 1–44. doi: 10.1007/S11831-021-09674-8.

24. Odusami, M., Maskeliūnas, R., & Damaševičius, R. (2023, July 8). Pareto optimized adaptive learning with transposed convolution for image fusion Alzheimer's disease classification. *Brain Sciences*, 13(7), 1045. doi: 10.3390/brainsci13071045. PMID: 37508977. PMCID: PMC10377099.

25. (2022). *Multi Class Alzheimer Disease Detection Using Deep Learning Techniques.* doi: 10.1109/dasa54658.2022.9765267.

26. Agnés, Pérez-Millan, Contador, José, Juncà-Parella, Jordi, Bosch, Beatriz, Borrell, Laia, Tort-Merino, Adrià, Falgàs, Neus, Sergi, Borrego-Écija, Bargalló, Núria, Rami, Lorena, Balasa, Mircea, Lladó, Albert, Sánchez-Valle, Raquel, & Roser, Sala-Llonch (2023). Classifying Alzheimer's disease and frontotemporal dementia using machine learning with cross-sectional and longitudinal magnetic resonance imaging data. *Human Brain Mapping.* doi: 10.1002/hbm.26205.

27. Abdullah Farid, Ahmed, Selim, Gamal, & Khater, Hatem A. (2020). Applying artificial intelligence techniques for prediction of neurodegenerative disorders: A comparative case-study on clinical tests and neuroimaging tests with Alzheimer's disease. doi: 10.20944/PREPRINTS202003.0299.V1.

28. Chunfeng, Lian, Mingxia, Liu, Yongsheng, Pan, & Dinggang, Shen (2020). Attention-guided hybrid network for dementia diagnosis with structural MR images. *IEEE Transactions on Systems, Man, and Cybernetics.* doi: 10.1109/TCYB.2020.3005859.

29. Andy, King, Istvan, Bodi, & Claire, Troakes. (2020). The neuropathological diagnosis of Alzheimer's disease-the challenges of pathological mimics and concomitant pathology. *Brain Sciences.* doi: 10.3390/BRAINSCI10080479.

30. Azar, Martina, Chapman, Silvia, Gu, Yian, Leverenz, James, B., Stern, Yaakov, & Cosentino, Stephanie. (2020). Cognitive tests aid in clinical differentiation of Alzheimer's disease versus Alzheimer's disease with Lewy body disease: Evidence from a pathological study. *Alzheimer's and Dementia.* doi: 10.1002/ALZ.12120.

31. Kang, Sung Hoon, Park, Yu Hyun, Lee, Daun, Kim, Jun Pyo, Chin, Ju Hee, Ahn, Yisuh, Park, Seong Beom, Kim, Hee Jin, Jang, Hyemin, Jung, Young Hee, Kim, Jaeho, Lee, Jongmin, Kim, Ji Sun, Cheon, Bo Kyoung, Hahn, Alice, Lee, Hyejoo, Na, Duk, L., Kim, Young Ju, & Seo, Sang Won (2019). The cortical neuroanatomy related to specific neuropsychological deficits in Alzheimer's continuum. *Dementia and Neurocognitive Disorders.* doi: 10.12779/DND.2019.18.3.77.

32. Iman, Beheshti, Norihide, Maikusa, & Hiroshi, Matsuda (2018). The association between "Brain-Age Score" (BAS) and traditional neuropsychological screening tools in Alzheimer's disease. *Brain and Behavior.* doi: 10.1002/BRB3.1020.

33. Cochrane, Courtney, Castineira, David, Shiban, Nisreen, & Protopapas, Pavlos (2020). Application of machine learning to predict the risk of Alzheimer's disease: An accurate and practical solution for early diagnostics. *arXiv: Quantitative Methods*: 2006.08702v1 [q-bio.QM] 2 Jun 2020, 1–14.

34. DeTure, Michael, & Dickson, Dennis W. (2019). The neuropathological diagnosis of Alzheimer's disease. *Molecular Neurodegeneration.* doi: 10.1186/S13024-019-0333-5.

35. Praveen, P., Srilatha, Koleti,, Sathvika, Masabathini, Nishitha, Edulapuram, & Nikhil, Madduri. (2023). Prediction of Alzheimer's disease using deep learning algorithms. Proceedings of the Second International Conference on Applied Artificial Intelligence and Computing (ICAAIC 2023) IEEE Xplore Part Number: CFP23BC3-ART.

36. Reeja, S.R., Mounika, Sunkar, & Mohanty, Sachi Nandan. *Biomarkers Classification for Various Brain Disease Using Artificial Intelligence Approach-A Study.* 12 June 2023, PREPRINT (Version 1) available at Research Square [https://doi.org/10.21203/rs.3.rs-3042717/v1].

37. Brindha, D.M., Geoff, Bevin, Dr Ebenezer, V., Dileep, B. Bethina, Selvaraj, E. Jackson, & Thirumalai Nambi, M. (2023). Classification and prediction of Alzheimer's disease using deep learning. Proceedings of the 7th International Conference on Intelligent Computing and Control Systems (ICICCS-2023) IEEE Xplore Part Number: CFP23K74-ART.

38. Visu, P., Smitha, P.S., Hemalatha, B., & Rajeshwari, P. (2023). Predictive diagnosis and IoT-based classification for effective management of spontaneous homeopathic syndrome through data mining and machine learning. *European Chemical Bulletin*, 12(6), 4579–4587.

39. Zofaghari, Samanesh, Suravee, Sumaiya, Riboni, Daniel, & Yordanova, Kristina. Sensor-based Locomototion data mining for supporting the diagnosis of Neurodegerative disorders: A survey. *ACM Computing Surveys*.

40. Masrani, Vaden, Murray, Gabriel, & Carenini, Giuseppa. (2017, August 4). Detecting dementia through retrospective analysis of routine blog posts by bloggers with dementia. Proceedings of the BioNLP 2017 Workshop. Association for Computational Linguistics, Vacouver, Canada, 232–237.

41. Mathkunti, N.M., & Rangaswamy, S. (2020). Machine learning techniques to identify dementia. *SN Computer Science*, 1(3), 118. doi: 10.1007/s42979-020-0099-4.

42. Deevyankar, Agarwal, Álvaro Berbís, Manuel, Luna, Antonio, Lipari, Vivian, Brito Ballester, Julien, & Torre Díez, Isabel de la. (2023). Automated medical diagnosis of alzheimer's disease using an efficient net convolutional neural network. *Journal of Medical Systems*. doi: 10.1007/s10916-023-01941-4[2222].

43. (2023). *Semantic Coherence Markers for the Early Diagnosis of the Alzheimer Disease.* doi: 10.48550/arxiv.2302.0102545.

44. Mirkin, Sophia, & Albensi, Benedict C. (2023). Should artificial intelligence be used in conjunction with neuroimaging in the diagnosis of Alzheimer's disease? *Frontiers in Aging Neuroscience*. doi: 10.3389/fnagi.2023.1094233.

45. Lopez-de-Ipiña, Karmele, Jesús B. Alonso, Nora Barroso, Marcos Faundez-Zanuy, Miriam Ecay, Jordi Solé-Casals, Carlos M. Travieso, Ainara Estanga, and Aitzol Ezeiza. (2012). "New approaches for Alzheimer's disease diagnosis based on automatic spontaneous speech analysis and emotional temperature." In Ambient Assisted Living and Home Care: 4th International Workshop, IWAAL 2012, Vitoria-Gasteiz, Spain, December 3–5, 2012. Proceedings 4, pp. 407–414. Springer Berlin Heidelberg.

4 Impact of Artificial Intelligence in Healthcare
Predictors of Multiple Sclerosis

Abhirup Bhattacharya and Zdzislaw Polkowski

4.1 INTRODUCTION

A variety of disorders affecting the nervous system exist today, which include the brain, spinal cord, and nerves. They are referred to as neurological diseases. These varied illnesses affect essential functions, resulting in deficits in motor, cognitive, or sensory abilities. These include ailments such as multiple sclerosis (MS), Parkinson's disease, epilepsy, and stroke. In particular, multiple sclerosis represents a complex neurological illness characterized by immune-mediated destruction to the sheath that surrounds nerve fibers, which acts as protection. Numerous neurological symptoms are caused by this immune attack's disruption of nerve transmission. As a representative neurological disease, multiple sclerosis highlights the complexity of disorders affecting the nervous system and the significant influence that immune system malfunction can have on neurological processes. Multiple sclerosis (MS) is a multifaceted and fatal ailment that affects the brain and the spinal cord, impairing nerve system-to-body communication. Inadvertent immune system assaults on the myelin sheath that covers nerve fibers result in a variety of symptoms and damage to the nerves. It affects the central nervous system (CNS). Multiple sclerosis presents with a wide range of unique symptoms, including fatigue, poor movement, vision problems, balance problems, limb weakness, and numbness. The location and extent of injury to the nerve fibers determine these symptoms [1]. Multiple sclerosis can manifest in diverse ways. For example, clinically isolated syndrome (CIS) is a term used to characterize a neurologic event that may be the initial clinical indication of MS; relapsing-remitting syndrome (RRMS) is the most common type of multiple sclerosis and is characterized by sporadic attacks of symptoms (relapses) interspersed with periods without clinical attacks (remissions); secondary progressive syndrome (SPMS) occurs due to a prolonged period with RRMS. In this, the relapses become less frequent and symptoms gradually worsen without relapses or remissions; and primary progressive (PPMS), in which there are no discernible relapses or remissions as the illness steadily worsens after exhibiting the early symptoms [2].

DOI: 10.1201/9781003464884-6

Diagnostic phases can be uncomfortable since getting a correct diagnosis frequently requires going through multiple stages, which leaves people uneasy. According to the National Multiple Sclerosis Society, over 2.8 million people have multiple sclerosis and the number of people living with MS had quadrupled from 1994 to 2017 in the United States [2]. Medical researchers are currently working on identifying various drugs that exist or must be prepared to either slow down the progression of MS or cure it. In 2021, it was found that simvastatin which is a medication that is frequently used to treat excessive cholesterol may also be used to delay the progression of secondary MS. A study that was conducted by utilizing information from normal blood tests on US military personnel discovered that the risk of developing MS was 32 times higher in those with Epstein-Barr virus (EBV) [3].

Artificial intelligence has a significant role to play in the field of medicine and healthcare as there exist multiple instances of technological solutions that have revolutionized the functioning of the health industry and it also supports diagnosis and advanced research in medicine and drugs. Tech-based solutions that employ artificial intelligence have also seen a boom in the medical and health industry because recently a mindfulness-based web program has been introduced for people with multiple sclerosis, which reduces the symptoms of depression and helps therapeutically [4]. Another group of researchers developed a novel antibody test to identify a particular kind of protein that is frequently present in the cerebrospinal fluid of MS patients. This test may provide a simpler diagnostic method than the more widely employed ones [5]. Studies have shown that the use of ML algorithms in MS is a rapidly developing subject that has expanded in recent years. Classifying disease subtypes, diagnosing MS in comparison to healthy individuals or patients with other illnesses, and forecasting treatment response or disease progression are the primary use cases for the field of machine learning. There are other research works as well that have concentrated on finding new indicators or refining methods to improve clinical assessment in terms of efficiency, affordability, and patient care [6]. In AI studies, various techniques have been developed to identify or segment MS lesions in MRI data and to predict the degree of disability in MS patients [7, 8]. Along with MRI, optical coherence tomography (OCT), motor data, and serological measures have all been employed [9, 10].

4.2 BACKGROUND

In this section, we w focus on the aspects of multiple sclerosis that drive the research, serve as a foundational framework, the complexities and challenges, and the imperative need for machine learning models. Understanding MS as a complex autoimmune disease of the central nervous system (CNS) emphasizes how important it is to identify predictors to improve patient outcomes, personalized treatment, and early identification. Nerve signal transmission is improved by the protective layer called myelin that surrounds neuronal axons. Similar to insulation on a wire, this insulating layer speeds up electrical impulses, allowing for effective neuronal communication throughout the nervous system, which is essential for healthy motor, sensory, and cognitive processes [11]. As there is no definite cause of MS, there can be multiple

TABLE 4.1

Symptoms of Multiple Sclerosis

Symptoms	Description
Vision Problems	Blurred or double vision, pain during eye movement, optic neuritis (inflammation of the optic nerve).
Fatigue	Profound exhaustion, unrelated to activity levels, impacting daily functioning.
Motor Issues	Weakness, tremors, muscle spasms, coordination difficulties, impaired balance.
Sensory Changes	Numbness, tingling, burning sensations, altered sensation in limbs or face.
Cognitive Impairment	Memory problems, difficulty concentrating, slowed thinking or processing speed.
Bowel and Bladder Problems	Incontinence, constipation, frequent urination, incomplete bladder emptying.
Emotional Changes	Depression, mood swings, anxiety, uncontrollable laughter or crying (pseudobulbar effect).
Pain	Chronic pain, is often in the form of neuropathic or musculoskeletal pain.
Speech and Swallowing Issues	Slurred speech, difficulty articulating words, and swallowing difficulties (dysphagia).
Heat Sensitivity	Exacerbation of symptoms in hot temperatures is known as Uhthoff's phenomenon.

factors that influence this disease and can contribute to its symptoms. Severe cases of multiple sclerosis may show symptoms such as paralysis and total loss of vision. In contrast, other regular symptoms include optic and motor impairments, tremors, trouble walking, balance disorders, speech difficulties, memory and attention issues, exhaustion, and more [12]. Table 4. 1 explains the symptoms in a detailed manner.

The progression of multiple sclerosis is highly unpredictable and varies from patient to patient in the initial stages due to which research on the first episode of neurological symptoms, which is known as clinically isolated syndrome (CIS), is in focus. Machine learning has a significant contribution to the cause because, with the use of AI techniques, it can be discovered which of the CIS is a better predictor of multiple sclerosis. Here, we have discussed a general trajectory of symptom development in multiple sclerosis [13].

- Initial Symptoms: The initial episode of neurological symptoms in multiple sclerosis frequently starts with a clinically isolated condition (CIS). The range of symptoms is broad and may include weakness, impaired coordination, sensory disturbances, visual issues (optic neuritis), or other conditions. Not every CIS patient advances to a definitive MS.

- Relapsing-Remitting MS (RRMS): It is characterized by sporadic relapses or flare-ups of symptoms interspersed with intervals of partial or whole recovery (remission). The frequency and intensity of these relapses can vary due to unpredictable onset and disappearance of symptoms.
- Secondary Progressive MS (SPMS): Some people with RRMS may go into a secondary progressive phase over time. Symptoms and impairment gradually develop throughout this period, frequently with fewer noticeable relapses and more consistent progression.
- Primary Progressive MS (PPMS): Some people may develop primary progressive MS from the beginning, which is defined by a consistent deterioration of symptoms without noticeable relapses or remissions. Compared to RRMS, this type of MS typically progresses more slowly.
- Maximal Disease Stage: When MS reaches its most advanced state, it can cause severe neurological impairment that affects vision, cognition, movement, and other essential skills. Severe motor deficits, loss of ambulation, extreme exhaustion, cognitive deterioration, and an increased dependence on assistive equipment are possible symptoms.

The progression of the disease faces challenges due to the nonexistence of clinical and imaging criteria and such uncertainties pose a limit to the efficiency of the medications as they depend on the disease phenotype. While some patients may see their disease advance quickly, others may spend a long time in the early stages. With the development of treatment techniques, the overall quality of life for MS patients is intended to be improved by managing symptoms and delaying the course of the disease. To lessen the effects of the condition and enhance long-term results, treatment approaches emphasize symptom management, lowering the risk of relapses, and maintaining neurological function.

As mentioned, multiple factors exist that contribute to the development of multiple sclerosis ranging from immune factors and genetic factors to infections. Theories and treatment results exist, which accept that immune alterations, bacterial infections, and family history are all responsible for the attack on nerve fibers and destruction of myelin [14–17]. Table 4. 2 goes into the details of various factors.

A complex web of interrelated elements contributes to multiple sclerosis, with each component having a major impact on the disease's genesis, progression, and symptomatology. The myriad of symptoms that MS patients encounter are caused by immune system dysfunction and chronic inflammation, which also cause demyelination, neuronal degeneration, and various neurological abnormalities. The complicated interplay between immunological, neurological, environmental, and genetic factors exacerbates these difficulties, resulting in a broad spectrum of clinical manifestations [18]. Environmental factors that affect disease progression and exacerbation, in addition to immunological and neurological issues, include stress, smoking, and vitamin D levels. These factors can also have an impact on relapse rates and the severity of the condition. Individual susceptibility to multiple sclerosis is influenced by genetic predispositions that involve genes such as TNFRSF1A, IL2RA, and HLA-DRB1. These genes are involved in immune modulation and inflammatory responses [19].

TABLE 4.2

Factors that Contribute to the Symptoms of Multiple Sclerosis

Factors	Effect on Multiple Sclerosis
Immune Attacks on Myelin	Impaired nerve signal transmission caused by demyelination of nerve fibers impairs sensory, motor, and cognitive functions.
Axonal Injury and Loss	Deficits in motor and sensory function result from damaged nerve axons, which compromise nerve conduction.
Grey Matter Atrophy	Cognitive functions are impacted by grey matter volume reduction, which can result in memory and processing issues.
White Matter Lesions	White matter integrity disruption impairs signal transmission and is linked to several neurological disorders.
Dopamine and Serotonin	Modified levels of neurotransmitters and hormonal changes affect how the mind regulates mood, which can lead to mood swings, anxiety, and sadness.
Cortisol	Changes brought on by stress have an impact on immune response regulation and symptom worsening.
Pro-inflammatory Cytokines	Elevated levels worsen neurological symptoms and lead to CNS inflammation.
Anti-inflammatory Response	Insufficient regulation affects disease progression and symptom severity.
Vitamin D Deficiency	Decreased levels are linked to a higher incidence of MS and worsening symptoms.
Smoking	Exacerbates disease progression and contributes to increased symptom severity.
Stress, Anxiety, and Depression	Worsen symptoms, cause relapses, and increase fatigue, which lowers general well-being and quality of life.
Gut Microbiome Dysbiosis	Affects immunological responses, which in turn may affect the change the course and signs of disease.
Human Leukocyte Antigen-DRB1	The gene that is strongly associated with increased MS risk.
Interleukin-2 Receptor Alpha	Linked to immune system regulation and increased MS risk.

Understanding these interactions is essential since they aggravate symptoms and the course of the disease. This knowledge serves as the foundation for the creation of individualized treatment plans that improve the quality of life for MS patients by reducing symptoms and delaying the course of the illness. Focused therapies seek to reduce the severity of symptoms and the progression of the disease by addressing these complex relationships; this holds promise for better outcomes and increased well-being for MS patients.

4.3 PREDICTORS OF MULTIPLE SCLEROSIS

Years of study have helped discover various predictors, which ensure that a patient is affected by multiple sclerosis. About 85% of patients with multiple sclerosis (MS) experience an acute clinical episode, often known as a clinically isolated condition.

Upon an individual's evaluation following a single episode of CNS inflammation, several follow-up decisions, including the decision to initiate therapy or not, must be made [20]. As a result, there is a growing need to determine the predictive variables that foretell CIS to MS conversion. A clinically isolated syndrome (CIS) is a state in which a person experiences their first neurological episode due to nerve tissue inflammation or demyelination. An episode might be multi-focal, meaning that symptoms appear at several different sites throughout the central nervous system, or mono-focal, meaning that symptoms only appear at one location. When there is sufficient paraclinical evidence, CIS can be regarded as a multiple sclerosis (MS) clinical stage [21]. When further data becomes available, it may also be retroactively identified as a form of multiple sclerosis. Clinically definite multiple sclerosis is referred to as CDMS. It describes a point in the multiple sclerosis (MS) diagnosis process when there is sufficient clinical evidence to establish the diagnosis based on particular standards established by neurological guidelines. After the first symptoms appear, it usually denotes a definitive diagnosis of multiple sclerosis (MS), frequently involving several neurological episodes suggestive of demyelination within the central nervous system (CNS). When typical neurological signs and symptoms are present, as well as when imaging studies and clinical evaluations support the diagnosis, MS is considered clinically definite [20].

Healthcare professionals may be able to use machine learning to categorize CIS patients into various risk groups for CDMS conversion, which would help with early intervention plans and individualized risk assessments. By using this predictive power, physicians may be able to provide patients who are more likely to develop CDMS with earlier and more individualized interventions or treatments, potentially changing the course of the disease and improving patient outcomes. Machine learning can be used to analyze datasets to gather information about various factors and use algorithms to determine patterns associated with the CIS that convert to CDMS or non-CDMS. Here we have conducted a study to extract which of the CIS are better predictors of multiple sclerosis and determine whether a patient falls into the group of CDMS or non-CDMS. For the study, a publically available dataset has been used and the attributes are presented in Table 4.3. This data had been gathered from a study done between 2006 and 2010 on Mexican mestizo patients who had just received a CIS diagnosis and had visited the National Institute of Neurology and Neurosurgery (NINN) in Mexico City [22]. From among the various CIS, our study determines which predictors are better for multiple sclerosis diagnosis as per analysis using machine learning techniques.

The methodology followed in this study includes:

i. Data Collection: The study utilized a publicly available dataset from Kaggle, focusing on Mexican patients diagnosed with CIS, providing a foundational dataset for investigating early MS indicators.

ii. Data Cleaning and Preprocessing: The initial dataset had limited missing values, with careful handling. Imputation methods addressed the missing values in 'Schooling' and 'Initial Symptoms.' However, due to a considerable number of missing values (148 out of 273) in 'initial EDSS' and

TABLE 4.3
Dataset Description

Factors	Effect on Multiple Sclerosis
ID	Patient identifier
Age	Age of the patient (in years)
Schooling	Time the patient spent in school (in years)
Gender	1 = male 2 = female
Breastfeeding	1 = yes 2 = no 3 = unknown
Varicella	1 = positive 2 = negative 3 = unknown
Initial Symptoms	1 = visual 2 = sensory 3 = motor 4 = other 5 = visual and sensory 6 = visual and motor 7 = visual and others 8 = sensory and motor 9 = sensory and other 10 = motor and other 11 = Visual, sensory, and motor 12 = Visual, sensory, and other 13 = Visual, motor, and other 14 = Sensory, motor, and other 15 = Visual, sensory, motor, and other
Mono or Polysymptomatic	1 = monosymptomatic 2 = polysymptomatic 3 = unknown
Oligoclonal Bands	0 = negative 1 = positive 2 = unknown
LLSSEP	0 = negative 1 = positive
ULSSEP	0 = negative 1 = positive
VEP	0 = negative 1 = positive
BAEP	0 = negative 1 = positive
Periventricular MRI	0 = negative 1 = positive
Cortical MRI	0 = negative 1 = positive
Infratentorial MRI	0 = negative 1 = positive
Spinal Cord MRI	0 = negative 1 = positive
Initial EDSS	?
Final EDSS	?
Group	1 = CDMS 2 = non-CDMS

'final EDSS,' these attributes were dropped to ensure data integrity during analysis.

iii. Data Analysis: Comprehensive scrutiny of dataset attributes involved detailed statistical analyses and visualization techniques, including graphs, to discern patterns, correlations, and distributions. This exploration aimed to identify significant predictors of MS and understand feature importance.

iv. Predictions: Leveraging classification models such as Random Forest and Decision Trees, the study aimed to predict the conversion of CIS to clinically definite multiple sclerosis (CDMS). Performance metrics like precision, recall, and F1-score were employed to assess and validate the model's predictive capability.

The entire analysis has been carried out using the Python programming language and Figure 4.1 illustrates the framework followed in this study.

The various predictors that we have determined in our study, which have been carried out using Python and machine learning techniques, have been discussed in detail in the following sections. All the results that have been presented in the following sections are the results that have been achieved or observed during our study.

4.3.1 Magnetic Resonance Imaging (MRI)

Magnetic Resonance Imaging is referred to as MRI. It is a noninvasive medical imaging method that creates finely detailed images of the body's internal components using radio waves, strong magnets, and a computer. A magnetic resonance imaging (MRI) scan generates high-definition images that offer details about the body's organs, tissues, and other structures [23]. These images are useful for both diagnosis and condition monitoring. To help with the diagnosis and treatment of multiple sclerosis (MS), magnetic resonance imaging (MRI) is widely used to see and identify lesions or areas of damage in the brain and spinal cord.

4.3.1.1 Periventricular MRI

Periventricular magnetic resonance imaging (MRI) is essential for both multiple sclerosis (MS) diagnosis and follow-up. Periventricular lesions, or regions of demyelination close to the brain's ventricles, are commonly shown on MRI images in MS patients. On T2-weighted MRI sequences, these lesions show up as bright or hyperintense patches and are suggestive of damage related to multiple sclerosis. Periventricular lesions seen by MRI imaging, including their size, number, and existence, are crucial diagnostic markers for multiple sclerosis (Table 4.4). Their placement close to the ventricles, which is indicative of MS pathology, helps neurologists distinguish MS from other disorders that impact the central nervous system. Additionally, the long-term MRI monitoring of periventricular lesions aids in evaluating the course of the disease and the effectiveness of treatment for MS patients. On MRI scans, variations in lesion size, quantity, or appearance over time can reveal information about the progression of the disease and the efficacy of treatments aimed at modifying it.

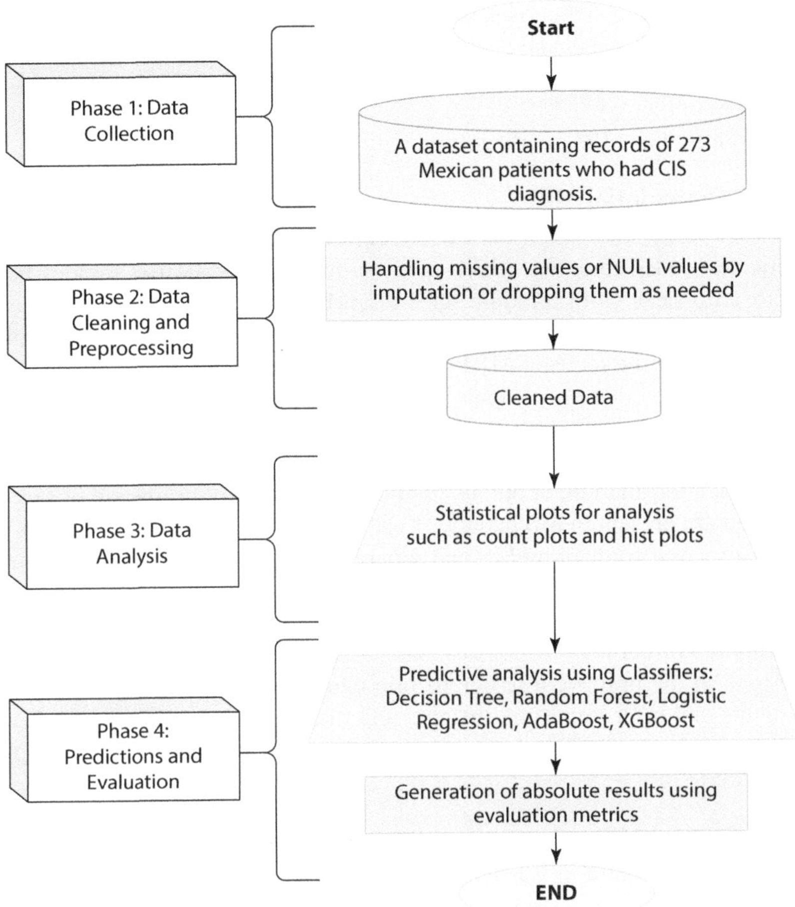

FIGURE 4.1 Framework followed in the study.

TABLE 4.4

Effect of Periventricular MRI on Multiple Sclerosis

Periventricular_MRI	Group	Percentage within the Group (%)
0	Non-CDMS	81.48
	CDMS	18.51
1	Non-CDMS	27.53
	CDMS	72.46

Periventricular magnetic resonance imaging plays a crucial role in the diagnosis of multiple sclerosis (MS) and is an invaluable instrument for evaluating the course and intensity of the disease, making informed treatment choices, and tracking the effectiveness of therapy in MS patients. According to our study, 72% of patients who have periventricular MRI are diagnosed with CDMS.

4.3.1.2 Infratentorial MRI

Multiple sclerosis (MS) diagnosis and treatment benefit greatly from infratentorial magnetic resonance imaging, which involves imaging the brain's regions beneath the tentorium. Lesions in multiple sclerosis (MS) can occur in many parts of the brain, such as the infratentorial area containing the cerebellum and brainstem. These regions are the focus of MRI scans, which aid in the identification and visualization of lesions that may impact balance, coordination, and other neurological functions related to the infratentorial structures. Evaluating infratentorial lesions using magnetic resonance imaging is especially crucial when balance problems, vertigo, poor coordination, or other symptoms suggestive of brainstem or cerebellar dysfunction are present in MS patients. Lesion detection in these regions aids in the diagnosis process, confirming MS and separating it from other illnesses with comparable symptoms. Furthermore, tracking alterations in infratentorial lesions over time with magnetic resonance imaging (MRI) facilitates the assessment of disease progression and treatment response. Changes in the size, shape, or development of new lesions in the brainstem or cerebellum can help inform treatment choices for MS patients and offer important insights into disease activity (Table 4.5). The current study shows that 78% of patients who have infratentorial MRI are diagnosed with CDMS.

4.3.1.3 Cortical MRI

Targeting the gray matter in particular, cortical MRI imaging focuses on the brain's cortical regions and is essential for understanding and diagnosing multiple sclerosis (MS) (Table 4.6). Although cortical lesions have been shown to have a substantial role in the pathophysiology of MS, white matter disease was traditionally thought to be the primary cause of MS. This has changed with recent research. Cortical lesions are regions of demyelination and destruction inside the brain's gray matter, and they are becoming more and more understood to be important factors in the development

TABLE 4.5

Effect of Infratentorial MRI on Multiple Sclerosis

Infratentorial_MRI	Group	Percentage within the Group (%)
0	Non-CDMS	67.87
	CDMS	32.12
1	Non-CDMS	21.25
	CDMS	78.75

TABLE 4.6
Effect of Cortical MRI on Multiple Sclerosis

Cortical_MRI	Group	Percentage within the Group (%)
0	Non-CDMS	63.87
	CDMS	36.12
1	Non-CDMS	41.52
	CDMS	58.47

of multiple sclerosis (MS). When it comes to white matter lesions, cortical lesions are frequently harder to find and see. To help with this, particular MRI sequences and sophisticated imaging methods are needed. In MS, the presence and size of cortical lesions shown on cortical MRI imaging are linked to a range of clinical symptoms and the advancement of the illness. They may be correlated with cognitive impairments that are frequent in MS patients, such as memory issues, processing speed deficiencies, and executive function difficulties.

Additionally, cortical MRI helps to distinguish MS from other neurological disorders and adds to a more thorough evaluation of the prognosis and severity of the disease. The identification and measurement of cortical lesions yield important data that can be used to forecast the course of the disease, comprehend the clinical variability of multiple sclerosis, and inform therapy choices. To diagnose and treat multiple sclerosis (MS), cortical MRI imaging is crucial because it sheds light on the severity of cortical lesions, improves our understanding of how the illness manifests and helps anticipate cognitive decline and the course of the disease in affected individuals.

4.3.1.4 Spinal Cord MRI

In the field of multiple sclerosis (MS), spinal cord magnetic resonance imaging (MRI) is a vital diagnostic and surveillance tool. This imaging modality clarifies the amount and type of neuroinflammatory processes in multiple sclerosis by enabling detailed visualization of lesions or areas of damage inside the spinal cord. These lesions' location and characteristics along the spinal cord play a crucial role in supporting the MS diagnosis, particularly when paired with results from contemporaneous brain imaging studies. Spinal cord MRI provides more than just diagnostic help; it offers a dynamic window into the course of disease. Variations in spinal cord lesions throughout multiple MRI scans provide information on how the disease is progressing, assisting in the formulation of treatment plans, and revealing the effectiveness of various approaches (Table 4.7).

Furthermore, spinal cord MRI is a valuable tool for explaining the neurological symptoms that people with MS encounter. Clinicians can better understand the range of neurological abnormalities patients experience when they are aware of the relationship between certain clinical symptoms, like motor weakness or sensory difficulties, and the sites of lesions along the spinal cord. The ability of this imaging

TABLE 4.7

Effect of Spinal Cord MRI on Multiple Sclerosis

Spinal Cord_MRI	Group	Percentage within the group (%)
0	Non-CDMS	58.28
	CDMS	41.71
1	Non-CDMS	45.34
	CDMS	54.65

modality to monitor lesion changes over time is useful for monitoring therapy response in addition to helping to evaluate how the illness is progressing. Reductions in the size or quantity of lesions shown on follow-up scans indicate possible therapeutic benefit, which influences how MS is managed throughout time and provides a thorough picture of the state of the illness and patient care.

4.3.2 Neurological Predictors Related to Visuals, Sensations, and Movements

The complex nature of neurological illnesses is reflected in the wide range of presentations of neurological symptoms that can influence vision, sensory perception, and motor function in the setting of conditions such as multiple sclerosis. The various symptoms have been discussed and Table 4.8 displays a collective result of the symptoms and their contribution to the determination of CDMS.

4.3.2.1 Sensory Symptoms

When discussing multiple sclerosis (MS), the term 'sensory symptoms' refers to symptoms involving the sensory nerve system. These symptoms, which can include the following, frequently involve unusual feelings that people with MS experience:

- Numbness or Tingling: These feelings, which are frequently felt in the limbs or other portions of the body, might be characterized as aberrant tingling, pins, and needles, or a lack of feeling altogether.

TABLE 4.8

Initial Symptoms that Act as Predictors of Multiple Sclerosis

Symptom(s)	CDMS Percentage (%)
Visual, sensory, and motor	90.00
Visual, motor, and others	90.91
Visual, sensory, and others	83.33
Sensory, motor, and others	78.57
Motor and others	53.33

- Hypersensitivity: Some MS patients may be extremely sensitive to pain, warmth, or touch in particular places.
- Itchy or Scorching Sensations: Unexplained prickling, burning, or itching sensations on the skin that are unrelated to outside influences.

4.3.2.2 Visual Symptoms

When it comes to multiple sclerosis (MS), visual symptoms include a wide range of disorders in vision and ocular function. Damage to the optic nerves, neural pathways, or parts of the brain involved in vision processing may be the cause of these symptoms in cases of multiple sclerosis. Typical MS visual symptoms include the following:

- Optic Neuritis: An inflammation of the optic nerve that can cause changes in color perception, pain while moving the eyes, blurred vision, or loss of vision in one eye (typically unilateral).
- Double Vision (diplopia): The perception of two images instead of one because the muscles controlling eye movement are out of alignment or weak.
- Blurred Vision: The result of a lack of focus or sharpness in the eyes, making vision fuzzy or confusing.
- Visual Field Defects: Blind spots and loss of peripheral vision are examples of visual field defects.

4.3.2.3 Motor Symptoms

A wide spectrum of anomalies in movement and muscular control are referred to as motor symptoms. When motor symptoms occur in the context of multiple sclerosis (MS), it is typically because of demyelination or lesions in the central nervous system that cause damage or disruption to the neurons that govern voluntary muscle movements. Typical motor symptoms of multiple sclerosis include:

- Paralysis or Weakness: Decreased muscle strength or the incapacity to move particular body parts are examples of weakness or paralysis. It may be difficult to carry out daily tasks due to limb weakness.
- Spasticity: An increase in muscle tone or stiffness that can cause cramping, tightness in the muscles, or trouble moving. Muscles that are spastic may stiffen up or become resistant to stretching.
- Tremors: Uncontrollably occurring rhythmic movements that usually affect the hands, arms, or legs. Mild to moderate MS tremors can make it difficult to do jobs requiring precise motor control.
- Challenges and Problems with Walking or Coordination: Difficulties with walking with grace, staying balanced, or coordinating motions because of weakened or compromised leg muscles.

The varied and distinctive expressions of visual, sensory, and motor problems make them all possible predictors or markers of multiple sclerosis (MS) [24]. Before a confirmed MS diagnosis, these symptoms may occasionally appear early in the course of the disease, even during the clinically isolated syndrome (CIS) phase. Their incidence could lead to more research and pathology-related MS surveillance. When these symptoms are present along with other neurological signs and symptoms, their nature helps neurologists rule out MS as a possible diagnosis. Certain symptoms are frequently linked to multiple sclerosis (MS) and may be included in the diagnostic criteria. Examples of these symptoms are optic neuritis, a visual symptom, numbness or tingling, a motor symptom, and weakness. Monitoring how these symptoms vary over time aids in determining how the disease is progressing. Treatment decisions may be impacted by the persistence, exacerbation, or emergence of new sensory, visual, or motor impairments that signify disease activity. Some symptom patterns, including the co-occurrence of ocular neuritis and sensory abnormalities or the coexistence of motor weakness and sensory abnormalities, may lead medical professionals to believe that MS-related pathology is present. The full examination of multiple sclerosis is aided by the total clinical presentation, which includes the combination and intensity of visual, sensory, and motor symptoms. Certain symptom clusters or patterns may give rise to suspicions of multiple sclerosis, hence requiring additional research and diagnostic evaluation.

Although these symptoms can lead to a suspicion of multiple sclerosis, they are not specific to the illness and can also arise in several other neurological or non-neurological conditions. Accurate MS diagnosis and management require a thorough review that includes clinical assessments, imaging studies (MRIs), and other diagnostic criteria. Furthermore, how these symptoms manifest, how severe they are, and how they change over time all matter in determining how the illness progresses and how best to treat MS patients.

The other symptoms that contribute to CDMS vary from patient to patient such as cognitive changes – difficulties with memory, attention, information processing, bladder dysfunction, etc.

4.3.3 Oligoclonal Bands

Immunoglobulin bands known as oligoclonal bands (OCBs) are observed in a patient's blood serum or cerebrospinal fluid (CSF) upon analysis. They are employed in the diagnosis of numerous blood and neurological conditions. In more than 95% of people with multiple sclerosis who have a clear clinical diagnosis, oligoclonal bands are found in the circulation [25]. For example, multiple sclerosis (MS) and other illnesses of the central nervous system may be indicated by oligoclonal bands (OCBs), a special finding in cerebrospinal fluid (CSF) analysis (Table 4.9). When CSF is examined, bands of immunoglobulins – more precisely, immunoglobulin G, or IgG – appear on electrophoresis. These are known as OCBs. The reason they are referred to as 'oligoclonal' is that, in contrast to the wide variety shown in typical immune responses, they reflect a small or restricted number of distinct antibodies.

CSF electrophoresis, a laboratory test that separates the proteins in the CSF and looks for the presence of these aberrant immunoglobulins, is used to identify these

TABLE 4.9
Effect of Oligoclonal Bands on Multiple Sclerosis

Oligoclonal Bands	Group	Percentage within the Group (%)
0	Non-CDMS	64.51
	CDMS	35.48
1	Non-CDMS	22.36
	CDMS	77.63

bands [26]. The existence of OCBs is a noteworthy discovery in MS and a component of the diagnostic standards. OCBs are suggestive of inflammation and immunological activity typical of multiple sclerosis (MS) and reflect an aberrant immune response inside the central nervous system (CNS). When absent from the blood, OCBs in the CSF suggest a particular immune response taking place inside the CNS, which helps validate the MS diagnosis. The presence of OCBs in the CSF aids in the overall assessment as well as neurologists in validating the diagnosis of MS when paired with clinical symptoms, MRI results, and other diagnostic procedures. OCBs indicate that a lumbar puncture is used to get cerebrospinal fluid, which is then used to detect OCB (spinal tap). After that, this CSF sample is examined using an analysis method known as electrophoresis, which divides proteins according to their size and electrical charge. An abnormal pattern of OCBs can be observed in some neurological disorders, such as multiple sclerosis (MS). This indicates that the CSF contains extra IgG bands that are absent from the blood. The presence of OCBs in the CSF can be an indication of inflammation in the central nervous system and is indicative of intrathecal (inside the CNS) antibody production. It is believed to be the outcome of the immune system's reaction to antigens unique to the central nervous system, such as myelin.

4.3.4 VISUAL EVOKED POTENTIAL (VEP)

A neurophysiological test called the visual evoked potential (VEP) is used to assess how well the visual pathway – more specifically, how well visual information is transmitted from the eyes to the brain's visual cortex – is functioning [27]. When determining the involvement of the optic nerve in the diagnosis of multiple sclerosis (MS), visual field testing (VEP) is highly helpful, especially when the patient has optic neuritis, an early-stage MS symptom that causes inflammation of the optic nerve and visual abnormalities (Table 4.10).

In VEP testing, the patient has electrodes applied to their scalp, frequently in particular spots over the visual cortex at the rear of the brain. Visual stimuli, such as flashing or patterned patterns like checkerboards or contrast-reversing black-and-white patterns, are presented to the patient. The electrical activity produced in reaction to the visual stimulus is recorded by the electrodes. 'Evoked potentials,' which are recorded reactions, are the electrical impulses that the brain produces in reaction

TABLE 4.10
Effect of VEP on Multiple Sclerosis

VEP	Group	Percentage within the Group (%)
0	Non-CDMS	61.37
	CDMS	38.62
1	Non-CDMS	38.09
	CDMS	61.90

to visual stimuli. The timing and amplitude of the evoked potentials are assessed by analyzing the recorded responses. Deviations from these metrics may point to anomalies in the visual pathway. When compared to normal values, longer latency (a delayed response time) or lower amplitude (a weaker signal intensity) is an example of abnormal VEP results in MS. These anomalies point to poor transmission of visual information via the optic nerves or the brain's visual pathways, which is suggestive of demyelination or injury to these structures, which is frequently observed in optic neuritis linked to multiple sclerosis.

4.3.5 Brainstem Auditory Evoked Potentials (BAEP)

Neurophysiological tests called Brainstem Auditory Evoked Potentials (BAEPs) are used to assess the health of the auditory circuits that connect the brainstem to the ear [28]. When evaluating the functioning of various neural pathways – especially the brainstem and auditory nerve pathways – BAEP is a useful tool in the context of multiple sclerosis (MS).

To conduct the test, electrodes are applied to the scalp across particular head regions during a BAEP test; occasionally, extra electrodes are applied to the earlobes. The patient listens to a sequence of tones or clicks while using headphones. The electrodes record the amount of time it takes for auditory signals to go from the ear to the brainstem by picking up the electrical responses that the brain produces in reaction to these noises. When comparing BAEP data in MS to normal values, anomalies such as extended delay or changed waveforms can be seen. These anomalies may point to decreased conduction along the auditory pathways, which may be indicative of demyelination or damage to the brainstem structures or auditory nerves, which are frequently observed in lesions related to multiple sclerosis. Even in the absence of overt auditory symptoms, BAEP abnormalities may be a predictor of MS and a sign of subclinical involvement of the auditory pathways. When it comes to MS, subclinical involvement describes neurological abnormalities that are picked up by tests such as the BAEP but may not yet show up as symptoms. Abnormalities in BAEP may manifest before the emergence of clinically noticeable symptoms, which could indicate damage to the auditory system caused by MS at an early stage (Table 4.11).

TABLE 4.11
Effect of BAEP on Multiple Sclerosis

BAEP	Group	Percentage within the Group (%)
0	Non-CDMS	54.90
	CDMS	45.09
1	Non-CDMS	44.44
	CDMS	55.55

4.3.6 Somatosensory Evoked Potentials (SSEP)

Somatosensory evoked potentials (SSEPs) are neurophysiological tests that measure how well sensory impulses are transmitted from peripheral nerves to the brain, as well as the health of the somatosensory pathways [29]. When used for multiple sclerosis (MS), SSEP is a useful tool for evaluating how well certain neural networks operate, especially when it comes to the brain's ability to receive sensory information.

To conduct the test, electrodes are positioned on particular regions of the scalp and occasionally on other body parts, like the wrists or ankles, during an SSEP test. A peripheral nerve, usually the tibial nerve in the ankle or the median nerve in the wrist, is stimulated mildly electrically. The electrodes record the time it takes for messages to reach the brain by picking up the electrical reactions the brain produces in response to these sensory stimuli. In MS, abnormal SSEP results could include waveform features that are delayed or different from usual. These anomalies may point to decreased conduction via the sensory pathways, which could be indicative of demyelination or injury to the nerves or neurological structures that are involved in the transmission of sensory information. Even before the manifestation of observable sensory symptoms, anomalies in SSEP can offer insights into the subclinical involvement of the somatosensory pathways. Subclinical involvement describes brain alterations that may not yet show up as overt symptoms but are identified by tests such as the SSEP. Abnormalities in SSEP may function as a preliminary marker of sensory system impairment associated with multiple sclerosis (Table 4.12).

When it comes to MS, SSEP testing helps with both diagnosis and understanding of the disease's etiology. It contributes to the understanding of how demyelination affects sensory conduction and offers important insights into the involvement and evolution of lesions connected to multiple sclerosis throughout the sensory pathways. Additionally, SSEP acts as an objective diagnostic tool for MS, combining objective neurological results with clinical symptoms. Its function as a quantitative, noninvasive test improves the accuracy of the diagnosis, especially in situations when the clinical symptoms may be unclear or equivocal.

Using OCB and evoked potentials such as VEPs, BAEPs, and SSEPs as predictors for MS diagnosis provides important information on subclinical brain involvement.

TABLE 4.12

Effects of Upper Limb and Lower Limb SSEP on Multiple Sclerosis

SSEP		Group	Percentage within the Group (%)
Lower Limb	0	Non-CDMS	63.69
		CDMS	36.30
	1	Non-CDMS	41.37
		CDMS	58.62
Upper Limb	0	Non-CDMS	61.62
		CDMS	38.37
	1	Non-CDMS	41.58
		CDMS	58.41

For a proper diagnosis and treatment plan, their interpretation – along with clinical and imaging data – remains crucial. By including these indicators, we can expand our diagnostic toolkit and gain a better understanding of the complex underlying causes of multiple sclerosis, which will facilitate early intervention.

The current study also looked into various machine learning models for the prediction of CDMS and non-CDMS. Multiple classifiers such as Logistic Regression, Decision Tree, Random Forest, Support Vector Machine, Gradient Boosting, and Extreme Gradient Boosting were utilized. These classifiers were selected for this study based on the criteria of diversity in algorithms to foster a comparative study as well as utilize the robustness of each classifier and understand their contribution toward the prediction of CIS that converts to CDMS or non-CDMS. A thorough investigation of dataset correlations is made possible by the use of varied classifiers, each of which has a specific underlying algorithm, providing distinctive modeling techniques. The best models for MS prediction can be found by comparing different classifiers and pointing out their advantages and disadvantages for various dataset settings. By evaluating prediction robustness across a range of models, one can increase confidence in identified predictors, guarantee dependable conclusions, and lower the possibility of biased results. Furthermore, a variety of classifiers shed light on the significance of features, which helps interpret clinically meaningful predictors for the advancement of MS. Table 4.13 presents the results and a comparative analysis of each classifier.

The analysis presents that Random Forest beats the other classifiers in terms of accuracy in classifying a patient into clinically definite multiple sclerosis (CDMS) or non-CDMS. It achieved an accuracy of 85% on the dataset used. Random Forest is an ensemble learning model that uses several decision trees. It uses random subsets of the dataset and features to create a variety of trees. Every tree produces a forecast on its own, and the outcome averages (for regression) or votes (for classification) these predictions together. Since each tree takes into account a distinct component of the data, this strategy reduces overfitting and increases accuracy. Random Forest is an effective method for handling big datasets, maintaining predictive accuracy,

TABLE 4.13
Results of Various Classifiers

Classifier	Accuracy Percentage (%)
Logistic Regression	82
Random Forest	85
Decision Tree	71
XGBoost	82
Gradient Boosting	74
AdaBoost	76
Support Vector Machine	66

and providing insights into feature relevance for improved model interpretation. It achieves these goals by mixing predictions from several trees to provide robust results.

4.4 CHALLENGES AND FUTURE SCOPE

The application of artificial intelligence (AI) to MS research holds great potential to transform our understanding and management of the disease. Personalized medicine is made possible by AI-driven predictive models that use a variety of datasets to anticipate how a disease will advance, how a treatment plan will work, and when a relapse may occur. Furthermore, AI's skill in image analysis speeds up the study of MRI scans, making it easier to identify lesions early on and precisely track structural alterations in the brain and the spinal cord. AI also helps with biomarker discovery, which finds important markers from different data sources for early MS diagnosis and customized treatments.

Future research avenues in MS include precision medicine; leveraging AI to categorize distinct MS subtypes based on genetic, molecular, and clinical profiles, thereby tailoring therapies to different MS phenotypes. AI's capacity to analyze extensive longitudinal data offers insights into disease progression, elucidating factors influencing disease variability and revealing potential therapeutic targets. Moreover, patient stratification through AI clustering of data aids in personalized treatment planning and predicting disease trajectories, enhancing individualized care.

Even with these developments, problems still exist. The current study worked with a dataset that has data limitations and does not include data related to geographical locations. Another drawback is that deep learning techniques such as neural networks, Generative Adversarial Network(GANs) etc. have not been utilized which could optimize the predictions and improve the accuracy. The efficient use of AI in MS research requires integrating and harmonizing a variety of data sources while maintaining data quality and standardization. To guarantee dependability and applicability in healthcare environments, bridging the gap between AI-driven research and clinical implementation necessitates thorough evaluation. Building trust between patients and clinicians requires ethical concerns, bias mitigation, and transparency in AI decision-making processes. Maximizing the impact of AI will require addressing obstacles, upgrading AI algorithms, and fostering collaborations. These actions will ultimately improve results and the quality of life for MS patients.

4.5 CONCLUSIONS

Artificial intelligence (AI) has revolutionized the field of multiple sclerosis (MS) research and healthcare by providing opportunities to improve disease understanding, diagnosis, and treatment. A new era of personalized approaches to addressing this complex neurological disorder is being ushered in by AI-driven predictive models, and precision medicine. Predictive models powered by AI are revolutionizing MS care by predicting treatment responses, identifying future relapses, and forecasting disease progression. These models draw from a variety of datasets including genetic, imaging, clinical, and environmental aspects. By enabling customized therapeutic interventions, this individualized knowledge helps MS patients achieve their best possible outcomes. AI's accuracy in quickly evaluating MRI data speeds up lesion diagnosis and provides accurate and timely information about anatomical changes in the brain and spinal cord. AI-driven research on multiple sclerosis (MS) has been greatly enhanced by visual evoked potentials (VEPs) and oligoclonal bands (OCBs). By evaluating visual pathway integrity, VEPs help identify lesions early and can predict optic neuritis associated with multiple sclerosis. AI models that use VEP data to track therapy responses and predict illness trajectories perform better. Important MS indicators, OCBs represent intrathecal immune responses. AI that examines clinical data and OCB patterns offers insights regarding prognosis and disease activity. Treatment plans are customized and prognostic accuracy is improved through the incorporation of OCB data into AI models. AI enhances predictive models to enable early MS detection, accurate prognostication, and customized therapy by utilizing VEPs and OCBs. By providing multifaceted insights into MS progression, these metrics optimize management approaches. Their incorporation strengthens AI's ability to improve diagnosis, forecast the course of the disease, and personalize care for MS patients.

In summary, AI's incorporation into MS research promises a paradigm shift in the treatment of the illness. Resolving obstacles, improving AI algorithms, encouraging cooperation, and maintaining moral principles are essential to achieving AI's promise to improve outcomes and quality of life for MS patients. These advancements signal a new age in multiple sclerosis diagnosis and therapy marked by previously unheard-of levels of precision, personalization, and creativity.

REFERENCES

1. Andorra, M., Freire, A., Zubizarreta, I., de Rosbo, N. K., Bos, S. D., Rinas, M., ... Villoslada, P. (2023). Predicting disease severity in multiple sclerosis using multimodal data and machine learning. *Journal of Neurology, 271*, 1–17.

2. Multiple Sclerosis Statistics Blog (2023) – singlecare.com

3. Research News Progress (2023) – nationalmssociety.org

4. Vázquez-Marrufo, M., Sarrias-Arrabal, E., García-Torres, M., Martín-Clemente, R., & Izquierdo, G. (2023). A systematic review of the application of machine-learning algorithms in multiple sclerosis. *Neurología (English Edition)*, *38*(8), 577–590. https://doi.org/10.1016/j.nrleng.2020.10.013

5. Bharucha, T., Gangadharan, B., Kumar, A., de Lamballerie, X., Newton, P. N., Winterberg, M., ... Zitzmann, N. (2019). Mass spectrometry-based proteomic techniques to identify cerebrospinal fluid biomarkers for diagnosing suspected central nervous system infections. A systematic review. *Journal of Infection*, *79*(5), 407–418.

6. Eshaghi, A., Young, A. L., Wijeratne, P. A., Prados, F., Arnold, D. L., Narayanan, S., Guttmann, C. R., Barkhof, F., Alexander, D. C., Thompson, A. J., Chard, D., & Ciccarelli, O. (2021). Identifying multiple sclerosis subtypes using unsupervised machine learning and MRI data. *Nature Communications*, *12*(1), 1–12. https://doi.org/10.1038/s41467-021-22265-2

7. Aslam, N., Khan, I. U., Bashamakh, A., Alghool, F. A., Aboulnour, M., Alsuwayan, N. M., ... Al Ghamdi, K. (2022). Multiple sclerosis diagnosis using machine learning and deep learning: Challenges and opportunities. *Sensors*, *22*(20), 7856.

8. Moazami, F., Lefevre-Utile, A., Papaloukas, C., & Soumelis, V. (2021). Machine learning approaches in study of multiple sclerosis disease through magnetic resonance images. *Frontiers in Immunology*, *12*, 700582.

9. Montolío, A., Martín-Gallego, A., Cegoñino, J., Orduna, E., Vilades, E., Garcia-Martin, E., & Del Palomar, A. P. (2021). Machine learning in diagnosis and disability prediction of multiple sclerosis using optical coherence tomography. *Computers in Biology and Medicine*, *133*, 104416.

10. Montolío, A., CEGONino, J. O. S. E., Garcia-Martin, E., & Pérez del Palomar, A. (2022). Comparison of machine learning methods using spectralis OCT for diagnosis and disability progression prognosis in multiple sclerosis. *Annals of Biomedical Engineering*, *50*(5), 507–528.

11. Dedoni, S., Scherma, M., Camoglio, C., Siddi, C., Dazzi, L., Puliga, R., ... Fadda, P. (2023). An overall view of the most common experimental models for multiple sclerosis. *Neurobiology of Disease*, *184*, 106230.

12. Multiple Sclerosis: Symptoms - Causes (2022) – mayoclinic.org

13. Zhang, H., Alberts, E., Pongratz, V., Mühlau, M., Zimmer, C., Wiestler, B., & Eichinger, P. (2019). Predicting conversion from clinically isolated syndrome to multiple sclerosis-An imaging-based machine learning approach. *NeuroImage. Clinical*, *21*, 101593. https://doi.org/10.1016/j.nicl.2018.11.003

14. Ghasemi, N., Razavi, S., & Nikzad, E. (2017). Multiple sclerosis: Pathogenesis, symptoms, diagnoses and cell-based therapy. *Cell Journal*, *19*(1), 1–10. https://doi.org/10.22074/cellj.2016.4867

15. Fymat, A. L. (2023). Multiple sclerosis: I. Symptomatology and etiology. *Journal of Neurology and Psychology Research*, *4*(1), 1–46.

16. Frau, J., Coghe, G., Lorefice, L., Fenu, G., & Cocco, E. (2023). The role of microorganisms in the Etiopathogenesis of demyelinating diseases. *Life*, *13*(6), 1309.

17. Lublin, F. D., Häring, D. A., Ganjgahi, H., Ocampo, A., Hatami, F., Čuklina, J., ... Bermel, R. A. (2022). How patients with multiple sclerosis acquire disability. *Brain*, *145*(9), 3147–3161.

18. Kuhlmann, T., Moccia, M., Coetzee, T., Cohen, J. A., Correale, J., Graves, J., ... Waubant, E. (2023). Multiple sclerosis progression: Time for a new mechanism-driven framework. *The Lancet Neurology*, *22*(1), 78–88.

19. Vasić, M., Topić, A., Marković, B., Milinković, N., & Dinčić, E. (2023). Oxidative stress-related risk of the multiple sclerosis development. *Journal of Medical Biochemistry*, *42*(1), 1.
20. López-Gómez, J., Enciso, B. S., Miró, M. C., & Pascual, M. Q. (2023). Clinically isolated syndrome: Diagnosis and risk of developing clinically definite multiple sclerosis. *Neurología (English Edition)*, *38*, 663–670.
21. Efendi, H. (2015). Clinically isolated syndromes: Clinical characteristics, differential diagnosis, and management. *Noro Psikiyatri Arsivi*, *52*(Suppl 1), S1–S11. https://doi.org/10.5152/npa.2015.12608
22. Conversion predictors of cis to multiple sclerosis – Kaggle.
23. Magnetic Resonance Imaging MRI – nibib.nih.gov
24. Filippi, M., Bar-Or, A., Piehl, F. *et al.* (2018). Multiple sclerosis. *Nature Reviews Disease Primers*, *4*, 43. https://doi.org/10.1038/s41572-018-0041-4
25. Graner, M., Pointon, T., Manton, S., Green, M., Dennison, K., Davis, M., Braiotta, G., Craft, J., Edwards, T., Polonsky, B., Fringuello, A., Vollmer, T., & Yu, X. (2020). Oligoclonal IgG antibodies in multiple sclerosis target patient-specific peptides. *PloS One*, *15*(2), e0228883. https://doi.org/10.1371/journal.pone.0228883
26. Protein Electrophoresis, Immunofixation Electrophoresis – testing.com
27. Sharma, R., Joshi, S., Singh, K. D., & Kumar, A. (2015). Visual evoked potentials: normative values and gender differences. *Journal of Clinical and Diagnostic Research: JCDR*, *9*(7), CC12–CC15. https://doi.org/10.7860/JCDR/2015/12764.6181
28. Brainstem Auditory Evoked Potential – sydneynorthneurology.com.au
29. Ghatol, D., & Widrich, J. (2023, July 24). Intraoperative neurophysiological monitoring. In: *StatPearls*. Treasure Island, FL: StatPearls Publishing; 2023 January. https://www.ncbi.nlm.nih.gov/books/NBK563203/

Part III

Medical Imaging Technologies and their Applications in Diagnosis and Treatment

5 Enhancing Patient Care with Modality-Based Image Registration in Modern Healthcare

*Abhisek Roy, Pranab Kanti Roy,
Anirban Mitra, Paramita Kundu Maji, Sraddha
Roy Choudhury, and Sheng-Lung Peng*

5.1 INTRODUCTION

Various facets of medical diagnosis, treatment, and research have been revolutionized by image processing, which has emerged as a crucial tool in contemporary healthcare. Healthcare experts are able to perceive and comprehend the underlying structures and abnormalities within the human body thanks to their ability to capture, analyze, and interpret medical images. The field of medical imaging has improved significantly in recent years thanks to the development of cutting-edge imaging modalities and sophisticated image processing algorithms. Medical imaging methods offer a noninvasive way to record precise anatomical and physiological data about the human body. These methods include, among others, positron emission tomography (PET), computed tomography (CT), magnetic resonance imaging (MRI), ultrasound, and imaging for nuclear medicine. For clinical diagnosis and decision-making, these modalities provide enormous amounts of data in the form of digital images, which must be processed and analyzed. Image processing is a collection of methods and algorithms used to enhance the quality of digital images, extract important information, and enable automated analysis. To alter and analyze the obtained images, these techniques apply concepts from many fields, such as mathematics, physics, signal processing, and computer science. Clinicians can gain insightful information and make wise judgments by using image processing techniques to enhance, segment, register, and classify medical images. The improvement of medical diagnosis accuracy, efficacy, and dependability is the main goal of image processing in healthcare. Clinicians can more precisely identify and interpret anatomical structures to improve the visual quality of medical pictures produced by image processing techniques. Additionally, image processing makes it easier to identify and classify abnormalities, facilitating early diagnosis and treatment

DOI: 10.1201/9781003464884-8

"

planning. Additionally, it is essential for image-guided interventions and surgical operations, giving the operating team real-time direction and feedback. Computer-aided diagnosis (CAD) is one of the primary fields where image processing has made substantial advances. Radiologists and clinicians are assisted in the interpretation and analysis of medical images by CAD systems, which use image processing algorithms in conjunction with machine learning and artificial intelligence approaches. These technologies can automatically spot potential anomalies and highlight them, reducing human error and increasing diagnostic precision. Detecting lung nodules in chest X-rays and breast cancer using mammography are two instances where CAD systems have proved to be extremely effective. Picture segmentation, which entails dividing a picture into useful sections or objects, also makes use of image processing techniques. For correctly recognizing and outlining anatomical features, lesions, tumors, and other anomalies in medical pictures, segmentation is essential. To identify and distinguish pertinent structures from the background or surrounding tissues, segmentation algorithms employ a variety of strategies, including thresholding, region-growing, level sets, and machine learning-based techniques. The quantitative study of disease development and treatment planning both depend heavily on segmentation. Another crucial component of image processing in healthcare is image registration. In order to evaluate and interpret changes in a patient's condition, it entails aligning many images taken using various modalities or at various times. Healthcare providers can combine complementary data from various imaging modalities, such as integrating MRI and CT pictures, by registering images, in order to get a more thorough understanding of a patient's anatomy and disease. To accurately align and fuse images, image registration algorithms employ a variety of methods, such as feature-based methods, intensity-based methods, and deformable models. The drive to improve patient care with modality-based picture registration is rooted in the quest to give the best treatment possible in the dynamic environment of contemporary healthcare. Clinicians can better understand a patient's condition by combining and aligning medical pictures from several modalities, such as CT and MRI scans. This makes it possible to arrange effective treatments and track patients' progress with accuracy. Healthcare providers can gain new insights thanks to modalities-based image registration, enabling tailored therapies. In the end, this innovation seeks to raise the general level of care in the healthcare sector, improve patient outcomes, and increase treatment efficacy. The novelty of the current study lies in its ability to fuse and synchronize medical images from diverse modalities. This advanced technology revolutionizes the diagnostic process, providing healthcare professionals with a comprehensive and accurate understanding of a patient's condition, leading to more precise and effective treatment strategies.

5.2   FUNDAMENTALS OF IMAGE REGISTRATION

Taking a moving image and transforming it such that it is spatially or temporally aligned with a target stationary image is the basic objective of an image registration algorithm. The sort of transformation that can be applied to the moving picture is determined by the transformation model, and a definition of appropriate alignment is defined by the similarity cost function between the two images. When an algorithm is iterative, an optimizer is also present and looks for ways to modify the transformation so that the cost function is minimized as effectively as possible. Normally, to do this, a model is used to estimate a transformation, which is then applied to the moving image. Finally, the cost function between the changed moving image and the fixed image is assessed. The algorithm then uses this cost to guide its estimation of a more precise transformation for the following iteration. Until the moving and fixed pictures are thought to be aligned (i.e. a local minimum in the cost function is reached) or a maximum iteration count is reached, the procedure is repeated and optimized. This iterative framework is depicted as a block diagram in Figure 5.1.

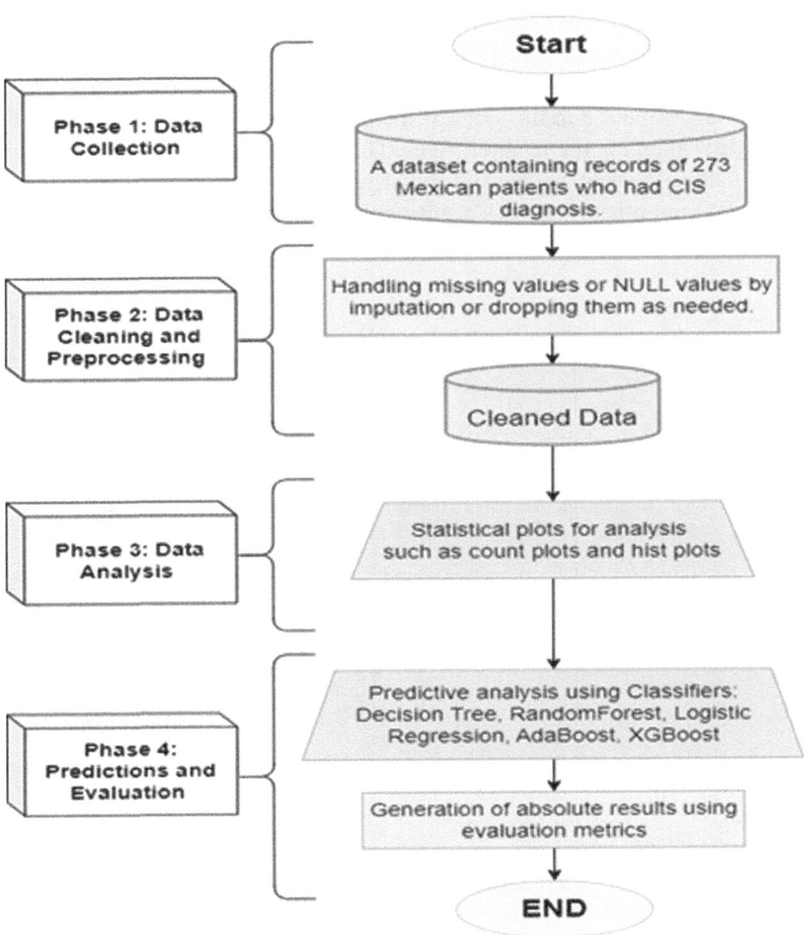

FIGURE 5.1 Image registration process flow diagram.

5.2.1 Transforms Used in Registration: Rigid, Affine, Deformable

A unique type of transformation called a stiff transformation preserves a figure's size and contour. We could assume that it is constructed of a solid object, such as metal or wood, which we can move, flip over, and spin, but which we cannot stretch or bend. A transformation that maintains the size and shape of a geometric figure is known as a rigid transformation (or isometry). When a pre-image is translated, reflected, rotated, or any combination of these three, for instance, this is an example of a stiff transformation. The three most fundamental stiff transformations are as follows: (1) Reflection: This transformation emphasizes how the object's position has changed, but its size and shape are unaltered. This transformation is an excellent illustration of a rigid transformation. The pre-image is 'slid' into the image, but the image's size and shape don't change. (2) Rotation: In rotation, the pre-image is kept in its original shape and size while being 'turned' around a specified angle and with regard to a reference point. Because of this, this transition is stiff. An affine registration is a collection of linear transformations (Figure 5.2). (3) Scaling: In scaling the object's size will be changed but shape will remain as it was.

Linear transformation in this context means maintaining the parallelism of existing lines while mapping them to new lines. The distance ratio is maintained while the pixels are mapped to new pixels. Additionally, satellite image processing, image data augmentation, and other processes require affine transformation. A matrix M is used to multiply various matrices to conduct affine registration. Different transformations

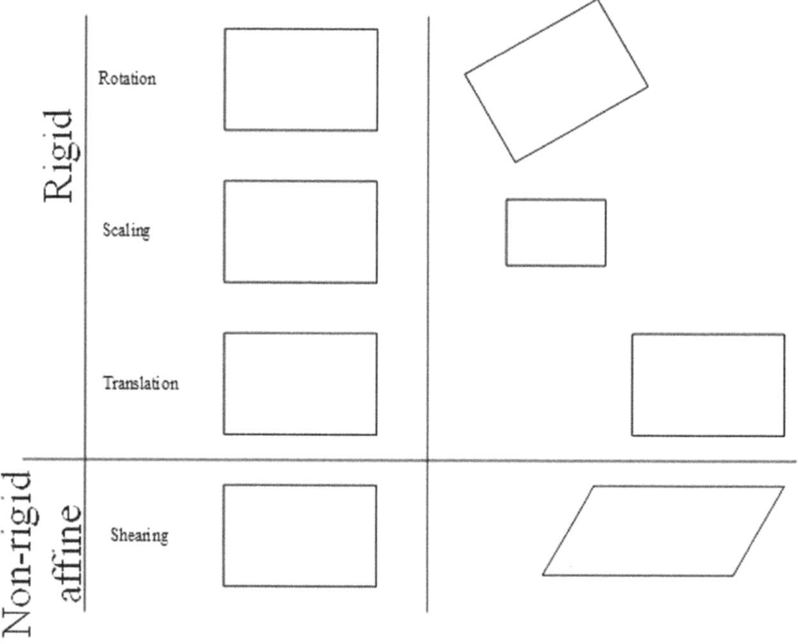

FIGURE 5.2　Rigid and affine registration.

call for various kernel matrices, which, when multiplied by the image matrix, result in the appropriate transformations. Scaling, Translation, Shear, and Rotation are just a few examples of the rigid and nonrigid transformations that make up the affine transformation. The image is tilted in either the x or y direction during shearing. Aligning two or more three-dimensional (3D) pictures into a single coordinate frame is known as deformable registration. This method of combining several photos quantifies changes in organ form, size, and location as specified by the image collection, giving doctors a deeper insight into the anatomy and function of their patients. Due to their adaptability and durability, spline-based deformable registration techniques are quite well-liked in the medical imaging community. However, they take a long time to compute in order to produce good results. The iterative demons approach for deformable registration alternates between updating the velocity vector field and Gaussian regularization, both of which require significant processing resources.

5.2.2 Types of Registration: Intensity-Based, Feature-Based, Hybrid

A crucial step in medical imaging is registration, which entails the alignment and fusion of various pictures or datasets to provide a coherent representation. Modern healthcare uses a variety of registration methods, including hybrid registration, feature-based registration, and intensity-based registration. Healthcare professionals have a variety of options depending on the particular requirements of their applications because each strategy has its own advantages and disadvantages. The examination of pixel intensities in the images being registered is the foundation of the commonly used approach known as intensity-based registration. To accomplish alignment, it entails optimizing a similarity metric, such as the sum of squared differences or mutual information. This approach can handle images with different modalities and is computationally efficient. However, images with considerable anatomical distortions or poor structural contrast may have trouble registering using the intensity-based method. On the other hand, feature-based registration focuses on locating and matching recognizable features in the photos. Anatomical landmarks or other recognizable patterns can be included in these elements. The registration method can ascertain the spatial change between the images by extracting and matching these features. When there are major anatomical variations between the images or when intensity-based approaches don't work because of poor contrast, feature-based registration is especially successful. This method, meanwhile, may be sensitive to noise and may not be effective when there aren't many distinguishing features to match. Combining the benefits of both intensity-based and feature-based approaches is the goal of hybrid registration techniques. These methods usually start with an intensity-based registration to get a rough alignment, then enhance it with feature-based registration to get a better alignment. Hybrid registration can manage a variety of image properties and deliver reliable and accurate alignment results by utilizing both intensity and feature information. Hybrid registration techniques, however, could be more computationally taxing and call for meticulous parameter adjustment to produce the best results. The properties of the images being registered, the needed level of precision, and the particular clinical application all play a role in the choice of registration technique. Because of its effectiveness and adaptability, intensity-based registration is frequently chosen over feature-based registration, which is helpful when distinct anatomical features are present. By striking a balance between the two, hybrid registration ensures reliable alignment in a range of situations. Overall, alignment and merging of medical pictures can be accomplished using intensity-based, feature-based, and hybrid registration strategies. Because each approach has its own advantages and disadvantages, it can be used in a variety of therapeutic situations. The selection of a registration method should be based on careful analysis of the unique specifications and properties of the images at hand, with the ultimate goal of achieving accurate and dependable registration results for enhanced patient care in contemporary healthcare.

5.3   REVIEW OF MEDICAL IMAGING MODALITIES

Medical imaging modalities are a diverse set of techniques and technologies used in the field of medicine for visualizing and diagnosing various medical conditions (Figure 5.3). They play a pivotal role in modern healthcare, aiding in the early detection, diagnosis, and treatment planning of diseases. In a clinical setting, radiology or 'clinical imaging' is typically used to describe medical imaging. The current section discusses image registration in various medical imaging and their modalities.

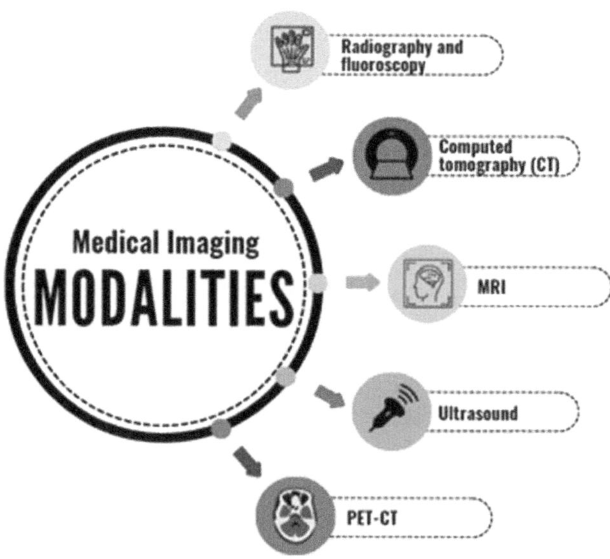

FIGURE 5.3   Modalities in medical imaging.

5.3.1 RADIOGRAPHY AND FLUOROSCOPY

Typically, radiology and the medical subdiscipline pertinent to the medical condition or field of medical science (neuroscience, cardiology, psychiatry, psychology) under inquiry do research into the application and interpretation of medical images. Zaidi briefly described various methods of medical imaging (Bushberg J. T. 2002) and discussed the current status and future perspective, division of nuclear medicine. Tian described the applications of wavelet transform [2] in medical image processing. X-rays are commonly used to visualize the internal structures of the body. This includes chest X-rays, bone X-rays, abdominal X-rays, and dental X-rays, among others. CT scans use X-rays to create detailed cross-sectional images of the body. They are invaluable for diagnosing conditions like tumors, fractures, and vascular diseases. X-ray mammography is used for breast cancer screening and the early detection of breast abnormalities in women. Real-time X-ray imaging is used during various medical procedures, such as barium studies of the gastrointestinal tract, catheter placement, and joint injections. X-ray guidance is also used for minimally invasive procedures, including angioplasty, stent placement, remobilization, and biopsies. These technologies have replaced traditional film-based X-rays, allowing for faster image acquisition and digital storage. X-rays are used in dentistry for diagnosing dental caries, gum disease, and planning dental procedures. X-ray imaging is used in children to diagnose congenital anomalies, injuries, and respiratory conditions. X-rays play a crucial role in diagnosing and monitoring bone and joint conditions, as well as guiding orthopedic surgeries. X-ray imaging is used in radiation therapy for treatment planning and ensuring precise targeting of cancerous tissues. Radiography and fluoroscopy are two essential medical imaging techniques that use X-rays to visualize and diagnose various medical conditions. Image registration in radiography and fluoroscopy plays a crucial role in diagnosis, treatment planning, and real-time medical interventions. It improves the accuracy and safety of procedures while minimizing radiation exposure to patients and healthcare providers. The choice of registration method depends on the specific clinical context and the modality used. Image registration plays a significant role in radiography and fluoroscopy by enhancing the accuracy and utility of medical imaging in various clinical applications.

A) *Diagnosis and Visualization*

- Multimodal Fusion: Radiography and fluoroscopy are often used alongside other imaging modalities such as CT, MRI, and ultrasound. Image registration allows for the fusion of images from different modalities, enabling clinicians to integrate complementary information for a more comprehensive understanding of a patient's condition.
- Time-Series Analysis: In fluoroscopy, especially during dynamic procedures, such as angiography or joint motion studies, image registration helps align and track changes in the images over time, aiding in the diagnosis of vascular abnormalities, joint disorders, and other dynamic conditions.

B) *Treatment Planning and Guidance*

- Preoperative Planning: In radiography, CT or MRI scans are used for detailed preoperative planning. Image registration facilitates the overlay of preoperative images onto live fluoroscopic images during surgery, helping surgeons accurately target specific structures or lesions and plan their approach.
- Minimally Invasive Interventions: During interventional procedures guided by fluoroscopy, image registration allows physicians to precisely position medical instruments or implants within the body, ensuring minimal damage to healthy tissues and effective treatment of the targeted pathology.

C) *Monitoring and Follow-Up*

- Comparative Analysis: Image registration is crucial for comparing current radiographic or fluoroscopic images with previous ones. This is valuable for tracking disease progression, monitoring the healing process of fractures, and assessing the effectiveness of treatments.

D) *Motion Compensation*

- Patient Motion Correction: Both radiography and fluoroscopy can be affected by patient motion, which can result in blurred or misaligned images. Image registration techniques can help correct patient motion, allowing for clearer and more accurate imaging.

E) *Quality Improvement*

- Image Enhancement In radiography, especially in cases of limited dose or challenging patient positioning, image registration can be used to improve the quality of radiographic images by aligning and averaging multiple exposures to reduce noise and enhance the overall image.

F) *Interventional Radiation Safety*

- Reducing Radiation Exposure: In interventional procedures using fluoroscopy, minimizing the duration and extent of X-ray exposure is essential to reduce radiation dose to the patient and healthcare providers. Accurate image registration can help streamline procedures, leading to reduced radiation exposure.

When a patient has suspected heart or lung problems, a chest X-ray (CXR) examination is nearly often ordered as the first imaging test. Through the application of a modest amount of X-ray energy, the chest is exposed during this noninvasive imaging method to produce a static projection image on the detector (Bushberg J. T. 2002). Another imaging modality that uses X-ray radiation to scan the heart is angiography. A radiocontrast agent is injected into the blood artery, and a low-dose X-ray beam is utilized to obtain real-time images of the heart using fluoroscopy (Moscucci 2013). Angiography can be utilized to identify the infarct location in ischemic heart disease, such as coronary artery disease (Timinger et al. 2005; Dauwe et al. 2014). Furthermore, this imaging approach is employed for the implantation of left ventricular (LV) (Dey et al. 2010) leads during cardiac resynchronization therapy for patients with heart failure (Auricchio et al. 2009; Manzke et al. 2010). Angiography can also help physicians guide patients with cardiac arrhythmias during cardiac electrophysiology procedures (Duckett et al. 2011; Ma et al. 2012). Angiography can also be used on patients with congenital heart disease during cardiac catheterization procedures (Wielandts et al. 2016; Glockler et al. 2013). In summary, image registration in radiography and fluoroscopy is integral to clinical decision-making, treatment planning, and real-time guidance during medical procedures. It improves diagnostic accuracy, helps optimize treatment strategies, and enhances patient safety by minimizing radiation exposure. The application of image registration techniques is diverse and highly beneficial across various aspects of medical imaging and intervention.

5.3.2 Computed Tomography (CT)

Computed tomography (CT) is a powerful medical imaging technique that uses X-rays and advanced computer processing to create detailed cross-sectional images, also known as tomographic slices, of the human body. CT scans are invaluable tools in medicine, providing high-resolution images of internal structures for diagnostic and therapeutic purposes. Here, the key aspects of CT imaging are explored:.

CT imaging is based on the principles of X-ray absorption. When X-ray beams pass through the body, different tissues and structures absorb varying amounts of X-rays. These X-rays are detected by an array of detectors positioned opposite the X-ray source. By rotating the X-ray source and detectors around the patient, multiple X-ray projections are obtained from different angles. The X-ray tube emits a focused beam of X-rays that passes through the body. The detector array, positioned opposite the X-ray tube, measures the intensity of X-rays that pass through the body at each angle. The gantry is the circular structure that houses the X-ray tube and detector array. It rotates around the patient during scanning. The patient lies on a movable table that can be repositioned to ensure accurate scanning of the desired body area. A powerful computer processes the data collected by the detectors and generates detailed cross-sectional images. CT imaging is used in various medical specialities for a wide range of applications. CT scans are essential for diagnosing conditions such as cancer, cardiovascular disease, traumatic injuries, and infectious diseases. CT scans provide detailed information about the size, location, and extent of tumors, aiding in cancer staging and treatment planning. In emergency medicine, CT scans are used to evaluate injuries to the head, chest, abdomen, and musculoskeletal system. CT angiography (CTA) is employed to visualize blood vessels and detect conditions like aneurysms, stenosis, and vascular malformations. CT is used for detecting and characterizing brain tumors, hemorrhages, and other neurological conditions. CT scans assist in orthopedic evaluations, especially for complex fractures and joint disorders. CT provides detailed images of both bones and soft tissues, making it useful for various medical conditions. Modern CT scanners can perform rapid scans, reducing the time patients need to remain still during the procedure. CT imaging is generally noninvasive, requiring no surgical procedures or contrast injections for routine scans. While CT scans are extremely valuable, they involve exposure to ionizing radiation, which carries some risk. Radiologists and medical professionals carefully weigh the benefits of the diagnostic information obtained against the potential risks of radiation exposure, particularly in children and pregnant individuals. Dose-reduction techniques and guidelines are followed to minimize radiation exposure. In conclusion, computed tomography (CT) is a vital medical imaging modality that plays a crucial role in diagnosing and monitoring a wide range of medical conditions. Advances in technology have improved image quality, reduced scan times, and enhanced the safety profile of CT imaging, making it an indispensable tool in modern healthcare. Image registration plays a crucial role in computed tomography (CT) imaging in a variety of applications, enhancing the utility and accuracy of CT scans. Here are some key roles of image registration in CT:

- *Multimodal Image Fusion*: CT scans are often combined with other imaging modalities like MRI, PET, or SPECT for a more comprehensive assessment of a patient's condition. Image registration allows for the fusion of these images, providing complementary information to aid in diagnosis and treatment planning.
- *Follow-Up and Longitudinal Studies*: In cases where patients require follow-up CT scans over time, image registration is used to align and compare images taken at different intervals. This helps track the progression or regression of diseases, assess treatment effectiveness, and monitor the healing process of fractures or surgical sites.
- *Dose Reduction*: In some situations, it's necessary to minimize the radiation dose delivered during CT imaging, particularly in pediatric patients or individuals who require repeated scans. Image registration can be used to reduce noise and artifacts in low-dose CT scans by aligning and averaging multiple scans, thereby improving image quality without increasing radiation exposure.
- *Respiratory Motion Compensation*: Image registration is essential for managing respiratory motion artifacts, which can degrade the quality of CT images. Techniques like 4D CT are used to acquire images at different phases of the respiratory cycle, and image registration is employed to align these images for accurate diagnosis and treatment planning in lung or abdominal cases.
- *Treatment Planning*: CT scans are widely used for radiation therapy planning. Image registration is crucial in aligning the patient's planning CT images with simulation scans, enabling the precise targeting of tumors and minimizing damage to healthy tissues.
- *Image-Guided Interventions*: During minimally invasive procedures and surgeries, CT image registration can overlay preoperative or planning CT scans onto real-time images, providing surgeons with guidance, and improving the accuracy of instrument placement.
- *Stitching for Large-Field Scans*: When capturing images of large anatomical areas (e.g. spine, extremities), multiple CT scans may be required. Image registration is used to stitch these images together into a seamless, comprehensive image for diagnostic purposes.

- ***Deformable Registration***: In cases where the anatomy undergoes changes between scans (e.g. due to tumor shrinkage or organ deformation), deformable image registration techniques are employed. These methods accommodate variations and provide more accurate alignment.
- ***Image Analysis and Research***: Image registration is fundamental for quantitative image analysis and research, enabling the comparison of different CT datasets, the measurement of anatomical changes, and the assessment of treatment outcomes.
- ***Image Quality Improvement***: Image registration techniques can be used to correct artifacts, such as patient motion during CT scanning, leading to clearer and more accurate images.

Volumetric brain registration methods are currently being used for general purpose registration on abdominal computed tomography (CT) scans. Human abdomens have a large variety of variants, which complicates registrations in comparison to the comparatively stable brain structure. Aside from intersubject variations (e.g. age, gender, stature, normal anatomical variances, illness state), soft anatomy within the abdomen deforms significantly within individuals (e.g. position, respiratory cycle). While larger errors can be predicted, caution should be exercised when using atlas-based abdominal segmentation in the setting of non-robust abdominal CT registrations. This necessitates a performance evaluation of existing registration systems on abdominal CTs, with a particular emphasis on atlas-based segmentation. Previously, Klein et al. (2019) used 14 nonlinear registration tools and one linear registration technique (Klein et al. 2009) on human brain MRIs to find the nonlinear deformation algorithms most suited for brain image registration. In their investigation, registrations were analyzed using the Valmet validation tool, and 3D object segmentations were validated using both volume- and surface-based metric criteria (Gerig et al. 2001). In summary, image registration is an essential tool in CT imaging, serving various clinical and research purposes. It enhances the diagnostic and therapeutic capabilities of CT scans, improves patient safety, and contributes to the advancement of medical knowledge and practice.

5.3.3 Magnetic Resonance Imaging (MRI)

Magnetic Resonance Imaging (MRI) is a noninvasive medical imaging technique that uses strong magnetic fields and radio waves to generate detailed images of the internal structures of the body. MRI is a versatile and powerful diagnostic tool that provides exceptional soft tissue contrast, making it invaluable in various medical specialities. Let's delve into the key aspects of MRI. MRI relies on the principles of nuclear magnetic resonance (NMR), where the nuclei of certain atoms, particularly hydrogen nuclei (protons), align themselves with a strong magnetic field. When exposed to radiofrequency (RF) pulses, these nuclei temporarily deviate from their alignment. As they return to their original alignment, they emit radiofrequency signals. The signals are collected and processed by the MRI scanner to create detailed images. Image registration seeks to geometrically match up images or image volumes for structure localization and difference detection. It has been widely employed in medical diagnostics, treatment planning and evaluation, illness and intervention monitoring, image-guided surgery, and therapy, and so on. This technique is commonly used to combine important information from several sources (e.g. CT, PET, SPECT, X-ray, ultrasound, and magnetic resonance imaging) (Maes et al. 1997; Nikou et al. 1998), or to register images received at different periods (Ritter et al. 1999). In this study, we discuss various commonly used image registration algorithms and their applications in magnetic resonance imaging (MRI). One main goal of image registration in MRI applications is to examine picture variations, which can range from intersubject anatomical comparisons of brain imaging (Castro et al. 2006; Collins et al. 1994) to intra-subject monitoring of disease development (Takao et al. 2005), to matching an observed image with a reference template (Castro et al. 2006; Collins et al. 1994). In the case of intra-subject or temporal variation registration, observed images could be a time series obtained in a short period of time on a single occasion or a time series acquired on multiple times. The changes between the reference and subsequent photos are largely object-related in the first scenario because noise patterns and other environment-related artifacts would be comparable. However, in the second example, this may not be the case. For example, noise patterns at different times may differ due to changing acquisition settings.

5.3.4 ULTRASOUND

Ultrasound, also known as ultrasonography, is a medical imaging technique that uses high-frequency sound waves to produce real-time images of the inside of the body. It is a non-invasive and safe imaging method widely used in various medical specialities for diagnostic and monitoring purposes. Here are the key aspects of ultrasound imaging: Ultrasound imaging is based on the principle of sending high-frequency sound waves (typically in the range of 2–20 megahertz) into the body and capturing the echoes as they bounce back from different tissues and structures. The echoes are used to create images in real time. Ultrasound waves can penetrate tissues and fluids, making it suitable for examining a wide range of body parts. The transducer is a handheld device that emits ultrasound waves and receives the echoes. It is placed on the skin in the area being examined. A gel is applied to the skin to ensure good contact between the transducer and the body. It also helps eliminate air pockets that can interfere with sound wave transmission. While generic image registration methods can be used to align ultrasound pictures, greater results are obtained when domain-specific knowledge is incorporated into the registration process. Speckle, an interference process caused by random backscattering in an ultrasonic beam resolution cell, corrupts ultrasound images. Speckle appears as a spatially associated noise pattern with a non-Gaussian intensity distribution. Indeed, in the envelope detected image, fully formed speckle has a Rayleigh distribution and in the log-compressed image, it has a Fisher-Tippett (doubly exponential) distribution (Dutt et al. 1996). Speckle is deterministic for scatterers in a fixed position relative to the ultrasound beam.

As a result, for minor displacements, the speckle is correlated from image to image, which has been employed in speckle tracking systems (O'Donnell et al. 1994). However, if the displacement is larger, or photos of the same location are acquired from other scans, transducers, etc., the correlation of the speckle will be lost. In such instances, registration algorithms based on pixel-to-pixel comparisons will struggle, because two similar pixels from the same anatomic structure can have extremely different intensity levels due to speckle intensity changes. It would be preferable to compare estimates from the distributions rather than samples of Fisher-Tippett distributions from one image to the next. This is how we address the problem. While there are studies on ultrasound registration in the literature (Ledesma-Carbayo et al. 2005), many of them employ generic registration algorithms. However, there are ultrasound-specific registration techniques in the literature (Cohen et al. 2002; Boukerroui et al. 2003), which are based on probability distributions derived from theoretical speckle models. Because of the randomness of speckle noise, the similarity metrics used in these publications rely on pixel-to-pixel intensity comparisons, which may not be acceptable in many applications. Unlike earlier work, our solution is distribution-based, which increases robustness to noise.

5.3.5 Nuclear Medicine and PET-CT Imaging

Nuclear medicine is a specialized medical imaging technique that uses small amounts of radioactive materials (radiotracers) to diagnose and treat various medical conditions. Positron emission tomography-computed tomography (PET-CT) is a hybrid imaging modality that combines the principles of nuclear medicine (PET) and computed tomography (CT) to provide both functional and anatomical information. Here, we will explore nuclear medicine and PET-CT imaging: Nuclear medicine imaging relies on the principle that certain radiotracers, when introduced into the body, accumulate in specific organs or tissues based on their metabolic or physiological activity. These radiotracers emit gamma rays, which are detected by a gamma camera or single photon emission computed tomography (SPECT) scanner. The collected data are then processed to create images that highlight areas of abnormal function. These are radioactive materials labeled with compounds that mimic naturally occurring substances in the body. Different radiotracers are used for various applications. These devices detect gamma rays emitted by the radiotracers in the body and create images of the distribution of the radiotracer. Nuclear medicine is used for various diagnostic and therapeutic purposes, including nuclear medicine is employed to identify and stage cancers, detect metastases, and assess the effectiveness of cancer treatments. Multimodality PET/CT of the liver can be conducted using an integrated (hybrid) PET/CT scanner or by fusing dedicated PET and CT software. Regardless of the method used, accurate anatomic correlation and acceptable image quality are crucial conditions. Breathing motion differences on PET and CT can affect registration accuracy, which can also affect (attenuation correction-related) artifacts, particularly in the upper abdomen. The impact of these difficulties was assessed for both hybrid PET/CT and software fusion, with an emphasis on liver imaging. Normal image registration quality-assurance methods for hybrid PET/CT were followed as stated by the manufacturer. It entailed utilizing a 'crossed-lines' phantom to align the PET and CT gantries after maintenance. Following scanning, no additional image registration optimization was attempted. Software image registration was carried out on a personal computer using in-house created image viewing and registration software based on the visualization toolkit VTK (Schroeder et al. 2003) and the insight segmentation and registration toolkit ITK (Ibanez et al. 2003). The process has previously been described in greater detail (Van et al. 2004). In summary, the software enables rigid-body image registration using three translation and three rotation parameters. On a 3D volume of interest containing liver, anatomic registration of PET emission images to CT was pursued using an implementation of the automatic mutual information approach.

5.4 IMAGE REGISTRATION TECHNIQUES IN CLINICAL SETTINGS

In clinical settings, a wide array of imaging modalities are essential tools that play a pivotal role in modern healthcare. Each imaging technique has its unique strengths and applications, making them valuable for diagnosing and monitoring various medical conditions. Whether it's obtaining detailed anatomical information, assessing functional aspects, or conducting minimally invasive procedures, these imaging modalities collectively contribute to improved patient care, better treatment planning, and enhanced disease management. The choice of imaging modality depends on numerous factors, including the nature of the medical condition, the body part to be examined, patient-specific factors such as age and medical history, and the clinical question at hand. Radiography and CT provide detailed views of bones and internal structures, while MRI excels in soft tissue contrast. Ultrasound is versatile, portable, and noninvasive, suitable for real-time imaging in various clinical scenarios. Nuclear medicine and PET offer valuable insights into both structure and function, aiding in cancer staging and organ assessment. Mammography remains a critical tool for breast cancer screening, and endoscopy enables direct visualization of internal organs. Continual advancements in imaging technology, such as improved resolution, reduced radiation exposure, and enhanced software processing, contribute to more accurate diagnoses and better patient outcomes. These innovations are complemented by the expertise of radiologists, technologists, and healthcare providers who interpret and utilize the imaging data to guide clinical decisions. In summary, the diverse range of imaging modalities available in clinical settings ensures that healthcare professionals have a comprehensive toolbox to diagnose, treat, and monitor medical conditions effectively. As technology continues to evolve, these imaging techniques will remain indispensable in delivering high-quality healthcare and improving patient well-being.

5.4.1 IMPORTANCE AND NECESSITY OF IMAGE REGISTRATION IN CLINICAL SETTINGS

Image registration techniques are fundamental tools in clinical settings, revolutionizing the field of medical imaging by enabling the integration and analysis of diverse imaging data. These techniques play a pivotal role in diagnosis, treatment planning, and patient monitoring, offering healthcare professionals a comprehensive view of anatomical and pathological changes. Image registration involves aligning and comparing images from various sources, such as different imaging modalities, time points, or patient positions. By bringing together these disparate pieces of information, clinicians gain valuable insights that enhance the accuracy of diagnoses and the effectiveness of medical interventions. In clinical practice, image registration serves as the bridge between different imaging modalities, allowing for the fusion of anatomical and functional data. It enables healthcare providers to precisely locate and evaluate abnormalities, assess treatment outcomes, and plan interventions with greater precision. Whether it's aligning preoperative and intraoperative images during surgery, tracking tumor growth, or monitoring changes in a patient's anatomy over time, image registration techniques are indispensable tools that contribute to improved patient care and outcomes. This exploration of image registration techniques in clinical settings will delve into various methods and applications, shedding light on how these techniques have become integral to modern healthcare. From rigid and affine transformations to nonrigid deformable registration and intensity-based or feature-based approaches, this overview will examine the principles, applications, and significance of these techniques in the medical field. We will explore how image registration contributes to the multidisciplinary efforts of healthcare providers, radiologists, surgeons, and researchers, ultimately enhancing our ability to understand, diagnose, and treat a wide range of medical conditions.

In the clinical evaluation of chronic kidney diseases (CKD), magnetic resonance imaging (MRI) methods have grown in significance (Selby et al. 2018). They permit the least invasive measurement of a range of parameters that may be crucial in the diagnosis and follow-up of renal disorders. This includes, among other things, measuring kidney volumes (Zöllner et al. 2012), assessing microstructure using diffusion-weighted imaging (Caroli et al. 2018), measuring hemodynamic parameters using arterial spin labeling (ASL) (Odudu et al. 2018), or using dynamic contrast-enhanced (DCE-) MRI (Jones et al. 2011). The 'emerging need of public databases of representative expert-annotated images and of validation protocol' and 'the rare use of registration in diagnostic clinical practice' are among Viergever et al.'s list of comments and observations (Viergever et al. 2016). Several strategies use breath-hold techniques in renal perfusion MRI to reduce kidney movement. These include regular shallow breathing (Brox 2007), holding your breath during the first pass of the contrast agent during a DCE-MRI, and holding your breath repeatedly, like in ASL (Robson et al. 2016). Image registration is utilized for later data analysis such as perfusion quantification interpolation or image-based post-processing. Since the data sampling is difficult to manage, prospectively gated acquisitions typically take longer to capture the required quantity of data and are rarely employed in dynamic imaging. As demonstrated by Attenberger et al. retrospective gating of renal perfusion MRI (Attenberger et al. 2010) is possible if the data are captured at a high temporal rate, allowing the remaining accepted data to adequately capture the signal change with time.

5.4.2 Overview of Different Image Registration Techniques in Clinical Practice

Finding conformity between two photos such that all of their points line up is known as image (Pipe et al. 1999) registration; specifically, by comparing the values of each pixel in the referred and sensed images. Images may have been taken at various times, from various views or angles, using various sensors or equipment, and then the various data sets may have been combined into a single coordinate system.

The image that serves as the foundation for all subsequent image transformations and alignments with respect to it is known as the referenced image. Many different sectors, including remote sensing, weather prediction, environmental monitoring, change detection, image mosaics, producing higher-resolution photos, and geographic information, can benefit from image registration (as shown in Figure 5.4). Image registration is a fundamental process that aligns and integrates multiple medical images, providing healthcare professionals with a more comprehensive and accurate understanding of a patient's condition. Here are several key reasons why image registration is crucial in clinical practice.

- *Multimodal Fusion*: Clinical settings often involve the use of multiple imaging modalities, such as MRI, CT, ultrasound, and PET. Each modality provides unique information about different aspects of a patient's anatomy or pathology. Image registration enables the fusion of these multimodal images, allowing clinicians to combine the strengths of each modality and obtain a more complete picture of the patient's health.
- *Improved Diagnosis*: Image registration enhances the accuracy of diagnoses by providing a consolidated view of anatomical and functional information. For example, combining structural MRI with functional MRI (fMRI) data can help pinpoint the exact location of brain abnormalities associated with neurological disorders.

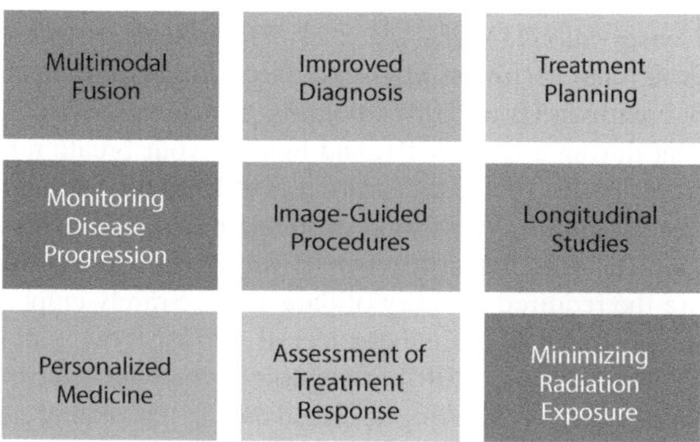

FIGURE 5.4   Different image registration techniques in clinical practice.

- ***Treatment Planning***: In radiation therapy and surgery, precise treatment planning is essential. Image registration ensures that treatment plans are based on the most up-to-date and accurate patient information. For example, in radiation therapy, it enables the precise targeting of tumors while sparing healthy tissues.
- ***Monitoring Disease Progression***: For chronic conditions or diseases that change over time (e.g. cancer), image registration is essential for monitoring disease progression. By aligning images from different time points, clinicians can track changes in tumor size, shape, and location, which informs treatment decisions.
- ***Image-Guided Procedures***: During minimally invasive procedures or surgeries, image registration guides surgeons by overlaying preoperative images onto real-time intraoperative images. This provides critical navigational information, improving the accuracy of procedures and minimizing damage to surrounding tissues.
- ***Longitudinal Studies***: Image registration supports research and clinical studies by enabling the comparison of images collected over time. This is particularly valuable for understanding disease development, treatment efficacy, and the impact of interventions.
- ***Personalized Medicine***: Image registration is essential in the emerging field of personalized medicine, where treatment plans are tailored to individual patients. By integrating various imaging data, healthcare providers can make more informed decisions regarding patient-specific therapies.
- ***Assessment of Treatment Response***: In oncology, image registration helps assess how tumors respond to treatments like chemotherapy or radiation therapy. Clinicians can compare pre-treatment and post-treatment images to determine the effectiveness of interventions.
- ***Minimizing Radiation Exposure***: In cases where repeated imaging is necessary (e.g. for monitoring chronic conditions), image registration can reduce the need for additional scans, thus minimizing patient exposure to ionizing radiation.

Image registration is a cornerstone of medical research. It enables the development of new imaging techniques, algorithms, and technologies, leading to continuous improvements in healthcare. In summary, image registration is a vital tool in clinical settings, facilitating accurate diagnoses, treatment planning, and patient monitoring. It empowers healthcare professionals with a comprehensive view of patient data, improves the precision of medical procedures, and supports advancements in research and personalized medicine. As technology continues to evolve, image registration techniques will play an increasingly pivotal role in enhancing patient care and outcomes. In clinical practice, different image registration techniques serve as indispensable tools for aligning and fusing medical images, contributing to more accurate diagnoses, effective treatment planning, and comprehensive patient monitoring. These techniques encompass a spectrum of approaches, each tailored to specific clinical scenarios. Rigid registration provides precise alignment through translations, rotations, and scaling, ideal for ensuring proper positioning during surgery and for comparing images at different time points. Affine registration extends this by including nonuniform scaling and shearing, accommodating geometric variations. Nonrigid registration, on the other hand, is essential when deformations are significant, making it invaluable for tracking tumor growth or monitoring organ motion during radiation therapy. The Demons algorithm offers a versatile nonrigid registration method by iteratively optimizing deformation fields. Intensity-based registration relies on the similarity of intensity patterns within images, crucial for aligning multimodal images. Feature-based registration employs distinctive landmarks for precise alignment during image-guided surgery. Demographic-driven registration leverages population-based atlases for comparative studies, particularly in neuroimaging. Lastly, free-form deformation (FFD) allows grid-based control point deformation to capture complex transformations, aiding image-guided radiotherapy and correction of image deformations. Together, these techniques empower clinicians to leverage the full potential of medical imaging, advancing healthcare and patient outcomes.

5.4.3 PREPROCESSING STEPS AND IMAGING PROTOCOL FOR REGISTRATION

Image registration in clinical practice involves a series of preprocessing steps and adhering to specific imaging protocols to ensure accurate and reliable results. These preparatory measures are critical to the success of the registration process, whether it's aligning images from different modalities, time points, or patients.

- *Image Quality Enhancement*: Before registration, it's essential to enhance the quality of the images. This may involve noise reduction, contrast enhancement, or artifact correction to improve the clarity of anatomical structures.
- *Resampling*: Images may have varying resolutions or voxel sizes. Resampling ensures that all images have the same spatial resolution, which is crucial for accurate alignment.
- *Image Cropping*: Removing irrelevant or empty regions from images can reduce computational complexity and enhance the registration process's efficiency.
- *Normalization*: Normalizing image intensities across different scans or modalities can be necessary to make them directly comparable. Histogram matching or intensity scaling techniques are often employed.
- *Deformation Field Initialization*: In nonrigid registration, initializing the deformation field with an appropriate starting point can expedite the convergence of registration algorithms.
- *Imaging Protocol for Registration*: Standardized Patient Positioning – to ensure consistency, patients should be positioned as closely as possible to a standardized orientation during image acquisition. Proper immobilization techniques can be used, especially for procedures requiring high precision.

- ***Contrast Agents***: In cases where contrast agents are used, the timing of their administration is crucial for accurate registration. Images should be acquired during the optimal contrast phase to capture the relevant information.
- ***Imaging Modality Selection***: Choose the appropriate imaging modality or sequence for the clinical question at hand. Consider factors like spatial resolution, tissue contrast, and the nature of the condition being investigated.
- ***Field-of-View (FOV) Consistency***: Maintaining consistent FOV across images is essential for accurate registration. Ensure that the relevant anatomical structures are entirely captured within the FOV.
- ***Slice Thickness and Gap***: Consistency in slice thickness and gap between slices is critical for 3D volumetric data, such as CT and MRI. Uniform slice thickness minimizes artifacts and simplifies registration.
- ***Imaging Parameters***: Ensure that imaging parameters, such as echo time (TE), repetition time (TR), and flip angle (for MRI) or X-ray exposure settings (for radiography and CT), are standardized to reduce variations.
- ***Patient Identification***: Properly label and associate images with patient identifiers, acquisition dates, and other relevant metadata. This helps prevent errors in data selection during registration.
- ***Data Transfer and Storage***: Maintain data integrity during image transfer and storage. Verify that images are not subject to corruption, loss, or compression that could affect registration quality. By adhering to these preprocessing steps and imaging protocols, clinicians and radiologists can optimize the image registration process, ensuring that it yields accurate, clinically valuable results.

These measures help provide a solid foundation for subsequent analyses, diagnoses, and treatment planning in a wide range of clinical applications.

5.5 MODALITY-BASED IMAGE REGISTRATION IN DIAGNOSTIC IMAGING

An imaging modality is an apparatus used to capture images. A single device is used to acquire a mono-modal image (see Figure 5.5); multimodality involves the use of numerous devices. More broadly, the word 'modality' is used to refer to various techniques and treatments in clinical medicine; for example, chemotherapy, radiotherapy, and surgery are examples of modalities of treatment for cancer. A vital technique in diagnostic imaging, modality-based image registration aligns medical pictures obtained from many modalities, including MRI, CT, and PET. It increases the clarity of images, increases the precision with which anomalies are identified, and facilitates treatment planning by combining data from various modalities. With the help of this approach, medical experts may diagnose patients more accurately and give them tailored therapies.

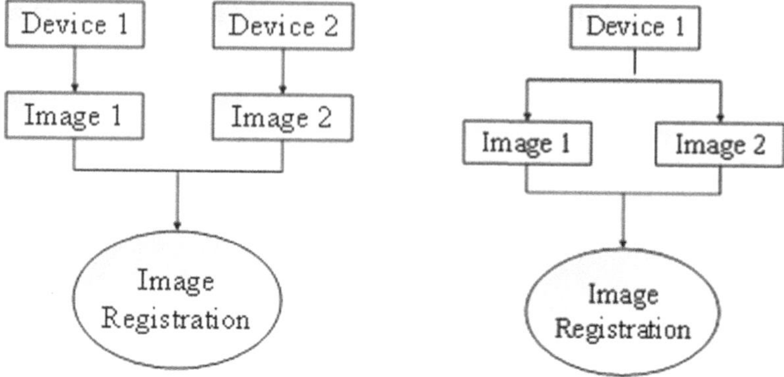

FIGURE 5.5   Multimodal (a) and monomodal (b) image registration.

5.5.1 PRINCIPLES OF DIAGNOSTIC IMAGE REGISTRATION

An essential aspect of diagnostic image registration in medical imaging is the comparison and alignment of various images of the same patient or anatomical area. It is essential to many medical applications, including disease diagnosis, planning of treatments, and tracking the progression of a disease. The technique of aligning and superimposing two or more medical photographs to provide a thorough study of the patient's health is known as diagnostic image registration. These images can be acquired using a variety of imaging techniques, including X-rays, CT scans, MRIs, and PET scans. Clinicians can compare and analyze these photos by aligning them to find changes or anomalies in the patient's anatomy or pathology.

The following essential ideas are central to the principles of diagnostic image registration:

a) *Deformable Image Registration (DIR)*: DIR is a method that enables the alignment of pictures with sizable anatomical variances. It accounts for the alterations and deformations that the patient's anatomy experiences between imaging sessions. DIR is very helpful in radiation therapy since it helps to account for anatomical deformations during the planning and administration of treatment.

b) *Image Alignment and Overlapping*: One of the main objectives of diagnostic image registration is to align and overlay several images that were taken at various periods or with various imaging modalities. With the help of this alignment, professionals can examine and compare images side by side to spot changes more easily in anatomy, disease, or therapeutic response.

c) *Feature Extraction and Matching*: Diagnostic image registration depends on locating similar features or landmarks in the pictures being registered. Anatomical landmarks like bones or organs as well as picture patterns can be considered among these aspects. These features are recognized and extracted using feature extraction methods, and matching algorithms are utilized to locate related features in other photos.

d) *Transformation Models:* Diagnostic image registration uses transformation models to straighten and reshape one image to fit another. The spatial relationship and distortion between images are described by these models. Rigid (translation, rotation, and scaling) and affine (including shearing) as well as nonrigid (deformations) transformation models are frequently used.

e) *Optimization Techniques*: Optimization algorithms help in the process of determining the best transformation parameters to align photos. By typically minimizing a cost function that measures the degree of dissimilarity between the photos, these algorithms seek to reduce the disparities between the registered images. Iterative algorithms for optimization, including gradient descent, as well as algorithms based on mathematical optimization methods are both possible.

f) *Evaluation and Validation:* To assure the accuracy and dependability of diagnostic image registration methods, evaluation and validation are crucial. The Dice coefficient or mean squared differences are two metrics used to measure the registration quality. Validation may entail contrasting registered photos with real-world information or professional annotations.

To simplify comparison and analysis, the principles of diagnostic image registration often involve aligning, overlaying, and deforming images. Important steps in this process include deformable image registration (DIR), feature extraction, transformation models, optimization techniques, and evaluation (Song et al. 2017). These principles are essential for many medical imaging applications because they help physicians diagnose patients correctly, plan therapies, and track the development of diseases. Multimodality fusion, longitudinal research, and population modeling are some of the significant uses of deformable image registration in medical image processing. Sotiras et al. (2013) gave a comprehensive review of deformable registration techniques with an emphasis on recent developments. The main elements of image registration methods were independently investigated, with a focus on methods used with medical pictures. The study contributed to a thorough understanding of registration procedures by methodically presenting the most recent strategies. Oliveira et al. (2014) [40] presented a review of automated image registration methodologies in the medical field, introducing the field, discussing different approaches, and covering key steps and assessment techniques like common geometric transformations, similarity measures, and accuracy assessment techniques. Guan et al. (2018) emphasized point features and point set matching algorithms (PMs), which were critical for medical image registration. The necessity of a thorough analysis of PMs in various clinical settings was discussed. The primary method of geometric transformation models and the individualized treatment plans. Maes et al. (1997) introduced mutual information (MI) as a matching criterion as a novel method for multimodality medical image registration. It was demonstrated that MI, which was accurate and reliable for aligning CT, MR, and PET scans, assessed the statistical dependence between matching voxels in various imaging. The technique was appropriate for clinical applications since it provided subvoxel accuracy without the need for prior segmentation or preprocessing processes. Hosseini et al. discussed the combination of X-ray mammography with vibro-acoustography (VA) for enhanced imaging (Hosseini et al. 2007). For image registration, an adaptable control-point selection method was applied, producing precise alignment. A color-based fusion technique was utilized to merge VA and X-ray images in the fused image in order to better visualize structural data. Bashiri et al. discussed the difficulties involved in aligning images taken using several modalities in multimodal image registration (Bashiri et al. 2018). The suggested strategy transformed multimodal to mono-modal that enabled accurate alignment using tried-and-true mono-modal registration methods. The technique focused on regaining scales, rotations, and translations among images. The findings of testing using real and simulated human brain pictures were encouraging, although the effectiveness of the suggested transformation method for aligning partially overlapped multimodal images needed more research, it was effective for aligning fully overlapped multimodal images. Diwakar et al. (2023) discussed the significance of modality-based registration techniques in diagnostic imaging and its clinical applications. Image improvement while keeping heterogeneous traits, better clarity and extended information for diagnosis and therapy, and adaptive identification of breakdown levels were all mentioned. The methods also assisted in keeping original data and color standards, as well as refining the input image. Overall, there are several clinical uses for modalities-based registration techniques in diagnostic imaging. They improve the precision and usefulness of medical imaging, empowering physicians to make wiser choices and deliver better patient care.

5.5.2   Image-Guided Interventions

Image-guided interventions use medical imaging tools to direct and support a range of treatments and procedures. An essential part of image-guided therapies, modalities-based image registration enables the alignment and integration of images from several modalities, including MRI, CT, ultrasound, and X-ray, to provide a thorough perspective of the patient's anatomy. These therapies have many advantages, such as improved patient outcomes, decreased invasiveness, and increased accuracy. Target structures or lesions must be precisely located within the patient's body for image-guided therapies to be effective. Physicians can more accurately navigate equipment or devices to the intended spot by employing real-time imaging to visualize the target area. This makes it possible to target tumors with greater accuracy, treat vascular problems, and insert tools like stents or catheters. Several medical specialities, including interventional radiology, cardiology, neurology, and oncology, have undergone revolutionary changes because of the use of image guidance. Percutaneous biopsies, tumor ablation methods (such as radiofrequency or cryoablation), angioplasty and stenting operations, and image-guided surgeries are a few examples of image-guided interventions. The outcomes and patient safety of these treatments have been greatly enhanced by the incorporation of imaging technologies. Image guidance minimizes the risk of problems, shortens hospital stays, and encourages quicker recovery periods by minimizing the invasiveness of procedures.

Image-guided therapies also improve overall success rates by enabling precise monitoring and alterations during procedures.

Cleary et al. (2010) discussed image-guided procedures, which used computer-based systems to offer virtual image overlays for exact visualization and targeting of surgical sites. It gave a historical review, talked about the underlying technologies, and looked at clinical uses in several medical specialities. The significance of clinical trials was stressed for establishing the effectiveness of image-guided systems. Abi-Jaoudeh et al. (2012) discussed the value of personalized cancer treatments as well as the function of multimodality image fusion in image-guided interventions and emphasized how additional information could be obtained during minimally invasive procedures using PET, MRI, and contrast-enhanced CT. The passage also cites the existence of picture fusion and device navigation techniques that may be purchased commercially. A review of current clinical applications for multimodality navigation was provided as a conclusion. Markelj et al. (2012) emphasized the significance of recording pre- and intra-interventional data throughout various medical operations. The main objective was to provide an overview of 3D/2D data registration techniques that made use of various imaging modalities. Aspects including picture modality, dimensionality, registration basis, geometric transformation, user interaction, optimization technique, subject, and object of registration were considered in the review. Peters et al. (2016) covered the efforts undertook to reduce surgical intervention invasiveness using medical imaging, surgical navigation, and visualization technology. But despite developments in these fields, image-guided therapies still did not enjoy broad acceptability. The study offered a summary of the current stage of development, discussed adoption obstacles, and suggested future research directions for the discipline. Uppot (2018) discussed the difficulties experienced by imaging departments while dealing with obese patients. It emphasized how the size of the patients made it challenging to obtain clear images and carry out image-guided procedures. In order to achieve good outcomes for obese patients, the necessity for appropriate accommodations, equipment modifications, and advanced preparation were highlighted. Image-guided interventions use cutting-edge imaging methods to direct minimally invasive operations, offering increased accuracy and better patient outcomes. These interventions have changed several medical professions and continue to be extremely important in providing secure and efficient medical care.

5.5.3 Image Fusion and Multimodality Imaging

Medical imaging uses the concepts of image fusion and multimodality imaging to mix and integrate data from several imaging modalities. To create a single, composite image, two or more imaging datasets are overlaid or integrated. Using many imaging modalities, like CT, MRI, PET, or ultrasound, to gather complementary data about a patient's anatomy or pathology is known as multimodality imaging. By utilizing the advantages of each imaging modality, image fusion and multimodality imaging aim to improve the visualization and comprehension of anatomical structures, functional data, and disease processes. Clinicians can get a more complete picture of the patient's state by combining images from various modalities, which enables more precise diagnosis, treatment planning, and monitoring. Across medical domains, these methods have a variety of therapeutic uses. For better tumor detection, characterization, and staging, multimodality imaging can be utilized in oncology to integrate anatomical information from CT or MRI with functional data from PET. By superimposing real-time imaging with preoperative or intraoperative pictures in interventional treatments, image fusion can help guide the accurate placement of equipment or devices, such as catheters or stents. Advanced image fusion and multimodality imaging approaches have been made possible by improvements in computer software and algorithms. In order to align and spatially match images, these techniques may use registration algorithms. They may also use mathematical techniques to mix and integrate data from several modalities. Patil et al. (2011) suggested an image fusion algorithm that combines pyramid decomposition and hierarchical PCA methods. Without employing a reference image, the method tried to improve the informative content of fused images. The study undertakes a qualitative analysis using a variety of measures and a quantitative analysis utilizing both expert and non-expert judgments. The suggested methodology outperforms other multimodal image fusion techniques using pyramid, wavelet, and PCA methods in comparison tests. The results of the fusion were assessed using observable inspection and quality parameters. Helck et al. (2012) examined the effectiveness of using ultrasound (US) image fusion to recognize and rank kidney abnormalities. They used contrast-enhanced US (CEUS) with image fusion and normal US to investigate 25 patients with 29 lesions. Compared to using cross-sectional images independently, image fusion enhanced the lesions' capacity to be identified and assessed. The study concluded that image fusion improved kidney lesions' detection and evaluation. Principal components analysis (PCA) and stationary wavelet transform (SWT) image fusion approaches were discussed by Bashir et al. (2019). These techniques were used to analyze different kinds of imagery, and the results revealed that PCA worked better with input images with varying contrast/brightness levels while SWT worked better with multimodal and multi-sensor images (Bashir et al. 2019). Maqsood et al. (2020) highlighted the significance of multimodal image fusion in the realm of medical imaging. A fusion approach based on sparse representation and two-scale picture decomposition was introduced. The plan included base and detail layer extraction, contrast amplification, and edge detection. An improved decision map and fusion procedure were employed to create the final fused image. The proposed scheme worked better than previous methods in both qualitative and quantitative analysis, according to experimental findings. Yadav et al. (2020) discussed the significance of image fusion in the medical industry, especially about multimodal medical images. The necessity for efficient methods that safeguard data without generating errors were emphasized. The application of numerous medical modalities, including MRI, PET, and CT (Huang et al. 2020) were examined. The use of wavelet transforms, ICA, and PCA for denoising and data dimension reduction were also covered. The prospects for the best multimodal medical image fusion techniques were covered in the review's conclusion. Huang and Hermessi presented an overview of multimodal medical image fusion techniques (Huang et al. 2020; Hermessi et al. 2021). The theory behind fusion procedures and related criteria for performance evaluation were explained. The current developments in fusion approaches, especially those based on deep learning, were discussed. Additionally, performance analysis and several imaging modalities were covered. The conclusion emphasized the importance of ongoing studies in medical image fusion as well as the difficulties that remained in the field. In conclusion, image fusion and multimodality imaging are important medical imaging techniques that allow the fusing of data from several imaging modalities. These methods improve diagnostic precision, treatment planning, and intervention guidance across a range of medical specialities by combining and utilizing the capabilities of diverse modalities.

5.5.4 Assessment of Treatment Response Using Image Registration

To compare and align medical photographs obtained before and after a therapy so as to assess the treatment's success, clinicians can precisely evaluate changes in tumor size, shape, and location by utilizing image registration, which is the act of spatially aligning images from several time points or modalities. To ascertain whether a treatment has the desired impact, such as reducing tumor size or slowing disease development, treatment response is evaluated using image registration. Clinicians can quantitatively analyze changes in tumor volume, metabolic activity, or other pertinent factors by comparing registered images. This method can be used to assess the effectiveness of chemotherapy, radiation treatment, or targeted therapies in oncology. Clinicians can evaluate whether a treatment is decreasing tumor, slowing disease growth, or causing other desired changes by precisely comparing photographs taken before and after a procedure. Additionally, image registration can be used to evaluate how well treatments are working in the fields of medicine like cardiology or neurology. Image registration, for instance, can help neurologists assess the efficacy of treatments for disorders like brain tumor or neurodegenerative diseases. Overall, the use of image registration for measuring therapy response provides clinicians with a useful tool for monitoring changes in anatomical structures or disease processes. It offers useful perceptions into the efficacy of therapies, assisting with future choices and perhaps enhancing patient outcomes. Schreibmann et al. (2013) created an automated system for evaluating PET imaging treatment response in cancer patients. To categorize voxels into response patterns based on signal reduction or amplification, the program used level-set mathematics. The technique was used on clinical data and was successful in identifying therapy mistakes as well as providing precise analysis of metabolic alterations. The automated method served as an effective tool for evaluating radiation treatment response. Tan et al. (2016) presented a novel image registration technique for evaluating the chemotherapeutic response of ovarian cancer patients. The findings indicated that this approach had a higher correlation with outcomes for progression-free survival at six months than the most recent clinical standard, RECIST. According to the results, future research might use the image registration method as a foundation for the creation of fresh quantitative image analysis methods. To forecast treatment response and recurrence-free survival, Jahani et al. (2019) examined DCE-MR scans from 132 patients who had locally advanced breast cancer. Voxel-wise analysis of tumor deformations and DCE-MRI characteristics enhanced outcome prediction, indicating its potential for early prediction in breast cancer treatment. Heiselman et al. (2023) explained the use of image registration, to evaluate therapy response in pancreatic ductal adenocarcinoma (PDAC). The findings demonstrated that registration-derived changes in tumor burden were superior to other evaluation techniques such as manual tumor segmentation and RECIST criteria as significant predictors of overall survival (OS) and recurrence-free survival (RFS). According to the study, longitudinal image registration-measured volumetric changes might serve as helpful biomarkers for assessing PDAC patients' treatment responses.

5.5.5 Diagnostic Accuracy and Performance Improvement Using Image Registration

The improvement of performance and diagnostic accuracy through picture registration have grown to be important topics of study in medical imaging. When aligning and comparing medical images to accurately measure therapy response and enhance diagnostic accuracy, image registration is essential. Studies have demonstrated that picture registration can improve the diagnosis accuracy of several imaging modalities when paired with AI algorithms. To analyze and comprehend registered images, AI algorithms can make use of the spatial alignment offered by image registration, which improves the identification and characterization of diseases. In a variety of medical specialities, including oncology, neurology, and cardiology, image registration has shown encouraging outcomes. Clinicians can objectively detect changes in tumor size, metabolic activity, or other important factors by accurately matching images taken before and after therapy, providing an accurate assessment of treatment response. Additionally, image registration can help deep learning models perform better overall. Images can benefit from spatial coherence and consistency by being aligned and preprocessed before being fed into deep learning algorithms. This improves model performance and yields predictions that are more correct.

Pontone et al. (2018) compared the diagnostic efficacy of coronary artery imaging and myocardial perfusion in a single stress dataset to invasive procedures as the reference standard. The feasibility of simultaneously evaluating the coronary arteries and myocardial perfusion was discovered after enrolling 130 symptomatic individuals. The sensitivity, specificity, negative predictive value, positive predictive value, and diagnostic accuracy of stress cCTA + stress CTP were all high, ranging from 92% to 98%. The acquisition of the stress protocol had a low total effective dosage of 2.5 ± 1.1 mSv. That technique had the potential to detect functionally significant stenosis in patients with intermediate to high CAD risk. Toyohara et al. (2022) investigated if deep neural network (DNN) models might increase the precision of preoperative MRI-based diagnosis for uterine sarcomas (Toyohara et al. 2022). MRI sequences from individuals with uterine sarcomas and leiomyomas were used to train the models. An accuracy of 91.3% was attained using axial T2WI, sagittal T2WI, and diffusion-weighted imaging. When given DNN data, radiologists' diagnosis accuracy also increased. According to the study, DNN models could improve diagnosis precision and close the clinical skills gap. Tang described how

AI algorithms had improved medical image analysis, particularly in radiology, especially for diagnostic and therapeutic purposes (Tang 2019). AIs capacity for quantitative evaluations and automatically identifying trends were emphasized. The difficulties and potential improvements in clinical application while examining the effects of AI in oncology were highlighted. Yang et al. (2020) reviewed the effectiveness of AI systems in identifying thoracic tumors, notably lung and esophageal cancer. To assess the sensitivity, specificity, and AUC of AI systems' diagnostic accuracy, the researchers performed a meta-analysis. To investigate heterogeneity, data synthesis was carried out with the aid of specialized tools, along with subgroup and sensitivity analysis. Kundeti et al. (2021) described a systematic review process that intends to assess the efficacy of artificial intelligence (AI) in identifying large-vessel occlusions (LVOs) and diagnosing acute ischemic stroke (AIS). The review followed predetermined procedures and included literature searches, data screening, and, if practical, meta-analysis. Enhancing patient outcomes and enabling precise tissue and vascular assessment were the objectives. Overall, there is a lot of potential for enhancing diagnostic performance and accuracy in medical imaging through the combination of image registration techniques with AI and deep learning methodologies. Clinicians can improve the quality of patient care by using spatial alignment to make diagnoses more precise, effectively tracking therapy response, and merging numerous imaging datasets.

5.6 MODALITY-BASED IMAGE REGISTRATION IN RADIATION ONCOLOGY

To increase the precision and efficacy of radiation therapy treatments, a key technique in radiation oncology called 'modality-based image registration' involves aligning and merging pictures from various imaging modalities. Target localization, adaptive radiation therapy, and treatment evaluation all heavily rely on it. Techniques for registering images include feature-based, intensity-based, and deformable registration. While feature-based registration matches anatomical landmarks or characteristics, intensity-based registration aligns images based on pixel values. Local anatomical changes and deformations are accounted for thorough deformable registration. Artificial intelligence (AI) and deep learning algorithms are being used to advance modality-based image registration.

5.6.1 PRINCIPLES OF RADIATION THERAPY DELIVERY IN MODALITY-BASED IMAGE REGISTRATION

The principles of radiation therapy delivery in modality-based image registration call for the precise planning and delivery of radiation therapy using a variety of imaging modalities, including CT, MRI, and PET. To merge images from several modalities and enable precise targeting and individualized therapy, image fusion and registration techniques are used. Functional imaging and MRI-based dosage calculation can be integrated into treatment planning thanks to deformable image registration techniques. By strengthening the target delineation and treatment planning procedures, these principles improve the precision and efficacy of radiation therapy (Rigaud et al. 2019). In radiation therapy, high-energy radiation is used to kill cancer cells and reduce tumor size. To ensure the safe and efficient delivery of radiation, a sophisticated process that incorporates multiple concepts must be followed. The theory of fractionation calls for dispersing the entire radiation exposure over a period in smaller, spaced-out doses. This lessens harm to neighboring tissues and enables healthy cells to regenerate in between treatments. The precise location and dimensions of the tumor and surrounding tissues are mapped out using imaging techniques as part of the simulation, a crucial stage in the delivery of radiation therapy. Using this data, a treatment strategy is created that delivers radiation precisely where it is needed to treat the tumor while exposing healthy tissues to it as little as possible. Treatment planning is creating a radiation treatment strategy that considers the patient's general health as well as the type, size, and location of the cancer. The aim of treatment planning is to minimize the radiation exposure to healthy tissues while providing the tumor with the highest amount of radiation. A technique called 3D conformal radiation therapy employs multiple radiation beams to deliver a highly targeted dosage of radiation to the tumor while limiting the damage to nearby healthy tissues. With intensity-modulated radiation therapy (IMRT), radiation beams are computer-controlled to provide a highly precise dose of radiation while changing their intensity to follow the contours of the tumor.

Zachiu et al. (2020) discussed the limitations of current manual approaches in determining tissue displacement during image-guided radiotherapy (IGRT) and proposed an anatomically adaptive variational multimodal deformable image registration (DIR) algorithm as a solution. This algorithm improved the accuracy and anatomical plausibility of estimated deformations across the field-of-view (FOV) compared to existing methods. It offered fast computational times and low input parameters, making it suitable for online adaptive applications. That anatomically adaptive approach could benefit future IGRT workflows by enabling precise contour propagation and dose accumulation in areas with significant anatomical variations. Brahme (1987) discussed the fourth generation of isocentric megavoltage external beam radiation therapy devices. High-quality scanning electron and photon beams were used in this generation, offering more flexibility in dose distribution. A radiotherapeutic computed tomography facility and dual dipole magnet scanning were among the features of the apparatus that provided improved radiation delivery strategies, dose accuracy, and beam shaping capabilities. Overall, the effectiveness of treatments had been greatly increased primarily due to these advances in radiation therapy technology. Baskar et al. (2012) illustrated the developments in our knowledge of cancer development and treatment. Cancer is becoming more common, but managing it clinically is still difficult. Radiation therapy, surgery, chemotherapy, immunotherapy, and hormone therapy were all available as treatment options. Approximately 50% of cancer patients received radiation therapy, which accounts for 40% of the curative course of action. Radiation therapy's main goal is to reduce the ability of cancer cells to proliferate. The biology of cancer cell responses was better understood, and radiation treatment methods are constantly being improved to increase survival rates and reduce adverse effects. Koushik et al. ((2013) emphasized the expanding significance of radiation medical knowledge, particularly for surgeons handling oncology situations. It highlighted the development of technology and our understanding of the physical, biological, and oncological concepts that improved the effectiveness of cancer treatments and how important it is for surgeons to comprehend the fundamentals and stay updated with modern developments like targeted treatment delivery and the fusion of radiation and immunotherapy. In the end, understanding radiation medicine helps surgeons work efficiently with radiation oncologists and give their patients the best care possible. Kamran et al. (2018) addressed the vital role radiation therapy plays in the management of solid tumor as well as the developments that have led to better patient outcomes. Although it recognized the advancements in our knowledge of tumor genetics, radiation oncology treatment decisions are still largely based on clinical and histopathologic considerations. The chapter analyzed the existing prospects and difficulties in applying precision oncology in radiation oncology and indicates that integrating genetic tools into radiation decision-making could optimize treatment regimens. In general, radiation treatment delivery principles aim to minimize harm to healthy tissues while ensuring the safe and effective delivery of radiation to malignant areas. The accuracy and efficacy of radiation therapy administration has significantly increased thanks to cutting-edge methods like IMRT and 3D conformal radiation therapy.

5.6.2 TUMOR LOCALIZATION AND TARGET VOLUME DELINEATION

In radiation therapy, image registration is essential for localizing tumors and defining target volumes. Accurate tumor diagnosis and localization within the body is made possible by aligning various medical imaging, including CT, MRI, and PET. Clinicians may more precisely define target volumes thanks to this exact registration, which guarantees that radiation therapy is given to the tumor with the least amount of damage to the surrounding healthy tissues. Additionally, image registration helps track how a tumor responds to therapy over time, allowing for necessary modifications to treatment programs. All things considered, image registration improves the precision and safety of target volume delineation and tumor localization in radiation therapy. A crucial component of planning radiation therapy is determining the target volume and localizing the tumor. For optimal treatment delivery and to minimize injury to healthy tissues, accurate localization of the tumor and exact delineation of the target volume are essential. The process of locating a tumor precisely within the body is referred to as tumor localization. For example, computed tomography (CT), magnetic resonance imaging (MRI), positron emission tomography (PET), or a combination of these methods, are frequently used to do this. Imaging methods give precise details on the tumor's dimensions, morphology, and location. They aid in accurate target volume delineation and the visualization of the tumor in relation to nearby structures. The gross tumor volume (GTV) may be influenced differently by various imaging modalities, allowing for a more thorough assessment of the tumor's features. Outlining the areas that require radiation therapy treatment is known as target volume delineation. It encompasses both the actual tumor as well as any surrounding regions that might have microscopic illness or be in danger of the tumor spreading (Giraud et al. 2002). The gross tumor volume (GTV), clinical target volume (CTV), and planned target volume (PTV) are typical divisions of the target volume. The gross tumor volume (GTV) is a measure of a tumor's observable extent as determined by imaging studies. It comprises the main tumor as well as any related metastases or lymph nodes. The clinical target volume (CTV) is an extension of the GTV that takes microscopic disease spread and possible tumor involvement into account. It is founded on knowledge of the behavior and spread patterns of tumor (Russo 2017). The planning target volume (PTV) is an augmentation to the CTV that takes organ motion, patient positioning, and therapy delivery uncertainty into account. It guarantees that the target volume will get a suitable amount of radiation during treatment (Bernstein et al. 2021). Burnet et al. (2004) described the need to precisely specifying tumor and target volumes for radiation planning. The GTV, CTV, and PTV, each performing a specific function in treatment planning, were highlighted. It additionally emphasized the significance of accurate imaging and the need to take important normal tissue structures known as organs at risk (ORs) into account. To guarantee that the tumor receives an adequate radiation dose while minimizing the damage to nearby healthy tissues, precise delineation of the target volume is essential. This is accomplished by carefully considering the anatomy of the patient, the location, size, and features of the tumor, as well as the intended outcomes of the treatment.

Accurate tumor localization and target volume delineation are crucial for a number of reasons. Accurate localization and delineation increase the likelihood that the tumor will be controlled and that the planned radiation dose will reach it. Accurate delineation aids in sparing healthy organs and tissues from harm, lowering the likelihood of radiation-induced problems and side effects. Accurate target volume delineation enables more exact treatment planning, allowing the radiation oncologist to customize the dose and delivery method. Accurate localization and delineation support repeatability of the treatment, ensuring that succeeding treatment sessions are administered accurately and consistently. Bussels et al. (2006) examined the role of RP nodes in oropharyngeal cancer. 16% of all patients and 23% of those with nodal illness in other neck locations had RP adenopathy. Specific neck levels that were involved predicted RP nodal involvement. For treatment planning, the study advised incorporating RP nodes in the target volume. Aslian et al. (2013) emphasized the importance of precision and consistency in target volume delineation for the likelihood of tumor control probability. In this research clinical target volumes (CTVs) were determined on brain MR images using a localized region-based active semi-automatic contouring method. Despite the segmentation method's considerable deformability, the results demonstrated a remarkable correlation with manual segmentation performed by radiation oncologists. Djan et al. (2013) compared the delineation produced by CT alone against CT-MRI image fusion and validated the CT-MRI image fusion approach. The results of 16 patients who had CT and MRI scans revealed that the target volume delineation produced by CT-MRI image fusion was more precise than CT alone. According to the study's findings, image fusion and registration techniques allowed for exact target localization, which enhanced disease management in radiation treatment planning. Den-Hartogh et al. (2014) evaluated the consistency of preoperative tumor delineation for breast-conserving radiation on CT and MRI. It was discovered that both imaging techniques produced reliable and precise identification of small target volumes. Tumor identification and irregularity visualization required the use of MRI. For tumor delineation, there were no appreciable changes in interobserver variability between CT and MRI. Valentini et al. (2016) [81] addressed the significance of creating global agreement guidelines for the definition of clinical target volume (CTV) in rectal cancer (RC) radiation. Existing guidelines were updated, RC cases with various clinical stages were chosen, and peer reviews were carried out to verify the outcome. The objective was to increase consistency in RC CTV delineation and enable future clinical trial results comparisons that would be more precise. Recent improvements in tumor localization and target volume delineation have been made possible by improvements in imaging technology and the application of artificial intelligence (AI). These developments have produced radiation therapy treatments that are more individualized and accurate, ultimately improving patient outcomes.

5.6.3 Adaptive Radiation Therapy in Modality-Based Image Registration

A treatment method known as adaptive radiation therapy (ART) tries to consider changes in a patient's anatomy that occur during radiotherapy. It entails adjusting the treatment strategy considering fresh imaging data obtained over the course of the therapy. The registration of images depending on their modalities is a crucial part of ART. The process of aligning images obtained from several imaging modalities, such as computed tomography (CT), magnetic resonance imaging (MRI), or positron emission tomography (PET), is known as 'modality-based image registration.' It entails identifying the spatial transformation that lines up the images, enabling precise comparison and the merging of data from several modalities. Modality-based image registration is essential to track alterations in a patient's anatomy during adaptive radiation therapy (ART). It allows for a comparison of the existing anatomy with the initial treatment plan by registering photographs taken at various periods in time. Patients may suffer morphological changes throughout treatment as a result of things like weight reduction, tumor shrinkage, or organ movement. The accuracy and efficacy of the first treatment strategy may be impacted by these modifications. By identifying and quantifying these changes, modality-based image registration enables the treatment plan to be modified to guarantee the target receives the best dosage possible while exposing healthy tissues to the least amount of radiation possible.

5.6.3.1 Benefits of Modality-Based Image Registration in Adaptive Radiation Therapy

Modality-based image registration, which aligns pictures from many modalities, aids in localizing the target volume accurately. This ensures that radiation is precisely delivered to the desired location. Image registration enables the observation of anatomical changes that may affect therapy effectiveness, such as tumor regression or organ movements. Clinicians can alter the treatment strategy to ensure optimal tumor coverage by recognizing these changes. By identifying changes in neighboring healthy tissues, modalities-based image registration makes it possible to modify the treatment strategy to reduce radiation exposure to these structures. This can lessen the possibility of typical tissue toxicity and adverse effects. Modality-based image registration can enhance treatment outcomes by ensuring that the radiation dose is precisely delivered to the target while sparing healthy tissues. This is done by changing the treatment plan considering new imaging data (Stanley et al. 2023). For example, nasopharyngeal carcinoma, cervical cancer, and head and neck cancer have all been treated with adaptive radiation treatment. It seeks to maximize radiation therapy's efficacy while minimizing harm to nearby healthy tissues.

Zhao et al. (2023) discussed about the creation of Patch-RegNet, a hierarchical deformable image registration framework for adaptive radiotherapy. In order to take both inter-modality and intra-modality registration into account, a modality agnostic neighborhood descriptor was chosen as the similarity measure in that model. To increase the precision and speed of CT-MR and MR-MR registration in head-and-neck procedures, that framework blends deep learning approaches with patch-based registration. The outcomes demonstrated better accuracy for MR-guided adaptive radiotherapy, with Patch-RegNet outperforming conventional approaches and a well-liked deep learning-based system. Castelli et al. (2018) discussed the use of ART in the management of head and neck cancer (HNC). It drew attention to the advantages of ART in adjusting dosage distribution to account for daily anatomical fluctuations. Different ART tactics and their clinical and dosimetric benefits were evaluated. According to the results, ART reduced toxicity, enhanced target coverage and homogeneity, and positive effects on xerostomia, quality of life, and local control. However, further randomized studies were required to support the widespread application of ART in the management of HNC. Morgan et al. (2020) discussed ART for head and neck squamous cell cancer (HNSCC). ART, a therapeutic strategy that was adapted for spatial and structural alterations brought on by radiotherapy. ART separated into two categories: anatomy-adapted (A-ART) and response-adapted (R-ART). While R-ART modified treatment in response to the patient's response, A-ART strived to decrease overdosage and enhance dose uniformity. Piperdi et al. (2021) highlighted the drawbacks and advantages of ART for the treatment of lung cancer. It drew attention to the lack of agreement over patient selection, timing, and techniques for plan modification. Widespread acceptance was hampered by the difficulty of the clinical workflow, however research suggested that mid-treatment plan change could reduce toxicity and enhance tumor dosage coverage. To achieve a more uniform application of ART, advancements in predictive modeling and workflow optimization were being undertaken.

5.6.4   TECHNIQUES FOR MULTIMODALITY IMAGE REGISTRATION INCLUDING CT, MRI, AND PET-CT

Using manual and computer-based methods, multimodality image registration techniques align and fuse pictures from several imaging modalities, including CT, MRI, and PET-CT. An emerging trend in multimodality imaging is trimodality PET/CT/MRI, and methods for multimodal deformable image registration are being explored. Accurate picture registration and image fusion employing strategies like mutual information (MI) are necessary for software approaches to integrating multimodality images. PET or SPECT combined with MRI has the potential to change clinical treatment and medical research. While software techniques enable precise rigid image registration of brain PET with CT and MRI, nonlinear techniques are used for whole-body image registration. These procedures can only be used with specialist technology and software, as well as by highly qualified medical personnel. Cherry (2009) examined the potential effects of merging several imaging modalities in clinical practice and medical research. It discusses the frequent usage of PET/CT and SPECT/CT, continuing research on PET or SPECT with MRI, and various combinations including CT/MRI and PET/optical imaging. It also investigated how to integrate instruments and create imaging agents for various modalities. The issue of whether PET and SPECT with CT was the best option or just a component of a larger trend in integrated imaging systems was raised. Slomka et al. (2009) discussed how multimodality imaging might integrate functional and anatomical data using hybrid imaging devices and software methodologies. The advantages of hybrid PET/CT systems for oncological imaging were discussed, as well as the function of software image co-registration for patient-specific and economically viable integrated imaging. Additionally, difficulties in verifying nonlinear registration of soft tissue organs and the requirement for proper infrastructure for effective picture integration were emphasized. Hybrid scanners were employed in conjunction with software image registration, which enabled their use in therapeutic settings. Wang et al. (2015) addressed the potential of concurrent CT-MRI imaging, stressing its medical uses in oncology and cardiovascular fields. It highlighted the limitations of current image registration methods and how synchronized data collection could minimize registration problems. It discussed enabling technologies and focused on the apparatus used with PET-CT, PET-MRI, and MRI-LINAC. Simultaneous CT-MRI was regarded as a key development that could integrate many imaging modalities for thorough and accurate medical imaging. Decazes et al. (2021) highlighted the importance of utilizing a trimodality strategy (PET/CT/MRI) in radiotherapy to solve the shortcomings of CT alone. The two procedures for trimodality imaging were described, and it was emphasized how crucial it was to conduct the procedures while the patient was receiving treatment. Additionally, the necessity for specialized tools and the possible clinical benefits of trimodality, particularly for head and neck cancers (HNC), brain tumor, prostate cancer, and cervical cancer were emphasized.

5.7　CHALLENGES AND FUTURE OF MODALITY-BASED IMAGE REGISTRATION IN MODERN HEALTHCARE

In radiation oncology, aligning and comparing medical images obtained using various imaging modalities or at various times is a crucial step in the image registration process. Planning treatments, defining targets, and keeping track of treatment outcomes all depend on it.

5.7.1 CHALLENGES OF MODALITY-BASED IMAGE REGISTRATION IN MODERN HEALTHCARE

The difficulties and possibilities related to image registration in radiation oncology are listed below:

a. *Deformable Registration*: Deformable image registration (DIR), which involves non-rigidly aligning pictures, is a difficult technique because of anatomical variances and organ deformations. For exact target delineation and treatment planning, accurate deformable registration is essential. Zhong et al. (2010) analyzed the potential issues in deformable image registration (DIR) using numerical phantoms. The accuracy of registration algorithms, such as Demons and B-Spline, was found to depend on parameter selection and intensity gradients of the images. The study cautioned that feature-based evaluation of DIR accuracy should be approached carefully, as DIR algorithms showed lower errors in heterogeneous lung regions compared to low-intensity gradient regions. Oh et al. (2017) discussed the use of DIR to align imaging data sets in radiation therapy. By determining spatial correspondence, DIR minimizes discrepancies between images. Numerous clinical uses and validation techniques exist for it.

b. *Image Data Complexity*: Imaging techniques used in radiation oncology include CT, MRI, PET, and ultrasound. Because each modality has unique qualities and difficulties, the registration process is complicated. Robust registration methods are needed for integrating and aligning data from many modalities.

c. *Reliability and Accuracy*: To ensure accurate target localization and treatment delivery, image registration algorithms need to be precise and dependable. Errors in registration can lead to suboptimal treatment outcomes and potential harm to patients.

d. *Efficiency of Computation*: Image registration techniques may be computationally demanding, needing a lot of time and processing power. Clinical workflows must be streamlined using effective algorithms that can handle massive datasets and offer real-time registration.

e. *Interobserver Variability*: Various doctors may interpret and annotate images in various ways, which might have an impact on image registration. To reduce variation and guarantee consistent registration results, standardization and quality-assurance procedures are required.

5.7.2 OPPORTUNITIES OF MODALITY-BASED IMAGE REGISTRATION IN MODERN HEALTHCARE

a) *Machine Learning and Artificial Intelligence (AI):* Deep learning-based techniques have shown promise in increasing the accuracy and effectiveness of picture registration. AI systems can reduce manual intervention and improve registration outcomes by learning from big datasets and automatically extracting key elements for registration.

b) *Radiomics and Quantitative Imaging:* Radiomics is a quantitative imaging approach that extracts and analyzes several image features. These characteristics can be used to describe tumors, gauge treatment effectiveness, and direct the development of individualized treatment plans. In order to align images for radiomics investigation, image registration is essential.

c) *Integration with Treatment Delivery Systems:* Real-time adaptive radiation therapy can be made possible by integrating image registration with treatment delivery devices like linear accelerators. Real-time registration can consider patient movement and anatomical changes as a treatment is administered, enhancing treatment precision, and lowering normal tissue toxicity.

d) *Integration with Treatment Delivery Systems:* Real-time adaptive radiation therapy can be made possible by integrating image registration with treatment delivery devices like linear accelerators. Real-time registration can consider patient movement and anatomical changes as a treatment is administered, enhancing treatment precision and lowering normal tissue toxicity.

e) *Clinical Decision Support*: Accurate image registration can give doctors important data to consider when prescribing a course of action. Target delineation, dose estimation, and treatment plan evaluation can all be aided by integrated registration technologies, resulting in more individualized and efficient radiation therapy.

Dowling et al. (2020) addressed how radiation therapy could employ computer technology to enhance treatment delivery and planning. Treatment planning software includes rigid and flexible image registration. A report on image registration methods and quality assurance was also suggested. Assessing the accuracy of commercial DIR tools and best practices for using them in head and neck cancer were focused. Hussein et al. (2021) discussed DIR's application in radiotherapy and pinpointed implementation issues. While some facilities were already utilizing DIR clinically, a survey of 71 radiation facilities in the UK found that further standards, instruction, and tools for commissioning and quality assurance were required. The study stressed the value of creating quantifiable measures and offering advice tailored to various DIR applications. In conclusion, there are difficulties with image registration in radiation oncology due to deformable registration, complicated image data, accuracy, computing efficiency, and interobserver variability. To address these issues and enhance patient outcomes in radiation oncology, there is potential to use quantitative imaging, improved imaging modalities, integration with treatment delivery systems, and clinical decision support.

5.8 CONCLUSIONS

Modality-based image registration has the potential to change the diagnosis process and enhance treatment outcomes, according to a review of how it can improve patient care in contemporary healthcare. The combination of several medical images enables more thorough insights, which results in accurate diagnosis, individualized treatment strategies, and improved patient care. For successful implementation, nevertheless, factors like cost, complexity of implementation, and specialist training must be taken into account. The use of modalities-based image registration in contemporary medicine has enormous potential to transform patient care. Clinicians may make better decisions by seamlessly integrating medical pictures from many modalities, which improves diagnostic precision, creates individualized treatment plans, and eventually improves patient outcomes. Modality-based image registration has benefits for improving patient care in contemporary healthcare, including greater diagnosis accuracy, individualized treatment plans, and improved patient outcomes. However, there may be drawbacks, such as higher costs, complexity in installation, and the requirement for specific training and experience to make efficient use of this technology. The potential for modality-based image registration to improve patient care in contemporary healthcare is encouraging. Technology advancements will probably result in better algorithms, quicker processing times, and greater accessibility. This will make adoption more widely available, improving diagnostic precision, therapeutic efficacy, and ultimately patient outcomes.

REFERENCES

Abi-Jaoudeh N, Kruecker J, Kadoury S, Kobeiter H, Venkatesan AM, Levy E, Wood BJ. Multimodality image fusion-guided procedures: Technique, accuracy, and applications. *Cardiovasc Intervent Radiol* 2012 Oct;35(5):986–998. doi: 10.1007/s00270-012-0446-5. Epub 2012 Aug 1. PMID: 22851166; PMCID: PMC3447988.

Aslian H, Sadeghi M, Mahdavi SR, BabapourMofrad F, Astarakee M, Khaledi N, Fadavi P. Magnetic resonance imaging-based target volume delineation in radiation therapy treatment planning for brain tumors using localized region-based active contour. *Int J Radiat Oncol Biol Phys* 2013 Sep 1;87(1):195–201. doi: 10.1016/j.ijrobp.2013.04.049. PMID: 23920396.

Attenberger UI, Sourbron SP, Michaely HJ, Reiser MF, Schoenberg SO. Retrospective respiratory triggering renal perfusion MRI. *Acta Radiol* 2010;51(10):1163–1171.

Auricchio A, Sorgente A, Soubelet E., et al. Accuracy and usefulness of fusion imaging between three-dimensional coronary sinus and coronary veins computed tomographic images with projection images obtained using fluoroscopy. *Europace*. 2009;11(11):1483–1490. doi: 10.1093/europace/eup237. in English.

Bashir R, Junejo R, Qadri N, Fleury M, Qadri M. SWT and PCA image fusion methods for multi-modal imagery. *Multimedia Tool Appl* 2019;78(2). doi: 10.1007/s11042-018-6229-5.

Bashiri FS, Baghaie A, Rostami R, Yu Z, D'Souza RM. Multi-modal medical image registration with full or partial data: A manifold learning approach. *J Imaging* 2018 Dec 30;5(1):5. doi: 10.3390/jimaging5010005. PMID: 34470183; PMCID: PMC8320870.

Baskar R, Lee KA, Yeo R, Yeoh KW. Cancer and radiation therapy: Current advances and future directions. *Int J Med Sci* 2012;9(3):193–199. doi: 10.7150/ijms.3635. Epub 2012 Feb 27. PMID: 22408567; PMCID: PMC3298009.

Bernstein D, Taylor A, Nill S, Oelfke U. New target volume delineation and PTV strategies to further personalise radiotherapy. *Phys Med Biol* 2021 Feb 25;66(5):055024. doi: 10.1088/1361-6560/abe029; PMID: 33498018; PMCID: PMC8208617.

Boukerroui D, Noble JA, Brady M. Velocity estimation in ultrasound images: A block matching approach. In: Taylor, C., Noble, J.A. (eds) *Information Processing in Medical Imaging. IPMI* 2003:2732:586–598. Springer, Berlin, Heidelberg. https://doi.org/10.1007/978-3-540-45087-0_49

Brahme A. Design principles and clinical possibilities with A new generation of radiation therapy equipment: A review. *Acta Oncol* 1987;26(6):403–412. doi: 10.3109/02841868709113708.

Brox I *Motion Correction of the Kidneys in Dynamic Contrast Enhanced MRI for Quantification of Renal Structure and Function*. Bergen: University of Bergen; 2007.

Burnet NG, Thomas SJ, Burton KE, Jefferies SJ. Defining the tumor and target volumes for radiotherapy. *Cancer Imaging* 2004 Oct 21;4(2):153–161. doi: 10.1102/1470-7330.2004.0054; PMID: 18250025; PMCID: PMC1434601.

Bushberg JT. *The Essential Physics of Medical Imaging*. Philadelphia, PA: Lippincott Williams & Wilkins; 2002. [Google Scholar]

Bussels B, Hermans R, Reijnders A, Dirix P, Nuyts S, Van den Bogaert W. Retropharyngeal nodes in squamous cell carcinoma of oropharynx: Incidence, localization, and implications for target volume. *Int J Radiat Oncol Biol Phys* 2006 Jul 1;65(3):733–738. doi: 10.1016/j.ijrobp.2006.02.034; PMID: 16751061.

Caroli A, Schneider M, Friedli I, Ljimani A, De Seigneux S, Boor P, Gullapudi L, Kazmi I, Mendichovszky IA, Notohamiprodjo M, Selby NM, Thoeny HC, Grenier N, Vallee JP Difusion-weighted magnetic resonance imaging to assess difuse. Magn Reson Mater Phys Biol Med 1 3 renal pathology: A systematic review and statement paper. *Nephrol Dial Transplant* 2018;33(Suppl_2):ii29–ii40.

Castelli J, Simon A, Lafond C, Perichon N, Rigaud B, Chajon E, De Bari B, Ozsahin M, Bourhis J, de Crevoisier R. Adaptive radiotherapy for head and neck cancer. *Acta Oncol* 2018 Oct;57(10):1284–1292. doi: 10.1080/0284186X.2018.1505053. Epub 2018 Oct 5. PMID: 30289291.

Castro FJS, Pollo C, Meuli R, Maeder P, Cuisenaire O, Cuadra MB, Villemure J-G, Thiran J-P. A cross validation study of deep brain stimulation targeting: From experts to atlas-based, segmentation-based and automatic registration algorithms. *IEEE Trans Med Imaging* 2006;25(11):1440–1450.

Cherry SR. Multimodality imaging: beyond PET/CT and SPECT/CT. *Semin Nucl Med* 2009 Sep;39(5):348–353. doi: 10.1053/j.semnuclmed.2009.03.001; PMID: 19646559; PMCID: PMC2735449.

Cleary K, Peters TM. Image-guided interventions: Technology review and clinical applications. *Annu Rev Biomed Eng* 2010 Aug 15;12:119–142. doi: 10.1146/annurev-bioeng-070909-105249; PMID: 20415592.

Cohen B, Dinstein I. New maximum likelihood motion estimation schemes for noisy ultrasound images. *Pattern Rec* 2002;35(2):455–463.

Collins DL, Neelin P, Peters TM, Evans AC. Automatic 3D intersubject registration of MR volumetric data in standardized Talairach space. *J Comput Assist Tomogr* 1994;18(2):192–205.

Dauwe DF, Nuyens D, De Buck S, et al. Three-dimensional rotational angiography fused with multimodal imaging modalities for targeted endomyocardial injections in the ischaemic heart. *Eur Heart J Cardiovasc Imaging.* 2014;15(8):900–907. doi: 10.1093/ehjci/jeu019. in English.

Decazes P, Hinault P, Veresezan O, Thureau S, Gouel P, Vera P. Trimodality PET/CT/MRI and radiotherapy: A mini-review. *Front Oncol* 2021 Feb 4;10:614008. doi: 10.3389/fonc.2020.614008; PMID: 33614497; PMCID: PMC7890017.

den-Hartogh MD, Philippens ME, van Dam IE, Kleynen CE, Tersteeg RJ, Pijnappel RM, Kotte AN, Verkooijen HM, van den Bosch MA, van Vulpen M, van Asselen B, van den Bongard HD. MRI and CT imaging for preoperative target volume delineation in breast-conserving therapy. *Radiatoncol* 2014 Feb 26;9:63. doi: 10.1186/1748-717X-9-63; PMID: 24571783; PMCID: PMC3942765.

Dey J, Segars WP, Pretorius PH., et al. Estimation and correction of cardiac respiratory motion in SPECT in the presence of limited-angle effects due to irregular respiration. *Med Phys* 2010;37(12):6453–6465. doi: 10.1118/1.3517836. in English.

Diwakar M, Singh P, Ravi V, Maurya A. A non-conventional review on multi-modality-based medical image fusion. *Diagnostics (Basel)* 2023 Feb 21;13(5):820. doi: 10.3390/diagnostics13050820; PMID: 36899965; PMCID: PMC10000748.

Djan I, Petrović B, Erak M, Nikolić I, Lucić S. Radiotherapy treatment planning: Benefits of CT-MR image registration and fusion in tumor volume delineation. *Vojnosanit Pregl* 2013 Aug;70(8):735–739. doi: 10.2298/vsp110404001d; PMID: 24069821.

Dowling JA, O'Connor LM. Deformable image registration in radiation therapy. *J Med Radiat Sci* 2020 Dec;67(4):257–259. doi: 10.1002/jmrs.446. Epub 2020 Oct 26. PMID: 33104276; PMCID: PMC7753986.

Duckett SG, Ginks MR, Knowles BR., et al. Advanced image fusion to overlay coronary sinus anatomy with real-time fluoroscopy to facilitate left ventricular lead implantation in CRT. *Pacing Clin Electrophysiol* 2011;34(2):226–234. doi: 10.1111/j.1540-8159.2010.02940.x.

Dutt V, Greenleaf J. Statistics of the LogCompressed envelope. *J Acoust Soc Am* 1996;99(6):3817–3825.

Dutt AK., Rao JM. Growth, distribution, and the environment: Sustainable development in India. *World Development* 1996;24(2):287–305.

Gerig G, Jomier M, Valmet CM. A new validation tool for assessing and improving 3D object segmentation. *Med Image Comput Comput Assist Interv MICCAI* 2001;2001:516–523.

Giraud P, Sabine E, Sylvie H, De Yann R, Vincent S, Carette FM, Alzieu C, Bondiau PY, Dubray B, Touboul E, Housset M, Rosenwald JC, Cosset JM. Conformal radiotherapy for lung cancer: Different delineation of the gross tumor volume (GTV) by radiologists and radiation oncologists. *Radiat Oncol* 2002 62(1):27–36. ISSN 0167-8140,https://doi.org/10.1016/S0167-8140(01)00444-3.

Glockler M, Halbfass J, Koch A, Achenbach S, Dittrich S. Multimodality 3D roadmap for cardiovascular interventions in congenital heart disease–a single-center, retrospective analysis of 78 cases. *Catheter Cardiovasc Interv* 2013;82(3):436–442. doi: 10.1002/ccd.24646. in English.

Guan SY, Wang TM, Meng C., et al. A review of point feature based medical image registration. *Chin J Mech Eng* 2018;31(1):76. doi: 10.1186/s10033-018-0275-9.

Hermessi H, Mourali O, Zagrouba E. Multimodal medical image fusion review: Theoretical background and recent advances. *Signal Processing* 2021;183:108036, ISSN 0165-1684. doi: 10.1016/j.sigpro.2021.108036.

Heiselman JS, Ecker BL, Langdon-Embry L, O'Reilly EM, Miga MI, Jarnagin WR, Do RKG, Horvat N, Wei AC, Chakraborty J. Registration-based biomarkers for neoadjuvant treatment response of pancreatic cancer via longitudinal image registration. *J Med Imaging (Bellingham)* 2023 May;10(3):036002. doi: 10.1117/1.JMI.10.3.036002. Epub 2023 Jun 2. PMID: 37274758; PMCID: PMC10237235.

Helck A, D'Anastasi M, Notohamiprodjo M, Thieme S, Sommer W, Reiser M, Clevert DA. Multimodality imaging using ultrasound image fusion in renal lesions. *Clin Hemorheol Microcirc* 2012;50(1–2):79–89. doi: 10.3233/CH-2011-1445; PMID: 22538537.

Hosseini HG, Alizad A, Fatemi M. Integration of vibro-acoustography imaging modality with the traditional mammography. *Int J Biomed Imaging* 2007;2007:40980. doi: 10.1155/2007/40980; PMID: 17710254; PMCID: PMC1893012.

Huang B, Yang F, Yin M, Mo X, Zhong C. A review of multimodal medical image fusion techniques. *Comput Math Methods Med* 2020 Apr 23;2020:8279342. doi: 10.1155/2020/8279342; PMID: 32377226; PMCID: PMC7195632.

Hussein M, Akintonde A, McClelland J, Speight R, Clark CH. Clinical use, challenges, and barriers to implementation of deformable image registration in radiotherapy - The need for guidance and QA tools. *Br J Radiol* 2021 Jun 1;94(1122):20210001. doi: 10.1259/bjr.20210001. Epub 2021 Apr 29. PMID: 33882253; PMCID: PMC8173691.

Ibanez L, Schroeder W, Ng L, Cates J. *The ITK Software Guide: The Insight Segmentation and Registration Toolkit: Version 1.4.* New York, NY: Kitware, Inc.; 2003.

Jahani N, Cohen E, Hsieh MK, Weinstein SP, Pantalone L, Hylton N, Newitt D, Davatzikos C, Kontos D. Prediction of treatment response to neoadjuvant chemotherapy for breast cancer via early changes in tumor heterogeneity captured by DCE-MRI registration. *Sci Rep* 2019 Aug 20;9(1):12114. doi: 10.1038/s41598-019-48465-x; PMID: 31431633; PMCID: PMC6702160.

Jones RA, Votaw JR, Salman K, Sharma P, Lurie C, Kalb B, Martin DR. Magnetic resonance imaging evaluation of renal structure and function related to disease: Technical review of image acquisition, postprocessing, and mathematical modeling steps. *J Magn Reson Imaging* 2011;33(6):1270–1283.

Kamran SC, Mouw KW. Applying precision oncology principles in radiation oncology. *JCO Precis Oncol* 2018 May 14;2:PO.18.00034. doi: 10.1200/PO.18.00034; PMID: 32914000; PMCID: PMC7446508.

KirthiKoushik AS, Harish K, Avinash HU. Principles of radiation oncology: A beams eye view for a surgeon. *Indian J Surg Oncol* 2013 Sep;4(3):255–262. doi: 10.1007/s13193-013-0231-1. Epub 2013 Mar 19. PMID: 24426732; PMCID: PMC3771048.

Klein A, Andersson J. Evaluation of 14 nonlinear deformation algorithms applied to human brain MRI registration. *NeuroImage* 2009;46(3):786–802.

Kundeti SR, Vaidyanathan MK, Shivashankar B, Gorthi SP. Systematic review protocol to assess artificial intelligence diagnostic accuracy performance in detecting acute ischaemic stroke and large-vessel occlusions on CT and MR medical imaging. *BMJ, (Open)* 2021 Mar 10;11(3):e043665. doi: 10.1136/bmjopen-2020-043665; PMID: 33692180; PMCID: PMC7949439.

Ledesma-Carbayo MJ, Kybic J, Desco M, Santos A, Suhling M, Hunziker P, Unser M. Spatio-¨temporal nonrigid registration for ultrasound cardiac motion estimation. *IEEE Trans Med Imaging* 2005;24(9):1113–1126.

Ma YL, King AP, Gogin N., et al. Clinical evaluation of respiratory motion compensation for anatomical roadmap guided cardiac electrophysiology procedures. *IEEE Trans Bio Med Eng* 2012;59(1):122–131. doi: 10.1109/tbme.2011.2168393.

Maes F, Collignon A, Vandermeulen D, Marchal G, Suetens P. Multimodality image registration by maximization of mutual information. *IEEE Trans Med Imaging* 1997 Apr;16(2):187–198. doi: 10.1109/42.563664; PMID: 9101328.

Manzke R, Bornstedt A, Lutz A., et al. Respiratory motion compensated overlay of surface models from cardiac MR on interventional X-ray fluoroscopy for guidance of cardiac resynchronization therapy procedures. In: Wong KH, Miga MI, editors. *Medical Imaging 2010: Visualization, Image-Guided Procedures, and Modeling.* San Diego, CA: International Society for Optical Engineering (SPIE); March 2010.

Maqsood S, Javed U. Multi-modal medical image fusion based on two-scale image decomposition and sparse representation. *Biomed Signal Process Control* 2020;57:101810, ISSN 1746-8094. doi: 10.1016/j.bspc.2019.101810.

Markelj P, Tomaževič D, Likar B, Pernuš F. A review of 3D/2D registration methods for image-guided interventions. *Med Image Anal* 2012 Apr;16(3):642–661. doi: 10.1016/j.media.2010.03.005. Epub 2010 Apr 13. PMID: 20452269.

Morgan HE, Sher DJ. Adaptive radiotherapy for head and neck cancer. *Cancers Head Neck* 2020 Jan 9;5:1. doi: 10.1186/s41199-019-0046-z; PMID: 31938572; PMCID: PMC6953291.

Moscucci M. *Grossman & Baim's Cardiac Catheterization, Angiography, and Intervention.* Philadelphia, PA: Lippincott Williams & Wilkins; 2013. [Google Scholar]

Nikou C, Heitz F, Armspach J-P, Namer I-J, Grucker D. Registration of MR/MR and MR/SPECT brain images by fast stochastic optimization of robust voxel similarity measures. *Neuroimage* 1998;8(1):30–43.

O'Donnell M, Skovoroda AR, Shapo BM, Emelianov SY. Internal displacement and strain imaging using ultrasonic speckle tracking. *IEEE Trans Ultrason Ferroelectr Freq Control* 1994;41(3):314–325.

Odudu A, Nery F, Harteveld AA, Evans RG, Pendse D, Buchanan CE, Francis ST, Fernandez-Seara MA. Arterial spin labelling MRI to measure renal perfusion: A systematic review and statement paper. *Nephrol Dial Transplant* 2018;33(Suppl_2):ii15–ii21.

Oh S, Kim S. Deformable image registration in radiation therapy. *Radiatoncol J* 2017 Jun;35(2):101–111. doi: 10.3857/roj.2017.00325. Epub 2017 Jun 30. PMID: 28712282; PMCID: PMC5518453.

Oliveira FP, Tavares JM. Medical image registration: A review. *Comput Methods Biomech Biomed Engin* 2014;17(2):73–93. doi: 10.1080/10255842.2012.670855. Epub 2012 Mar 22. PMID: 22435355.

Peters TM, Linte CA. Image-guided interventions and computer-integrated therapy: Quo vadis? *Med Image Anal* 2016 Oct;33:56–63. doi: 10.1016/j.media.2016.06.004. Epub 2016 Jun 14. PMID: 27373146; PMCID: PMC7609169.

Pipe JG. Motion correction with PROPELLER MRI: Application to head motion and free-breathing cardiac imaging. *Magn Reson Med* 1999;42(5):963–969.

Piperdi H, Portal D, Neibart SS, Yue NJ, Jabbour SK, Reyhan M. Adaptive radiation therapy in the treatment of lung cancer: An overview of the current state of the field. *Front Oncol* 2021 Nov 29;11:770382. doi: 10.3389/fonc.2021.770382; PMID: 34912715; PMCID: PMC8666420.

Pontone G, Baggiano A, Andreini D, Guaricci AI, Guglielmo M, Muscogiuri G, Fusini L, Soldi M, Del Torto A, Mushtaq S, Conte E, Calligaris G, De Martini S, Ferrari C, Galli S, Grancini L, Olivares P, Ravagnani P, Teruzzi G, Trabattoni D, Fabbiocchi F, Montorsi P, Rabbat MG, Bartorelli AL, Pepi M. Diagnostic accuracy of simultaneous evaluation of coronary arteries and myocardial perfusion with single stress cardiac computed tomography acquisition compared to invasive coronary angiography plus invasive fractional flow reserve. *Int J Cardiol* 2018 Dec 15;273:263–268. doi: 10.1016/j.ijcard.2018.09.065. Epub 2018 Sep 20. PMID: 30268383.

Rigaud B, Simon A, Castelli J, Lafond C, Acosta O, Haigron P, Cazoulat G, de Crevoisier R. Deformable image registration for radiation therapy: Principle, methods, applications and evaluation. *Acta Oncol* 2019 Sep;58(9):1225–1237. doi: 10.1080/0284186X.2019.1620331. Epub 2019 Jun 3. PMID: 31155990.

Ritter N, Owens R, Cooper J, Eikelboom RH, Saarloos PP. Registration of stereo and temporal images of the retina. *IEEE Trans Med Imaging* 1999;18(5):404–418.

Robson PM, Madhuranthakam AJ, Smith MP, Sun MR, Dai W, Rofsky NM, Pedrosa I, Alsop DC. Volumetric arterial spin-labeled perfusion imaging of the kidneys with a three-dimensional fast spin echo acquisition. *Acad Radiol* 2016;23(2):144–154.

Russo AL. Chapter 13. The role of radiation in uterine cancer. In: Birrer MJ, Ceppi L, editors, *Translational Advances in Gynecologic Cancers.* Academic Press; 2017, pp. 241–259. doi: 10.1016/B978-0-12-803741-6.00013-6.

Schreibmann E, Waller AF, Crocker I, Curran W, Fox T. Voxel clustering for quantifying PET-based treatment response assessment. *Med Phys* 2013 Jan;40(1):012401. doi: 10.1118/1.4764900; PMID: 23298110.

Schroeder W *The Visualization Toolkit: An Object-Oriented Approach to 3D Graphics.* 3rd ed. New York, NY: Kitware, Inc.; 2003.

Selby NM, Blankestijn PJ, Boor P, Combe C, Eckardt KU, Eikefjord E, Garcia-Fernandez N, Golay X, Gordon I, Grenier N, Hockings PD, Jensen JD, Joles JA, Kalra PA, Kramer BK, Mark PB, Mendichovszky IA, Nikolic O, Odudu A, Ong ACM, Ortiz A, Pruijm M, Remuzzi G, Rorvik J, de Seigneux S, Simms RJ, Slatinska J, Summers P, Taal MW, Thoeny HC, Vallee JP, Wolf M, Caroli A, Sourbron S. Magnetic resonance imaging biomarkers for chronic kidney disease: A position paper from the European cooperation in science and technology action PARENCHIMA. *Nephrol Dial Transplant* 2018;33(Suppl_2):ii4–ii14.

Slomka PJ, Baum RP. Multimodality image registration with software: State-of-the-art. *Eur J Nucl Med Mol Imaging* 2009 Mar;36(Suppl_1):S44–S55. doi: 10.1007/s00259-008-0941-8; PMID: 19104803.

Song G, Han J, Zhao Y, Wang Z, Du H. A review on medical image registration as an optimization problem. *Curr Med Imaging Rev* 2017 Aug;13(3):274–283. doi: 10.2174/1573405612666160920123955; PMID: 28845149; PMCID: PMC5543570.

Sotiras A, Davatzikos C, Paragios N. Deformable medical image registration: A survey. *IEEE Trans Med Imaging* 2013 Jul;32(7):1153–1190. doi: 10.1109/TMI.2013.2265603. Epub 2013 May 31. PMID: 23739795; PMCID: PMC3745275.

Stanley DN, Harms J, Pogue JA, Belliveau JG, Marcrom SR, McDonald AM, Dobelbower MC, Boggs DH, Soike MH, Fiveash JA, Popple RA, Cardenas CE. A roadmap for implementation of kV-CBCT online adaptive radiation therapy and initial first year experiences. *J Appl Clin Med Phys* 2023 Jul;24(7):e13961. doi: 10.1002/acm2.13961. Epub 2023 Mar 15. PMID: 36920871; PMCID: PMC10338842.

Takao M, Sugano N, Nishii T, Miki H, Koyama T, Masumoto J, Sato Y, Tamura S, Yoshikawa H. Application of 3D-MR image registration to monitoring diseases around the knee joint. *J Magn Reson Imaging* 2005;22(5):656–660.

Tan M, Li Z, Qiu Y, McMeekin SD, Thai TC, Ding K, Moore KN, Liu H, Zheng B. A new approach to evaluate drug treatment response of ovarian cancer patients based on deformable image registration. *IEEE Trans Med Imaging* 2016 Jan;35(1):316–325. doi: 10.1109/TMI.2015.2473823. Epub 2015 Aug 27. PMID: 26336119; PMCID: PMC5161344.

Tang X. The role of artificial intelligence in medical imaging research. *BJR Open* 2019 Nov 28;2(1):20190031. doi: 10.1259/bjro.20190031; PMID: 33178962; PMCID: PMC7594889.

Timinger H, Kruger S, Dietmayer K, Borgert J. Ultrasonic diaphragm tracking for cardiac interventional navigation on 3D motion compensated static roadmaps. In Galloway RL, Cleary KR, editors. *Medical Imaging 2005: Visualization, Image-Guided Procedures, and Display, Pts 1 and 2*. Bellingham, WA: International Society for Optical Engineering (SPIE); 2005, Vol. 5744, pp. 290–298. Proceedings of the Society of Photo-Optical Instrumentation Engineers. [Google Scholar]

Toyohara Y, Sone K, Noda K et al. Development of a deep learning method for improving diagnostic accuracy for uterine sarcoma cases. *Sci Rep* 2022;12(1):19612. doi: 10.1038/s41598-022-23064-5.

Patil U, Mudengudi U. Image fusion using hierarchical PCA. International Conference on Image Information Processing, Shimla, India, 2011, pp. 1–6. doi: 10.1109/ICIIP.2011.6108966.

Uppot RN. Technical challenges of imaging & image-guided interventions in obese patients. *Br J Radiol* 2018 Sep;91(1089):20170931. doi: 10.1259/bjr.20170931. Epub 2018 Jun 5. PMID: 29869898; PMCID: PMC6223172.

Valentini V, Gambacorta MA, Barbaro B, Chiloiro G, Coco C, Das P, Fanfani F, Joye I, Kachnic L, Maingon P, Marijnen C, Ngan S, Haustermans K. International consensus guidelines on clinical target volume delineation in rectal cancer. *Radiother Oncol* 2016 Aug;120(2):195–201. doi: 10.1016/j.radonc.2016.07.017. Epub 2016 Aug 12. PMID: 27528121.

van Dalen JA, Vogel W, Huisman HJ, Oyen WJ, Jager GJ, Karssemeijer N. Accuracy of rigid CT-FDG-PET image registration of the liver. *Phys Med Biol.* 2004;49(23):5393–5405.

Viergever MA, Maintz JBA, Klein S, Murphy K, Staring M, Pluim JPW. A survey of medical image registration— under review. *Med Image Anal* 2016;33:140–144.

Wang G, Kalra M, Murugan V, Xi Y, Gjesteby L, Getzin M, Yang Q, Cong W, Vannier M. Vision 20/20: Simultaneous CT-MRI--Next chapter of multimodality imaging. *Med Phys* 2015 Oct;42(10):5879–5889. doi: 10.1118/1.4929559; PMID: 26429262.

Wielandts JY, Buck SD, Michielsen K., et al. Multi-phase rotational angiography of the left ventricle to assist ablations: Feasibility and accuracy of novel imaging. *Eur Heart J Cardiovasc Imaging* 2016;17(2):162–168. doi: 10.1093/ehjci/jev120. in English.

Yadav SP, Yadav S. Image fusion using hybrid methods in multimodality medical images. *Med Biol Eng Comput* 2020 Apr;58(4):669–687. doi: 10.1007/s11517-020-02136-6. Epub

Yang Y, Jin G, Pang Y, Wang W, Zhang H, Tuo G, Wu P, Wang Z, Zhu Z. The diagnostic accuracy of artificial intelligence in thoracic diseases: A protocol for systematic review and meta-analysis. *Medicine (Baltimore).* 2020 Feb;99(7):e19114. doi: 10.1097/MD.0000000000019114. PMID: 32049826; PMCID: PMC7035064.

Zachiu C, de Senneville BD, Willigenburg T, van Zyp JV, de Boer JCJ, et al. Anatomically-adaptive multi-modal image registration for image-guided external-beam radiotherapy. *Phys Med Biol* 2020;65(21):215028. ff10.1088/1361-6560/abad7dff.ffhal-03453538f.

Zhao Y, Xinru C, McDonald B, Cenji Y, Abdalah MSR, Clifton FD, Laurence CE, Tinsu P, He W, Xin W, Jack P, Jinzhong Y. A transformer-based hierarchical registration framework for multimodality deformable image registration. *Comput Med Imaging Graph* 2023;108:102286, ISSN 0895-6111. doi: 10.1016/j.compmedimag.2023.102286.

Zhong H, Kim J, Chetty IJ. Analysis of deformable image registration accuracy using computational modeling. *Med Phys* 2010 Mar;37(3):970–979. doi: 10.1118/1.3302141; PMID: 20384233; PMCID: PMC3188658.

Zöllner FG, Svarstad E, Munthe-Kaas AZ, Schad LR, Lundervold A, Rorvik J. Assessment of kidney volumes from MRI: Acquisition and segmentation techniques. *AJR Am J Roentgenol* 2012;199(5):1060–1069.

6 Fashionable and Disposable Electrochemical Sensors as Modern Healthcare Appliance

Pranabi Maji and Shrabani Mondal

6.1 INTRODUCTION

One type of sensor that can both identify and measure bioanalytics is called a biosensor. The electronic configuration of a biosensor is composed of receptors (adsorption sites or immobilized bioreceptor), transducer (converts chemical/biological reaction to readable physical/electronic signal), and display [1]. Biosensors find enormous application not only as healthcare devices but also in the areas of food quality monitoring, environmental safety, and industry. Expanded linear detection range, high sensitivity, quick response, and specific/selective nature toward a target in the presence of many other interfering molecules evaluate the goodness of a sensor. Precisely, electrochemical biosensors are a favorite owing to their reliability, miniaturized and portable design amongst the sensor family [2]. In the modern age, people are looking for disposable sensors with great functionality and environment-friendly devices so that huge masses can afford and use them without hesitation of spreading infection [3]. For effectively achieving the conditions of disposability high performance, the nature of the material used for sensor designing plays a key role and hence a vital area to be taken care of. As a consequence, more and more research and development in the field of material science is an inherent part of sensor technology.

At an early age of sensors, most of them are fabricated using semiconductor or ceramic-based materials, which lack flexibility. Polymer-based substrates, viz. plastic or cellulose, have proven as first-line applicants for the base material of paper-based sensors. This paper-based technology has hugely paved the way for disposable sensors. The aforementioned unique materials satisfy almost all the required terms like flexibility, abundance, biodegradability, transparency, and biocompatibility opening up a fascinating applications of modern-day sensors [4]. Even everyone's familiar newspaper is also successfully applied as DES [5]. To these substrates, the

DOI: 10.1201/9781003464884-9

decoration of functional nanomaterials of various architectures pushes further the functionality of these sensors. Members of the carbon family, especially 2D graphene nanosheets possess synergistic properties owing to which it holds multifaceted applications. At the same time, it plays the role of base material and conductive layer and could be modified with proper bioreceptors during DES fabrication [6].

Biomolecules serve a crucial role in maintaining a healthy and fruitful life. Excess, deficiency or absence of these biomolecules leads any living organism to fatal destiny or life risks. Complicated diseases like Alzheimer's, Parkinson's, and osteoporosis, impediment in pregnancy, heart attack etc. can be caused by disorders of biological molecules. In such a scenario, to take primary control of the deadliest diseases, biosensors help enormously to get a balanced body system. A few amongst the popular DES in healthcare applications are the blood sugar monitoring device, uric acid sensors, blood ammonia sensing device, sensors for monitoring bioanalytes (protein, lipid, enzymes), reproductive health detection kit (pregnancy test kit) etc. Overall, this chapter explores the working and designing strategies of the most popular DES applied in modern healthcare.

6.2 POINT OF CARE (POC) DETECTION

The World Health Organization (WHO) has well-defined criteria for POC devices by an abbreviation ASSURED. The whole term can be explained sequentially as cheap, equipment-free, fast, robust, sensitive, specifics, and accessible to end users [7]. POC devices are trending in recent years and have effectively beaten the tedious analysis methods run in the laboratories with power consuming, huge equipment, and trained operators. The following paragraphs highlight some of the application areas of POC devices in healthcare. Typical POC analysis protocol has been cited in Figure **6.1.**

6.2.1 PATHOGEN AND INFECTIOUS DISEASE DETECTION

The one and only way to construct a strong and efficient healthcare system is rapid and POC detection of pathogens (virus/bacteria/parasites) at its early stage, so that effective measures can be undertaken for prevention from further spread. Moreover, quick medical decisions could be taken to attend to the affected patients as an outcome of an early-stage diagnosis [8]. The most recent pandemic (COVID-19) once again emphasized these facts. Outbreaks of any infectious disease not only cause vivid/drastic effects but also hamper the socioeconomic scenario. Records elucidate that infectious diseases such as Tuberculosis (TB), malaria, HIV etc. cause 10 million deaths annually on a global scale. Cancer, one of the leading life-threatening diseases, has over 200 varieties. Reports suggest that due to ovarian cancer and breast cancer alone, more than 151,000 death counts are recorded every year [9]. This battle against morbidity can be avoided if early-stage diagnosis is possible. Cancer detection is strongly based on the principle of identifying anomalies in some particular biomarkers viz., proteins, nucleic acid, cytogenetic parameters, metabolites, whole cell, and cytokinetic parameters [10]. For conventional devices to monitor these aforementioned in low concentration is a huge challenge and the

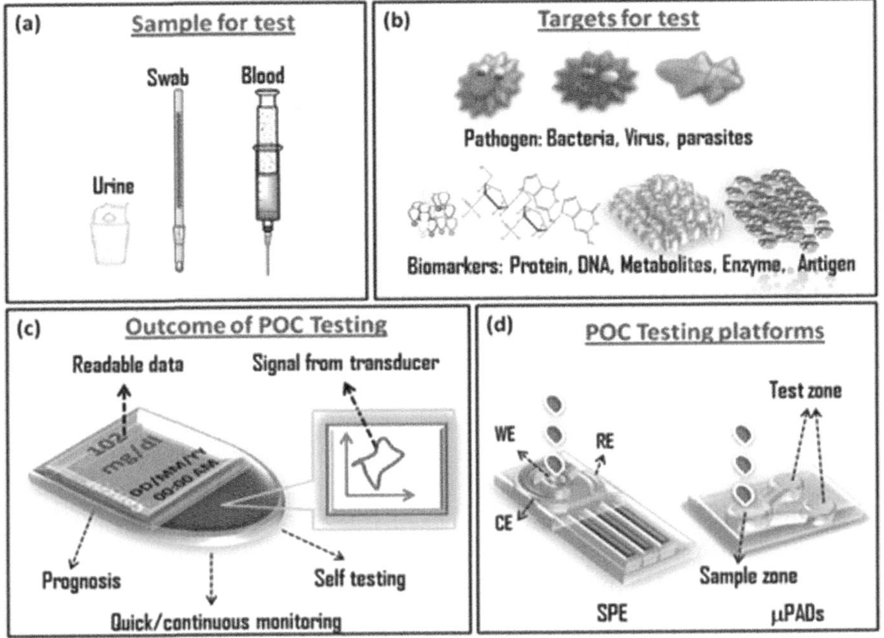

FIGURE 6.1 Typical POC testing protocol: (a) types of sample required, (b) target analyte, (c) & (d) data recording process during detection by various DES platforms.

number of such devices is almost insignificant. The current situation thus demands the new age early monitoring POC testing cancer devices with affordable as well as easily operated modes. Researchers' contributions toward developing these kinds of devices using nanotechnology are very briefly discussed later. Mosayebi et al. have developed a sensor to identify the aggregation of cancer cells in a specific area of blood vessels indicating peculiarity/abnormal growth of cardiovascular structure [11]. The device basically detects the emission and production profile of biomarkers. In another report silicon nanochannels were applied to detect single molecules for detecting breast cancer [12].

Not only cancer but the spread of pathogens play a crucial role in causing adverse situations to humans. It is undoubtedly an accepted fact that vaccination is the best way for the complete removal of infectious disease, yet we all must agree that early detection of infection is beneficial for saving lives. In addition, pathogenic contamination is of utmost importance in food safety, biodefense, forensic science, and in also clinical applications. Rapid and on-spot pathogen diagnosis is in continuous demand especially in isolated or rural places where proper clinical setup is not available. The conventional pathogen monitoring system is based on either cell culture method or immunological diagnosis. Biosensors beat both methods in terms of POC testing. Bioreceptors built in the sensor identify a very small amount of antigen or microorganism and transform it into an identifiable signal with the aid of a suitable transducer. Continuous development of nano- and micro-material research further improves the sensor sensitivity by integrating multiple arrays of pathogen/micro-organism-detecting platforms. Some successful examples of pathogen-detected electrochemical biosensors are Salmonella, L. Monocytogens, E. Coli etc. sensors. Detection of the most recent vividly significant trouble-causing few diseases is sited later. H1N1, influenza virus detection by microfluidic chip-based electrochemical biosensor as graphene oxide base material is reported by Wu and coworker [2]. MERS-CoV and H-CoV coronavirus were successfully detected using square wave voltammetry technique (SWV) with the aid of cysteamine-immobilized gold nanoparticles decorated with carbon electrodes. This fabricated sensor possesses LOD as low as pg/ML range [13]. Kogaki and group have designed an immunosensor capable of detecting SARS-CoV antigen from nasal swab within 15 minutes of sample collection. The sensor is composed of arrays of enzymes [14].

6.2.2 BIOMOLECULE DETECTION

As biomolecules are an essential part of any living system, for proper maintenance of organs and metabolism, the detection of these is vital. Routinely monitoring biomarkers levels in body fluid allows the person in the timely management of the disease and to fight against it. Personalized healthcare is mostly dependent on POC testing. Various disposable electrodes are modified or functionalized in order to detect the desired bioanalytes. Most of the bioanalytes are electrochemically active and hence the electrochemical detection method is most appropriate. Uric acid, ascorbic acid, creatinine, dopamine etc. are successfully detected by biosensors and also well matched with clinical test reports [15, 16]. The detection process can be accomplished both in solid and liquid phases. Exhaled breath, saliva secretion, urine vapor etc. serves the goal as a sample. A suitable bioreceptor is to be embedded in the sensor platform for biomolecule identification when interfering factors are present and without any further processing. The choice is strictly dependent on the purpose of analysis, type of the bioanalyte, and transducer. To name a few, various bioreceptors are categorized as antibody-based, synthetic protein-based, aptamer-based, enzyme-based, microorganism and tissue-based. Antibody-based sensors need special storage conditions and are costly as production and maintenance of antibodies are quite difficult. On the contrary, synthetic protein-based bioreceptors are favored owing to their small chemical structure, ability of reversible reaction with antigens, stability, and cost-effectiveness. The only drawback is of its use in in-vivo analysis. An aptameter is composed of a double helical structure of nucleotides performing as a bioreceptor. Enzymatic biosensors can be of long-run use as the bioreceptors (enzymes) take part only as a catalyst in reaction and are not even consumed during the process. These bioreceptors can be effectively adjusted to electrochemical transducers. Glucose oxidase-based enzymatic glucose biosensors is a common name in the field of enzymatic electrochemical sensors. Another good example of a catalytic bioreceptor is microorganisms and organs. Monitoring of biomolecules can be done by studying the metabolic product during the receptor's respiratory performance.

Amongst all bioreceptors, though tissue-based are the inexpensive ones, their selectivity over a wide range limits their applications.

In many developing countries, to minimize the cost of the device, paper-based lateral flow assay (LFA) type biosensors are hugely employed. The most popular and convenient example of LFA is the human chorionic gonadotropin (hcg)-sensing device (common name, pregnancy test kit). This comes with a Yes/No direct result just by viewing presence/absence or number of colored lines on the kit. Whitesides and his group first introduced a new type of paper-based biosensing technology named microPADs [17]. Micro channels are fabricated onto paper substrates using physical or chemical methods. These micropads are incorporated into an electrochemical device for the detection of specific targets. For example, in a glucose monitoring micropad when human blood is inserted, glass fiber filter paper extracts the red blood cell and plasma is only allowed to pass through the channel. The microchannels are fabricated using Cu compound and glucose oxidase which after reaction quantify glucose in the body by readable signals [18].

6.3 DES DESIGNING STRATEGIES

6.3.1 DISPOSABLE PAPER-BASED SENSORS FOR POC TESTING

A paper-based disposable POC testing device uses paper as a testing platform and a reasonable medium for creating an ultralight biodegradable analytical device which overthrows conventional testing materials in terms of accessibility, price, and simplicity of disposal. Moreover, hydrophilicity alongside its porous structure further retains its demand in varieties of applications. This unique feature makes it possible to initiate the flow of fluid (sample) without any external pumping. Proper functionalization of the paper surface such as conductivity, reactivity, and hydrophilicity is achieved due to the exclusive structures of the cellulose. However, it is really important to choose the appropriate paper to fit the specific application as the sensor performance is solely dependent on the pore size, thickness, and materials of any PAD. In recent years chromatographic filter papers have been frequently employed in microfluidic device fabrication for their affinity to wick liquid [19]. A lot of research has been devoted to the standard Whatman® filter paper (made up of cellulose) having medium retention, high porosity, and sufficient flow rate. Despite its wide range of applications, filter paper occasionally lacks the required physical properties. Therefore, research into various forms of paper and paper modification is still an emerging area of PADs. Hydrophobic nitrocellulose membranes are well adapted to immobilize the biomolecules including enzymes, protein, and DNA for their huge amount of nonspecific interaction with these biomolecules [20]. Glossy paper has been proposed as an alternative platform for PADs as replacement of filter paper. Flexible, nonbiodegradable glossy paper is a kind of substrate having smooth surface unruffled of cellulose fiber incorporated by inorganic filler [21]. In addition, cellulose acetate filter paper, drawing paper, commercial paper, and PVDF filter film are appealing candidates used in PADs. Approaches adopted in

PAD sensing are surface plasmon resonance, electrochemical, colorimetric, fluorescent, photo-electrochemical etc. However, the electrochemical techniques enable the preparation of extremely sensitive and quantitative assessment of microelectrodes and nanomaterial-based electrocatalysts. Sensitive electrochemical signals from PADs may be extracted using a variety of diverse electrochemical techniques such as amperometry, potentiometry, coulometry, and sophisticated pulse voltametry. Results demonstrate a good level of sensitivity as well as selectivity and comparable to the findings of traditional methodologies such as areliquid/gas chromatography, UV-VIS spectroscopy, and inductively coupled plasma-mass spectrometry. In addition to all aforementioned facts, PADs enable multifaceted monitoring of several analytes concurrently using the same platform. Being free from any pretreatment procedures of the sample viz. collection, separation, extraction, and concentration a single multiplexed platform is quick, cost-effective, and highly advantageous for clinical diagnosis. Varieties of conducting ink, the primary electrode carbon, and other nanostructured materials may be used as electrodes in PADs. Elaborately, to fabricate WE and RE Ag/AgCl ink is recurrently applied whereas carbon-based electrodes for the reference electrode are modified with synthetic/natural/biological generated chemicals. As the molecule (analyte) recognition process occurs on WE surface, nanostructured materials, electrocatalysts are being functionalized to extend the sensitivity and selectivity of DES. The surface of the transducer is also often modified to provide selective molecular sensing using antibodies, DNA, aptamers, immobilized enzymes, molecular imprinted polymers, and other substances [22]. Enzymatic biosensors have been created for measuring uric acid, lactate, and glucose in biological samples by integrating the oxidase enzyme onto the working electrode [23]. With paper-based microfluidic technology, this analytical technique shows how an electrochemical sensor may be integrated for portable, miniature POC analysis. It's important to mention that the CE was designed in a bigger shape than both the WE and RE in order to lower resistance in the circuit. Additionally, the WE should be placed close to the reference electrode to reduce the resistance between them.

To detect and immobilize CA125 antibody (anti-CA125) Fan et al. have designed electrochemical biosensor based on paper. This sensor is very useful for POC testing of tumor biomarkers [24]. Boonkaew et al. have introduced an electrochemical PAD paired with a label-free immunoassay for the simultaneous measurement of three crucial biomarkers for cardiovascular diseases (CVDs), namely C-reactive protein (CRP), procalcitonin (PCT), and troponin I (cTnI) in serum sample [25]. In response to outbreaks of the HIV p24 antigen and CR3022 antibody associated with the protein spike S1 of SARS-CoV-2 as a marker for COVID-19 in human serum, Li et al. have constructed paper-based disposable ZnO-NW-enhanced EIS (electrochemical impedance spectroscopy) biosensor (LOD down to 0.4 pg/ml) [26]. In order to detect different types of biomarkers, Liu and his group offer a versatile paper-based electrochemical sensing system where DNA is added to paper and labeled with a signal molecule. These testing methods may also be used to find the target in samples of spiked serum, showing the possibility for clinical sample monitoring at the POC testing [27]. The lack of knowledge about how these electrochemical PADs would function in the real world is one of the challenges behind the commercialization of these PADs. Multidisciplinary teams should work together to evaluate the features of PADs in the field of medical science since the data obtained from this work would be extremely helpful for further implementation of POC testing.

6.3.2 Disposable Screen-Printed Sensors for POC Analysis

The manufacturing of electrochemicals and biosensors by screen printing has gained widespread acceptance as an effective approach. Analytical chemistry has a strong emphasis on the removal of heavy materials and equipment from the analytical technique. For the measurement of numerous analytes, disposable biosensors with an immobilization mechanism for enzymes on screen printing electrodes (SPEs) have been employed extensively. In contrast to more conventional solid electrodes, SPEs have the advantage of being disposable sensor strips for one usage, which eliminates the need to frequently smooth or polish the electrode surface. The primary electrode systems, used in SPEs including working electrode (WE), reference electrode (RE), and counter electrode (CE) are patterned on an inert substrate. The screen-printing technology is the best available approach for the mass manufacture of disposable electrodes made of a flat substance. The complete fabrication process is composed of three to four steps: screen-printing the electrode, modifying its surface to increase sensitivity and selectivity, and using it as a sensor. At the time of printing onto a solid surface in the screen-printing process, the substrate's surface must be coated with ink or paste. [28]. The inks used to create screen-printed electrodes are made up of particles, a polymeric binder with other additives for better printing, adhesion, and dispersion. One excellent example of how this production approach could be utilized to make commercial devices for diabetes is the personal glucose biosensor, which accounts for a billion-dollar annual global market [29]. Screen-printed electrodes are extensively studied for ion-selective membrane-based potentiometric sensors, aptamer-based immunosensors, and enzyme-based amperometric sensors. Due to its great sensitivity and versatility, amperometric detection is one of the widely employed electrochemical sensing methods. In light of their selectivity, enzymes are the preferred biological component to employ in biosensor manufacture for SPEs modification. They quickly bind to the substrate in specific ways [30]. For the analysis of a wide range of chemical compounds including triglycerides, glucose-6-phosphate, phenobarbital, and organophosphorus compounds biosensors with different modified (SPEs) based on immobilized enzymes have recently been developed. Three main applications for enzyme-based sensors include offline, online, and in vivo detectors. All commercially available glucometers function as offline detectors; the screen-printed strips test the level of the glucose content of a droplet of blood from a diabetic patient, while the blood sugar level is shown on the handheld devices. Measuring the concentrations of glucose and cholesterol in the body is essential for the identification of the possible risks of various major diseases, including hypertension, cerebral thrombosis, arteriosclerosis, coronary artery disease, and diabetes mellitus. Chronic effects of diabetes mellitus include kidney failure, vision loss, and cardiac arrest. A biomarker's level is continuously monitored in the body using in vivo biosensors. The concentration of free biomarkers that do not belong to anything in the extracellular fluid is continually measured using online detectors that are incorporated into a channel originating from a sample collector within the human body or living substance. Recently, nanostructured electrically conductive substances have been employed on electrodes to increase the electrochemically active surface area and enzymatic sensor sensitivity. MWCNTs and palladium are used to create a composite material for a disposable glucose sensor as described by Guzsvány et al. The enzymatic sensor printed on screens functioned well with a LOD in the sub-millimolar concentration range of 0.14 mM [31]. Pt-Pd bimetallic nanoclusters that resemble snowflakes were generated by Niu et al. and modified on a gold nanofilm electrode by screen printing [32]. When GOx is immobilized, the biosensor displays favorable capabilities toward glucose and outstanding electrocatalytic activity toward H_2O_2. Modern medical diagnostic techniques emphasize on the rapid detection of biomarkers from entire blood samples, including glucose, lactate, tumor markers, and many more. The entire blood is a complex fluid made up of a variety of elements including protein, glucose, hormones, and inorganic ions. Kong et al. reported the customization of the electrode using graphene, polyaniline, AuNPs, and Gox and developed a portable single-use glucose sensor with screen-printed electrode and a paper disk [33]. The test revolves on the direct electrochemistry of two cofactors flavin adenine dinucleotide (FAD) molecules which can restore enzymatic activity. Phetsang et al. reported the techniques to develop a platinum/ reduced graphene oxide (rGO)/poly (3-aminobenzoic acid) film on a SPE and used for the accurate amperometric detection of glucose and cholesterol [34]. The effectiveness of sensors based on enzymes is primarily dependent on the functioning of the immobilized enzyme. It is challenging to maintain environmental variables and situations that affect the enzyme's stability such as temperature, pH, and moisture, which have a substantial impact on enzyme stability over time. Additionally, a lack of oxygen affects the effectiveness of enzyme sensors. Contrarily, nonenzymatic sensors generate electrical currents by reducing the analyte on the electrode surface without requiring oxygen. The nonenzymatic sensors' performance is quite consistent and pH or temperature have little impact on it. Dayakar et al. developed a nonenzymatic glucose sensor with a limit detection 0.019 µM, the screen-printed electrode was modified with CeO_2 @CuO core-shell nanostructures [35]. A screen-printed graphene electrode (SPGNE) was used in differential pulse voltammetry to measure uric acid in urine samples [36]. On the basis of surface-modified SPCE, a disposable strip amperometric sensor was developed for fast detection of paracetamol in urine [28]. Anzar et al. reported an innovative method to covalently connect paper-based screen-printed carbon electrodes with nanoparticles in order to specifically detect bilirubin, a key biomarker for jaundice. Bilirubin oxidase was immobilized on electrodes treated with AgNPs to produce an electrochemical biosensor [37]. For rapid POC testing, Malla et al. described an easy electrochemical approach to identify the COVID-19 spike protein in serum, urine, and saliva using SPE with magnetic beads (MBs) [38]. These analytical devices' possible capabilities include easy operation, affordability, and the ability to be miniaturized down into portable electrochemical sensors. This makes it possible to create controlled POC testing systems for the immediate analysis of several biomarkers.

6.3.3 INKJET PRINTED DISPOSABLE SENSORS

In addition to the aforementioned techniques another effectively faster proto type is Inkjet DES, recently being used as high-resolution, low-cost disposable biosensors for POC detections and therapy. In inkjet, printing ink consists of colloidal suspensions of a large amount of conducting nanomaterials and its composites and is printed directly on the flexible substrate for multifunctional applications. Various substrates including paper, glass, PMMA, Silicon, Polyethylene terephthalate, Polyethylene naphthalate, Polyimide, and 3D structures are the most common uses for inkjet printing technology. In comparison to conventional substrate printing technology, inkjet printing does not involve any sophisticated equipment like photo masks, stencils or other physiological aids and it can be printed without any ink loss. On the contrary, printing inks have to satisfy extremely crucial rheological benchmarks in terms of viscosity as well as surface tension. Typical values set for these parametersare 1-30 cP and 25-40 m/N [39]. Furthermore, ink sintering temperature and pretreatment of the substrate surface are important for producing stable printed traces as well as enhanced ink adhesion. However, the requirement of high temperatures for metal nanoparticle-based inks provides difficulties since many commonly used plastic substrates become unstable at high temperatures [40]. These are the main obstacles impeding the broad acceptance of technology in today's world. As a consequence of this, practically all of the efforts devoted thus far included directly producing one or more inks [39]. An inkjet printed PAD for diabetes monitoring has been developed by Määttänen et al. [41]. On a paper substrate, a three-electrode system is generated by inkjet printing the WE, CE using gold nanoparticles (AuNPs) and the RE using silver nanoparticles (AgNPs). Silver nanoparticles were employed for inkjet printing to make flexible biosensor devices by Abadi et al. [42] as it is less expensive than noble metals like Au and Pt and has a higher surface-to-volume ratio [43]. The disposable aptamer inkjet printing sensor is designed by Fernandez et al. [44] to measure salivary cortisol levels and has been improved by functionalized magnetic nanoparticles. This is helpful for POC monitoring of patients with obstructive sleep apnea. Petani et al. developed two typical impedimetric and amperometric inkjet-printed sensors using biocompatible materials to monitor the amount of ozone dissolved during ozone-oxygen-injection treatment [45].

6.3.4 DISPOSABLE LASER-INDUCED GRAPHENE (LIG) SENSORS

Research on graphene-based biosensors is still a priority for clinical diagnosticsas it can provide early diagnosis of many fatal diseases. LIG-based disposable sensors are composed of 3D-porous carbon nanomaterial made by directly printing on polymer with carbon dioxide (CO_2) lasers. Additionally, it is known as laser-scribed graphene (LSG), laser-ablated graphene (LAG), and laser-derived graphene (LDG) [46]. Apart from the infrared CO_2 laser, the LIG has been constructed using ultraviolet laser [47] and visible laser [48]. LIG has properties including flexibility, resistance to chemical agents, and porosity that make it suitable as an electrode material in microfluidic systems. In addition, there are several ways to modify the surface characteristics of the LIG, one of which is by coating solvents on the surface in order to produce multifunctional surfaces and improve hydrophobicity. To prepare the LIG, polyimide (PI) and its derivatives are frequently used. Polysulfone (PSU), wood, potato, coconut, skin cork, and polyetherimide (PEI) are specified for 3D porous graphene printing. The direct printing on PI is a porous, three-dimensional, conductive carbon structure with an extensive number of defects and edge-planes, which are advantageous for electrochemical-sensing processes. It is an excellent candidate for both physical and biological sensors. The prospect of using these sensors to monitor the body's regular functions is quite promising. An enzyme-free and highly sensitive glucose sensor using LIG treated with Cu NCs (copper nanocubes) with LOD 250 nM was prepared by Tehrani and his group. The sensor was shown to have remarkable effectiveness in detecting glucose in urine, sweat, tears, and saliva [49]. A LIG-based pH sensor was developed by Mamleyev et al. for the detection of urea. The sensor is adjustable and operates on catheters. Within 1 minute of response time, it can accurately identify urea upto 10^{-4} M of concentration [50]. Dopamine (DA) is a vital information carrier of the central nervous system in the mammalian. For the purpose of monitoring the DA in human urine and in a neutral solution Hui et al. reported a LIG/PDMS (polydimethylsiloxane) electrode functionalized with Pt-Au nanoparticles (NPs) with LOD 75 nM[51]. The concentration of NH_4^+ and K^+ ion in urine samples was successfully detected by Kucherenko et al. using an LIG ion-selective electrode with high stability over a broad pH range [52]. The potential of LIG electrodes to function as a capacitance-based transducer to detect thrombin in buffer and serum medium was reported by Yagati and coworkers [53]. We are still in the early phases of exploring this field of study. It still poses difficulties. It is a nonequilibrium, nonlinear, multi-scale phenomenon when lasers interact with polymer materials. The mechanism regarding the interaction of lasers with polymer materials remains unresolved at this time. A comparison of recently reported results has been cited in **Table 6.1**.

6.4 CHALLENGES AND FUTURE SCOPE

So far, every technology demonstrated in designing DES has its own flaws, still each one has proven advantageous in particular fields. New and improved technology is being adopted to overcome the challenge. In brief, the sensitivity and selectivity issue of analytical methods has significantly enhanced through the usage of disposable *screen-printed electrodes*, especially when it comes to the identification of certain environmental analytical compounds that were previously hard to analyze using conventional approaches. On the other hand, the usage of disposable screen-printed electrodes is still expanding and finding new uses. Future research is anticipated to concentrate on introducing nanomaterials into the screen-printed electrodes in order to increase the electron transfer rates and hence improve the sensors' analytical efficiency. A printed *paper-based analytical device* needs to overcome several challenges during fabrication, including excessive roughness, inadequate barrier

TABLE 6.1

Recently Reported Disposable Electrochemical Sensors as Modern Healthcare appliance

Type of Target	Target	Sensing Platform	Designing Technology	LOD	Linear Range	Reference
Biomarkers	cancer antigen 125 (CA125)	rGO/Thi/AuNPs nanocomposites	Paper-based	0.01 U mL^{-1}	0.1 U mL^{-1} to 200 U mL^{-1}	[24]
	CRP), (cTnI), and (PCT)	A wax-patterned paper and a transparency film	PADs	0.38 ng mL^{-1} for CRP, 0.16 pg mL^{-1} for cTnI, and 0.27 pg mL^{-1} for PCT	0.001–100 µg mL^{-1} for CRP, 0.001–250 ng mL^{-1} for cTnI and 0.5 pg mL-1 to 250 ng mL^{-1} for PCT	[25]
	HIV p24 antigen	ZnO-NW	Paper-based	0.4 pg ml^{-1}	–	[26]
	microRNAs (miRNA), Alkaline phosphatase (ALP), and Carcinoembryonic antigen (CEA)	Paper	Paper-based	–	1 fM to 1 µM (miRNA), 1 to 10^5 mU L^{-1} (ALP), 1 to 1500 fg mL^{-1} (CEA)	[27]
	Glucose	GOx/Pd-MWCNT-SPCE and GOx-Au/Pd-MWCNT-SPCE	SPE	0.04 mM for GOx/Pd-MWCNT-SPCE and 0.02 mM for GOx-Au/Pd-MWCNT-SPCE	0.16 mM–0.97 mM (GOx/Pd-MWCNT-SPCE) and 0.16 mM–0.72 mM (GOx-Au/Pd-MWCNT-SPCE)	[31]
	H$_2$O$_2$	SPGFE/Pt–PdBNC	SPE	804 mA M^{-1} cm^{-2}	0.005 to 6 mM	[32]
	Glucose and cholesterol	Platinum/reduced graphene oxide/poly(3-aminobenzoic acid decorated film	SPE	44.3 µM (glucose) and 40.5 µM (cholesterol)	0.25–6.00 mM for glucose and 0.25–4.00 mM for cholesterol	[34]
	Glucose	CeO2@CuO core-shell nanostructure	SPE	0.019 µM	1 to 8.9 µM	[35]
	Glucose	Paper-based chips	Inkjet	0.1 mM	0–20 mM	[41]
	Lactate	Silver nanoparticle	Inkjet	–	1~25mM/L	[43]
	Salivary cortisol	Magnetic nanoparticles	Inkjet	10 pM	100 pM to 50 nM	[44]
	Glucose	Copper nanocubes (CuNCs)	Laser-induced graphene	250 nM	25 µM–4 mM	[49]
	Urea	Polyimide (Kapton) sheets	Laser-induced graphene	10^{-4} M	10^{-4}–10^{-1} M	[50]
	Dopamine	Pt-Au nanoparticles (Pt-AuNPs)	Laser-induced graphene	75 nM	5 - 30 µM	[51]
	Urine samples to determine human hydration levels	Polyimide	Laser-induced graphene	30 µm (NH^{4+}) and 100 µm (K$^+$)	0.1 –150 mm (NH^{4+}) and 0.3 –150 mm (K$^+$)	[52]
	Thrombin	Carboxy group bearing polymeric nanoparticles or liposomes	Laser-induced graphene	0.12 pM in PBS, 1.3 pM in serum	0.01 nM–1000 nM	[53]

(Continued)

TABLE 6.1
(Continued)

Type of Target	Target	Sensing Platform	Designing Technology	LOD	Linear Range	Reference
	Dopamine and uric acid	$GO/Fe_3O_4@SiO_2$	SPE	8.9×10^{-8} M (dopamine) and 5.7×10^{-7} M (uric acid)	0.1 to 600.0 µM (dopamine) and 0.75 to 300.0 µM (uric acid)	[54]
	C-reactive Protein (CRP)	AuNPs/G	SPE	15 ng mL^{-1}	0.05 µg mL^{-1}–100 µg mL^{-1}	[55]
	Glucose	Polyimide /Graphene	Inkjet	0.3 mg/dL	0–40 mg/dL	[56]
Pathogen	Protein spike S1 of SARS-CoV-2 and HIV p24 antigen	ZnO-NW	Paper-based	0.4 pg ml^{-1}) in detecting p24 antigen		[26]
	Spike protein of COVID-19	Magnetic beads (MBs)	SPE	0.20 ng mL^{-1} (human saliva), 0.31 ng mL^{-1} (human urine), and 0.54 ng mL^{-1} (human serum)	3.12–200 ng mL^{-1}	[38]
	Salmonella typhimurium	Polyimide	Laser-induced graphene	13 ± 7 CFU mL^{-1}	25 to 10^5 CFU mL^{-1}	[57]
	SARS-COV-2 virus	Paper strips	PADs (LFA)	–	–	[58]
	E.Coli	Biotin	SPE	10^5cfu/mL for the general assay and 10^6 cfu/mL for the immunoassay	–	[59]
	Bacillus anthracis	Carbon	SPE	10^4 cfu/mL for 50-µL samples	10^2 to 10^8cfu/mL	[60]

*SPE: Screen-Printed Electrode; PADs: Paper-based analytical devices; LFA: Lateral Flow Array; Thi: thionine qualities, absorbency, moisture absorption, and opaqueness. Contrarily, smooth, dimensionally inert, and nonabsorbing substrates are necessary for high functional devices. Several approaches have been employed to overcome this problem, but even the latest research investigations do not completely study the impact of substrate pretreatment and its effect on the sensor's performance. The inherent high porosity and roughness of paper make it difficult to craft an electrochemical *inkjet-printed sensor* on it. Controlling the surface wettability is also crucial to preserve the printed pattern's quality. The easy accessibility of functional substances and accurate post-processing technique are critical to the continued adoption of inkjet method in the sensor-manufacturing industry. The creation of metallic inks with low sintering temperatures for inkjet printing methods that are suitable for a variety of flexible substrates is one of the most significant challenges. The glass-transition temperature for a large number of these substrates has a value lower than 130°C. But a lot of research has been done into developing conductive polymer inks which have the potential to get this restriction. The chemical interaction with photons and electrons or lattices needs to be described in *LIG*. Furthermore, because the LIG's graphene is porous, a generally high voltage or laser can damage it, making it an inadequate substrate for electrophoretic coating for different characterization techniques. There are several methods to broaden this field of research. Further, it is possible to enhance the robustness, conductivity, and electrochemical performance of LIG by modifying its shape, porosity, and surface functionalization.

All of these obstacles, therefore, offer an enormous challenge for the research community. Ensuring the future research and discovery of novel electrochemical sensors and their transmission from advanced laboratories to users in the pharmaceutical sector, environmental, and medical fields will be the century's challenge. With these, researchers are also facing enormous challenges in fabricating DES due to a lack of infrastructure and annual funding dedicated to the research sector of health and medicine. Even if the DES is manufactured, circulation and awareness in society especially in urban areas where healthcare facilities are inadequate is a prime fact to deal with. Under this circumstance, in spite of the successful application of POC devices in health management, as discussed in detail earlier in the chapter, implementation on a mass scale to doctor personnel is still challenging for the device manufacturing companies as they hardly believe in laboratory-based test results.

As the future scope of the work, along with finding new and improvised material as sensing platforms and efficient technology, integration of observed test data from POC test to personal electronic devices like smartwatches, mobiles, tablets etc. is the goal to achieve. Also, the country has now moved to form a strong and reliable telemedicine facility for which, the storage of these multiple recorded test data in the server is mandatory. Telemedicine facility is demanding, but at the same time it is truly challenging.

6.5 SUMMARY

In the current stage where a large number of people's lives are at stake because of harsh lifestyle and polluted environment, building a strong healthcare facility is a prime need. Specially home-based biosensing devices of low cost, ease of operation, miniaturized design, and quick response could be the pillars of the system. POC devices draw additional attention to the applicability of rural patients and regular monitoring as well as self-health management. Blooming area of nanotechnology has paved the way for new kinds of disposable biosensors and in some cases has broken the traditional lab-based tedious test concepts. Screen printing, microfluidic channels, laser printing etc., the type of technologies used on abundant and flexible paper substrates, have made overall progress in disposable biosensors. Detecting bio-markers with the help of suitable bioreceptors and conversion of biological response to readable data using transducers has effectively helped medical professionals in prognosis as well as an outbreak of disease management. Even by virtue of modern technologies simultaneous detection of more than one bioanalyte is successfully achieved. Overall, in this chapter a variety of disposable biosensors and their designing technologies have been brought into focus which would definitely draw the reader's attention in understanding the current scenario along with the need of the present field.

REFERENCES

1. Pandikumar, A., & Devi, K. S. (Eds.). (2021). *Disposable Electrochemical Sensors for Healthcare Monitoring: Material Properties and Design* (Vol. 21). Royal Society of Chemistry.
2. Wu, Z., Zhou, C. H., Chen, J. J., Xiong, C., Chen, Z., Pang, D. W., & Zhang, Z. L. (2015). Bifunctional magnetic nanobeads for sensitive detection of avian influenza A (H7N9) virus based on immunomagnetic separation and enzyme-induced metallization. *Biosensors and Bioelectronics, 68*, 586–592.
3. Killard, A. J. (2017). Disposable sensors. *Current Opinion in Electrochemistry, 3*(1), 57–62.
4. Kim, J. H., Mun, S., Ko, H. U., Yun, G. Y., & Kim, J. (2014). Disposable chemical sensors and biosensors made on cellulose paper. *Nanotechnology, 25*(9), 092001.
5. Yang, M., Jeong, S. W., Chang, S. J., Kim, K. H., Jang, M., Kim, C. H., ... Lee, K. G. (2016). Flexible and disposable sensing platforms based on newspaper. *ACS Applied Materials and Interfaces, 8*(51), 34978–34984.
6. Zhang, M., Halder, A., Hou, C., Ulstrup, J., & Chi, Q. (2016). Free-standing and flexible graphene papers as disposable non-enzymatic electrochemical sensors. *Bioelectrochemistry, 109*, 87–94.
7. Vashist, S. K. (2017). Point-of-care diagnostics: Recent advances and trends. *Biosensors, 7*(4), 62.
8. Kosack, C. S., Page, A. L., & Klatser, P. R. (2017). A guide to aid the selection of diagnostic tests. *Bulletin of the World Health Organization, 95*(9), 639.
9. Jayson, G. C., Kohn, E. C., Kitchener, H. C., & Ledermann, J. A. (2014). Ovarian cancer. *The Lancet, 384*(9951), 1376–1388.
10. Mishra, A., & Verma, M. (2010). Cancer biomarkers: Are we ready for the prime time? *Cancers, 2*(1), 190–208.
11. Mosayebi, R., Ahmadzadeh, A., Wicke, W., Jamali, V., Schober, R., & Nasiri-Kenari, M. (2018). Early cancer detection in blood vessels using mobile nanosensors. *IEEE Transactions on Nanobioscience, 18*(2), 103–116.
12. Mohanty, P., Chen, Y., Wang, X., Hong, M. K., Rosenberg, C. L., Weaver, D. T., &Erramilli, S. (2014). Field effect transistor nanosensor for breast cancer diagnostics. *arXiv Preprint ArXiv:1401.1168.*

13. Layqah, L. A., & Eissa, S. (2019). An electrochemical immunosensor for the corona virus associated with the Middle East respiratory syndrome using an array of gold nanoparticle-modified carbon electrodes. *Microchimica Acta, 186*(4), 1–10.

14. Kogaki, H., Uchida, Y., Fujii, N., Kurano, Y., Miyake, K., Kido, Y., … Okada, M. (2005). Novel rapid immunochromatographic test based on an enzyme immunoassay for detecting nucleocapsid antigen in SARS associated coronavirus. *Journal of Clinical Laboratory Analysis, 19*(4), 150–159.

15. Tsai, T. H., Thiagarajan, S., & Chen, S. M. (2010). Detection of melamine in milk powder and human urine. *Journal of Agricultural and Food Chemistry, 58*(8), 4537–4544.

16. Chen, J. C., Kumar, A. S., Chung, H. H., Chien, S. H., Kuo, M. C., & Zen, J. M. (2006). An enzymeless electrochemical sensor for the selective determination of creatinine in human urine. *Sensors and Actuators B: Chemical, 115*(1), 473–480.

17. Martinez, A. W., Phillips, S. T., Whitesides, G. M., & Carrilho, E. (2010). Diagnostics for the developing world: Microfluidic paper-based analytical devices. *Analytical Chemistry, 82,* 3–10.

18. He, R. Y., Tseng, H. Y., Lee, H. A., Liu, Y. C., Koshevoy, I. O., Pan, S. W., & Ho, M. L. (2019). Based microfluidic devices based on 3D network polymer hydrogel for the determination of glucose in human whole blood. *RSC Advances, 9*(56), 32367–32374.

19. Apilux, A., Dungchai, W., Siangproh, W., Praphairaksit, N., Henry, C. S., &Chailapakul, O. (2010). Lab-on-paper with dual electrochemical/colorimetric detection for simultaneous determination of gold and iron. *Analytical Chemistry, 82*(5), 1727–1732.

20. Lu, Y., Lin, B., & Qin, J. (2011). Patterned paper as a low-cost, flexible substrate for rapid prototyping of PDMS microdevices via "liquid molding". *Analytical Chemistry, 83*(5), 1830–1835.

21. Arena, A., Donato, N., Saitta, G., Bonavita, A., Rizzo, G., & Neri, G. (2010). Flexible ethanol sensors on glossy paper substrates operating at room temperature. *Sensors and Actuators. Part B,: Chemical, 145*(1), 488–494.

22. Mohanan, V. M. A., Kunnummal, A. K., & Biju, V. M. N. (2018). Selective electrochemical detection of dopamine based on molecularly imprinted poly (5-amino 8-hydroxy quinoline) immobilized reduced graphene oxide. *Journal of Materials Science, 53*(15), 10627–10639.

23. Lee, V. B. C., Mohd-Naim, N. F., Tamiya, E., & Ahmed, M. U. (2018). Trends in paper-based electrochemical biosensors: from design to application. *Analytical Sciences: The International Journal of the Japan Society for Analytical Chemistry, 34*(1), 7–18.

24. Fan, Y., Shi, S., Ma, J., & Guo, Y. (2019). A paper-based electrochemical immunosensor with reduced graphene oxide/thionine/gold nanoparticles nanocomposites modification for the detection of cancer antigen 125. *Biosensors and Bioelectronics, 135,* 1–7.

25. Boonkaew, S., Jang, I., Noviana, E., Siangproh, W., Chailapakul, O., & Henry, C. S. (2021). Electrochemical paper-based analytical device for multiplexed, point-of-care detection of cardiovascular disease biomarkers. *Sensors and Actuators. Part B,: Chemical, 330,* 129336.

26. Li, X., Qin, Z., Fu, H., Li, T., Peng, R., Li, Z., … Liu, X. (2021). Enhancing the performance of paper-based electrochemical impedance spectroscopy nanobiosensors: An experimental approach. *Biosensors and Bioelectronics, 177,* 112672.

27. Liu, X., Li, X., Gao, X., Ge, L., Sun, X., & Li, F. (2019). A universal paper-based electrochemical sensor for zero-background assay of diverse biomarkers. *ACS Applied Materials and Interfaces, 11*(17), 15381–15388.

28. Mohamed, H. M. (2016). Screen-printed disposable electrodes: Pharmaceutical applications and recent developments. *TrAC Trends in Analytical Chemistry, 82,* 1–11.

29. Singh, S., Wang, J., & Cinti, S. (2022). An overview on recent progress in screen-printed electroanalytical (bio) sensors. *ECS Sensors Plus, 1*(2), 023401.

30. Renedo, O. D., Alonso-Lomillo, M. A., & Martinez, M. A. (2007). Recent developments in the field of screen-printed electrodes and their related applications. *Talanta*, *73*(2), 202–219.

31. Guzsvány, V., Anojčić, J., Radulović, E., Vajdle, O., Stanković, I., Madarász, D., ... &Kalcher, K. (2017). Screen-printed enzymatic glucose biosensor based on a composite made from multiwalled carbon nanotubes and palladium containing particles. *Microchimica Acta*, *184*(7), 1987–1996.

32. Niu, X., Chen, C., Zhao, H., Chai, Y., & Lan, M. (2012). Novel snowflake-like Pt–Pd bimetallic clusters on screen-printed gold nanofilm electrode for H2O2 and glucose sensing. *Biosensors and Bioelectronics*, *36*(1), 262–266.

33. Kong, F. Y., Gu, S. X., Li, W. W., Chen, T. T., Xu, Q., & Wang, W. (2014). A paper disk equipped with graphene/polyaniline/Au nanoparticles/glucose oxidase biocomposite modified screen-printed electrode: Toward whole blood glucose determination. *Biosensors and Bioelectronics*, *56*, 77–82.

34. Phetsang, S., Jakmunee, J., Mungkornasawakul, P., Laocharoensuk, R., &Ounnunkad, K. (2019). Sensitive amperometric biosensors for detection of glucose and cholesterol using a platinum/reduced graphene oxide/poly (3-aminobenzoic acid) film-modified screen-printed carbon electrode. *Bioelectrochemistry*, *127*, 125–135.

35. Dayakar, T., Rao, K. V., Bikshalu, K., Malapati, V., & Sadasivuni, K. K. (2018). Nonenzymatic sensing of glucose using screen-printed electrode modified with novel synthesized CeO2@ CuO core shell nanostructure. *Biosensors and Bioelectronics*, *111*, 166–173.

36. Ping, J., Wu, J., Wang, Y., & Ying, Y. (2012). Simultaneous determination of ascorbic acid, dopamine and uric acid using high-performance screen-printed graphene electrode. *Biosensors and Bioelectronics*, *34*(1), 70–76.

37. Anzar, N., Suleman, S., Kumar, R., Rawal, R., Pundir, C. S., Pilloton, R., & Narang, J. (2022). Electrochemical sensor for bilirubin detection using paper-based screen-printed electrodes functionalized with silver nanoparticles. *Micromachines*, *13*(11), 1845.

38. Malla, P., Liao, H. P., Liu, C. H., Wu, W. C., & Sreearunothai, P. (2022). Voltammetric biosensor for coronavirus spike protein using magnetic bead and screen-printed electrode for point-of-care diagnostics. *Microchimica Acta*, *189*(4), 168.

39. Manjushree, S. G., & Adarakatti, P. S. (2023). Recent advances in disposable electrochemical sensors. *Recent Developments in Green Electrochemical Sensors: Design, Performance, and Applications*, *1*, 1–21.

40. Moya, A., Gabriel, G., Villa, R., & del Campo, F. J. (2017). Inkjet-printed electrochemical sensors. *Current Opinion in Electrochemistry*, *3*(1), 29–39.

41. Määttänen, A., Vanamo, U., Ihalainen, P., Pulkkinen, P., Tenhu, H., Bobacka, J., & Peltonen, J. (2013). A low-cost paper-based inkjet-printed platform for electrochemical analyses. *Sensors and Actuators B: Chemical*, *177*,153–162.

42. Abadi, Z., Mottaghitalab, V., Bidoki, M., & Benvidi, A. (2014). Flexible biosensor using inkjet printing of silver nanoparticles. *Sensor Review*, *34*(4), 360–366.

43. Abrar, M. A., Dong, Y., Lee, P. K., & Kim, W. S. (2016). Bendable electro-chemical lactate sensor printed with silver nano-particles. *Scientific Reports*, *6*(1), 30565.

44. Fernandez, R. E., Umasankar, Y., Manickam, P., Nickel, J. C., Iwasaki, L. R., Kawamoto, B. K., ... Bhansali, S. (2017). Disposable aptamer-sensor aided by magnetic nanoparticle enrichment for detection of salivary cortisol variations in obstructive sleep apnea patients. *Scientific Reports*, *7*(1), 17992.

45. Petani, L., Wehrheim, V., Koker, L., Reischl, M., Ungerer, M., Gengenbach, U., &Pylatiuk, C. (2021). Systematic assessment of the biocompatibility of materials for inkjet-printed ozone sensors for medical therapy. *Flexible and Printed Electronics*, *6*(4), 043003.

46. Lahcen, A. A., Rauf, S., Beduk, T., Durmus, C., Aljedaibi, A., Timur, S., ... Salama, K. N. (2020). Electrochemical sensors and biosensors using laser-derived graphene: A comprehensive review. *Biosensors and Bioelectronics*, *168*, 112565.

47. Carvalho, A. F., Fernandes, A. J., Leitão, C., Deuermeier, J., Marques, A. C., Martins, R., ... Costa, F. M. (2018). Laser-induced graphene strain sensors produced by ultraviolet irradiation of polyimide. *Advanced Functional Materials*, *28*(52), 1805271.

48. Zhang, Z., Song, M., Hao, J., Wu, K., Li, C., & Hu, C. (2018). Visible light laser-induced graphene from phenolic resin: A new approach for directly writing graphene-based electrochemical devices on various substrates. *Carbon*, *127*, 287–296.

49. Tehrani, F., & Bavarian, B. (2016). Facile and scalable disposable sensor based on laser engraved graphene for electrochemical detection of glucose. *Scientific Reports*, *6*(1), 27975.

50. Mamleyev, E. R., Heissler, S., Nefedov, A., Weidler, P. G., Nordin, N., Kudryashov, V. V., ... Sharma, S. (2019). Laser-induced hierarchical carbon patterns on polyimide substrates for flexible urea sensors. *NPJ Flexible Electronics*, *3*(1), 2.

51. Hui, X., Xuan, X., Kim, J., & Park, J. Y. (2019). A highly flexible and selective dopamine sensor based on Pt-Au nanoparticle-modified laser-induced graphene. *Electrochimica Acta*, *328*, 135066.

52. Kucherenko, I. S., Sanborn, D., Chen, B., Garland, N., Serhan, M., Forzani, E., ... Claussen, J. C. (2020). Ion-selective sensors based on laser-induced graphene for evaluating human hydration levels using urine samples. *Advanced Materials Technologies*, *5*(6), 1901037.

53. Yagati, A. K., Behrent, A., Beck, S., Rink, S., Goepferich, A. M., Min, J., ... Baeumner, A. J. (2020). Laser-induced graphene interdigitated electrodes for label-free or nano-label-enhanced highly sensitive capacitive aptamer-based biosensors. *Biosensors and Bioelectronics*, *164*, 112272.

54. Beitollahi, H., Nejad, F. G., & Shakeri, S. (2017). GO/Fe 3 O 4@ SiO 2 core–shell nanocomposite-modified graphite screen-printed electrode for sensitive and selective electrochemical sensing of dopamine and uric acid. *Analytical Methods*, *9*(37), 5541–5549.

55. Boonkaew, S., Chaiyo, S., Jampasa, S., Rengpipat, S., Siangproh, W., & Chailapakul, O. (2019). An origami paper-based electrochemical immunoassay for the C-reactive protein using a screen-printed carbon electrode modified with graphene and gold nanoparticles. *Microchimica Acta*, *186*(3), 1–10.

56. Pu, Z., Wang, R., Wu, J., Yu, H., Xu, K., & Li, D. (2016). A flexible electrochemical glucose sensor with composite nanostructured surface of the working electrode. *Sensors and Actuators B: Chemical*, *230*, 801–809.

57. Soares, R. R., Hjort, R. G., Pola, C. C., Parate, K., Reis, E. L., Soares, N. F., ... Gomes, C. L. (2020). Laser-induced graphene electrochemical immunosensors for rapid and label-free monitoring of Salmonella enterica in chicken broth. *ACS Sensors*, *5*(7), 1900–1911.

58. Huang, C., Wen, T., Shi, F. J., Zeng, X. Y., & Jiao, Y. J. (2020). Rapid detection of IgM antibodies against the SARS-CoV-2 virus via colloidal gold nanoparticle-based lateral-flow assay. *ACS Omega*, *5*(21), 12550–12556.

59. Mittelmann, A. S., Ron, E. Z., &Rishpon, J. (2002). Amperometric quantification of total coliforms and specific detection of Escherichia c oli. *Analytical Chemistry*, *74*(4), 903–907.

60. Shabani, A., Zourob, M., Allain, B., Marquette, C. A., Lawrence, M. F., & Mandeville, R. (2008). Bacteriophage-modified microarrays for the direct impedimetric detection of bacteria. *Analytical Chemistry*, *80*(24), 9475–9482.

Part IV

Infectious Diseases Detection and Treatment Planning

7 Smart Healthcare Systems in Combating Infectious Diseases Outbreaks

Maheswata Moharana,
Prakash Chandra Maharana, Fahmida Khan,
and Subrat Kumar Pattanayak

7.1 INTRODUCTION

Smart healthcare systems play an imperative role in the fight against infectious diseases by utilizing cutting-edge technologies and data analytics to enhance outbreak management, identification, treatment, and prevention [1]. The current pandemic condition worldwide is indicative of an increased occurrence of infectious diseases caused by microorganisms [2]. The well-being of the general population, and possibly the economy is in risk due to the faster and relatively rapid spread of infectious diseases [3]. Smart healthcare systems can track and examine health information continually from a variety of sources, including wearable technology [4], electronic health records [5], and different social media platforms [6]. These technologies can aid in the early detection of epidemics by spotting trends and anomalies, and enabling healthcare officials to act quickly to stop the spread of diseases. Smart healthcare systems can foresee the probable spread of infectious diseases using machine learning (ML) algorithms [7]. This lessens the impact of the outbreak by enabling healthcare professionals and public health organizations to properly allocate resources and undertake preventive actions in high-risk locations. Remote patient monitoring and telemedicine consultations are made possible by smart healthcare technologies [8], which lowers the risk of disease transmission in medical institutions. Without physically visiting a hospital, patients can receive medical advice and care, which is important during infectious disease outbreaks. To locate and alert individuals who had direct contact with infected patients, smart healthcare systems can use contact tracing tools [9]. This aids in serving the line of transmission and stops the disease from spreading further. Smart healthcare systems make it easier for hospitals, public health organizations, and academics to share real-time data [10]. This information sharing improves coordination and allows for greater awareness of the diseases,

DOI: 10.1201/9781003464884-11

157

resulting in more accurate assessments and actions. Smart healthcare systems can help in the development of individualized treatment programmes by analysing the data on each unique patient. By ensuring that patients receive the best possible care, this strategy improves outcomes and lessens the spread of infectious diseases [11]. Modern healthcare systems can help ensure that vaccines are distributed effectively during outbreaks. Additionally, they may keep on checking the rate of vaccination administration and adverse reactions, allowing healthcare administrators to quickly address any security issues [12]. AI can be used by sophisticated healthcare systems to speed up the drug discovery process [13]. The discovery of novel medicines can be accelerated by using AI algorithms to analyse enormous volumes of biological data and identify prospective medication candidates to target certain infectious pathogens. Smart healthcare systems are capable of providing the general population with accurate and current information regarding infectious diseases [14]. This encourages preventive measures, invalidates myths, and raises awareness, all of which improves public health outcomes. Optimization of resources is important because healthcare resources may be constrained during infectious disease epidemics. In order to make sure that hospital beds, medical supplies, and staff are used effectively where they are most needed, smart healthcare systems can help optimize resource allocation [15]. Smart healthcare systems greatly develop our capacity to effectively combat infectious diseases and safeguard public health by merging data-driven and cutting-edge technologies. The potential advantage of these systems must be weighed against issues related to security, privacy, and ethics.

7.2 INFECTIOUS DISEASES

Human health has been significantly hampered by contagious diseases. These diseases are caused by microbes including viruses, fungi, bacteria, and parasites. They can spread from person to person through several methods [16]. Despite enormous advances in medicine and healthcare infectious diseases still present risk to global health [17]. The tendency of infectious diseases to spread quickly among populations is one of their key traits [18]. Depending on the particular microorganism involved, the ease of transmission varies. When an infected individual coughs, some infections, including the common cold and influenza, spread by respiratory droplets [19]. Other infections, like human immunodeficiency virus (HIV) and hepatitis B are mostly spread by contact with infected blood and fluids [20, 21]. Furthermore, insect-borne diseases like malaria and Lyme diseases are spread by mosquitos and ticks, respectively [22]. It can have a variety of effects, from minor discomfort to serious illness and even death [23]. Some infections, however, can result in chronic problems or long-term effects, whereas many infections cause self-limiting illnesses [24]. For instance, untreated sexually transmitted infections can raise the chance of developing certain carcinomas or cause infertility [25]. Additionally, infectious diseases have the potential to have wider-reaching effects on society, such as decreased productivity, increased healthcare expenses, and stress on the healthcare systems during outbreaks [26].

The detection, diagnosis, and treatment of infectious diseases have greatly benefited from modern scientific and medical developments. One of the best methods for preventing infectious diseases has been vaccination [27]. Smallpox has been eradicated because of vaccination [28], and other infections like polio and measles have seen sharp declines in prevalence [29]. Resistance to vaccines and vaccine hesitancy have emerged as obstacles to attaining total control over some illnesses. Outbreaks of infectious diseases continue to draw attention on a global scale. The continued threat posed by infectious diseases is highlighted by the appearance of novel infectious agents, such as the severe acute respiratory syndrome coronavirus-2 (SARS-CoV-2), which caused the COVID-19 [30–33]. Due to their potential to start pandemics, zoonotic diseases, which originate in animals and can spread to humans, have also drawn more attention [34]. In the past year, researchers discovered nearly 1,500 new unidentified pathogens of animal origin, including the human immunodeficiency virus, Ebola virus, and influenza virus [35]. To stop outbreaks from turning into major global health emergencies, public health officials must continue to be on the lookout for them and act quickly when they do [36]. A variety of strategies are usually used in the prevention and management of infectious diseases, such as immunization, proper personal hygiene, antimicrobial drugs, vector control, and public health initiatives. Furthermore, the burden of many infectious diseases has significantly decreased in developed nations due to advancements in public health and medical science.

7.3 DIAGNOSTIC ASPECTS FOR TREATING INFECTIOUS DISEASES

Identification of bacterial pathogens, infection causes, diagnostics, treatment, healthcare costs, and minimizing illness impacts are all included in the concept of infection management [37]. Assessment of microbial infection is the first step in disease management, followed by deliberate choices about the treatment of chronic patients. Sometimes an infectious disease outbreak goes untreated for a while, allowing the virus to spread covertly and cause severe epidemics. Therefore, in order to serve as efficient detectors and first-line responders, clinical awareness and the pertinent understanding of diagnostic instruments are extremely needed. Most essentially, the best method to stop the spread of these infections and lessen their effects is through early and precise diagnosis in the fight against emerging infections. The common diagnostic methods rely on the types of infectious diseases and microbial species [38]. Aptamers, antibodies, entire pathogens, and the molecular components of infectious agents (such as proteins and nucleic acids) are examples of common disease biomarkers. Traditional techniques that are widely used and regarded to be efficient diagnostics for infectious diseases include microscopy and culture [39]. However, there are a number of difficulties with these methods when trying to detect viral markers, including the limited sensitivity of microscopy techniques, and the requirement for highly qualified persons and techniques in order to perform accurate tests. Additionally, due to culturing and drug susceptibility testing, these traditional diagnostics also take longer for clinical interpretations. Due to their higher sensitivity and quicker infection detection than traditional methods, molecular technologies have also enhanced laboratories' throughput [40]. Among various molecular techniques, enzyme-linked immunosorbent assay [41], nucleic acid amplification [42], colorimetric [43], and other advanced biotechnological technologies are gaining popularity and are frequently used in clinical microbiology laboratories. However, these techniques have a number of drawbacks, including the fact that they are labour-intensive, time-consuming, and too expensive for regular clinical diagnosis. The World Health Organization (WHO) even recommends the use of automated diagnostic tools like proteome chips, microfluidic, colorimetric assay, and other advanced molecular approaches for usage in emergency and remote situations due to the ongoing evolution of these technologies [44]. The choice of an acceptable diagnostic method is based on a number of factors, including sensitivity, selectivity, cost, duration of time needed for the diagnosis, and accessibility to diagnostic equipment. Rapid diagnostic techniques can aid in more effective, dependable, and cost-effective management of infectious disease transmission. A breakthrough idea called "smart healthcare" uses cutting-edge technology to turn conventional medical procedures into highly effective and individualized experiences for both patients and healthcare professionals [45]. The healthcare sector is leading this change into the digital era as the world moves forward, forwarding the way for a more efficient and inclusive approach to healthcare. The potential of smart healthcare to revolutionize medicine and benefit humanity is explored in this chapter along with its many facets.

The Internet of Things (IoT) and wearable technology are essential components of smart healthcare [46]. Through the use of these networked devices, patients and medical professionals can remotely monitor a variety of health factors [47]. People can monitor their heart rate, sleep habits, physical activity, and more with wearable technology like smartwatches, fitness trackers, and health monitors. This constant flow of information enables people to make smart lifestyle choices that will protect their health and enhance their general well-being [48]. The IoT is a cutting-edge technology that is utilized for biometric measurements including blood pressure, heart rate, and glucose levels [49]. Due to the widespread availability of smartphones [50] nowadays, IoT-based healthcare systems leveraging mobile computing may readily access the data they want from consumers. The IoT-based home hospitalization systems, cloud computing, and fog computing are the three most significant technologies that have made a substantial contribution to the growth of the healthcare sector. The IoT-supported fog safety monitoring system can be used to monitor Aedes mosquito outbreaks in vulnerable places and assists governmental organizations with dengue prevention and control because there is no reliable method for straight monitoring or detecting Aedes mosquitoes that transmit viral infections [51].

Medical diagnosis and therapy have been transformed through the application of ML and AI in the healthcare industry [52]. Large volumes of medical data, including patient records and research papers, can be analysed by AI algorithms, leading to more precise and quicker diagnosis [53]. Additionally, ML-driven personalized treatment plans are created to meet the needs of each patient, maximizing therapy effectiveness and reducing side effects [54]. Chatbots and virtual assistants powered by AI also improve patient–doctor contact and offer round-the-clock help and guidance in the medical field [55]. Ancient myths and stories that included mechanical

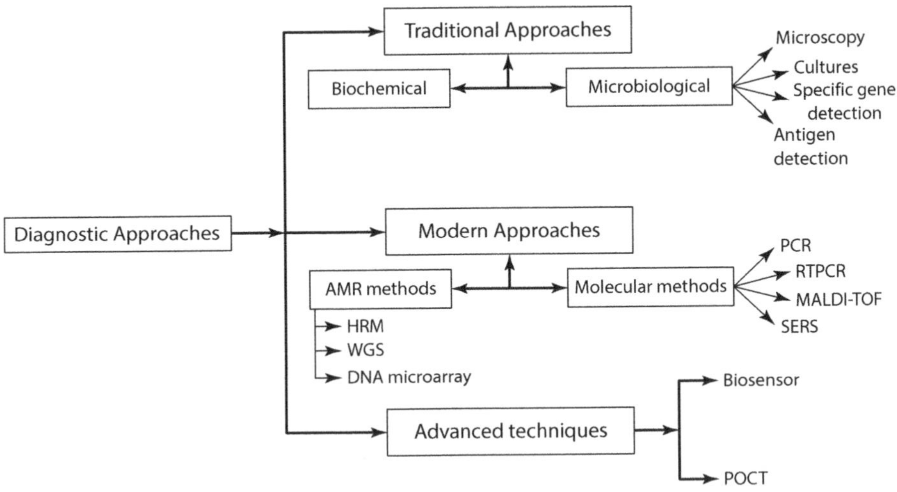

FIGURE 7.1   Different diagnostic approaches to combat infectious diseases.

beings and intelligent inventions predate modern times and predate the concept of artificial intelligence (AI) by centuries. However, AI didn't really start to develop as a field of study until the 20th century. Turing Test is a standard for determining whether a machine can demonstrate intelligence comparable to that of a person [56], which served as the starting point for AI study and motivated a generation of researchers to work towards the goal of building intelligent machines [57]. AI programmes like the logic theorist and general problem solver showed that robots were capable of carrying out human-like activities [58]. But as a result of failed expectations and financial issues, an "AI winter" in the 1970s and 1980s quickly replaced the original enthusiasm [59]. The 1990s witnessed the rebirth of AI, driven by improvements in computing power, the accessibility of enormous amounts of data, and modernizations in algorithms and machine learning methods [60]. The back propagation method and the progress of neural networks have enabled substantial advancements in pattern recognition and data processing. During this time, applications for AI in speech recognition, picture processing, and natural language comprehension began to appear [61] (Figure **7.1**).

7.4 KEY CONCEPTS AND APPLICATION OF ARTIFICIAL INTELLIGENCE

Machine learning is a branch of artificial intelligence that focuses on allowing computers to learn from data and develop over time without explicit programming. The three basic categories of machine learning methodologies are supervised, unsupervised, and reinforcement learning [62]. The goal of AI-driven robotics is to build machines that can work independently or in combination with people. AI is transforming the robotics industry, from surgical robots to industrial automation [63].

Using computer vision, it is possible for machines to comprehend and interpret visual data from the outside world exactly like people do [64]. Applications for this topic can be found in robots, autonomous cars, facial recognition, and medical imaging. Artificial neural networks are used in deep learning, a specialized type of machine learning, to process and interpret complex data. It has completely changed fields like speech recognition, natural language processing, and computer vision [65]. The ability of machines to recognize, decipher, and produce human language is known as natural language processing [66].

The crucial element of AI is the control strategy adopted by the agent, which describes how inputs from sensors are converted to actuators, or more simply, how the sensors are mapped to actuators [67]. This is made possible by a function within the agent. AI aims to provide machine intelligence similar to that of humans [68]. However, achieving such a goal is possible because of learning algorithms that imitate how the human brain learns. Machine learning, a discipline that developed from artificial intelligence, is crucial because it enables machines to develop intelligence comparable to that of humans without explicit programming [69]. However, AI programmes handle the more fascinating tasks, like email spam detection, photo tagging, and web search [70, 71]. Therefore, machine learning was developed as a new computing capability, and it now has an impact on several industrial sectors as well as in fundamental research.

Recently, the agriculture industry has seen the application of AI. To increase production, the agricultural industry must overcome a number of obstacles, including poor soil management, insect and disease infestation, the need for large amounts of data, low output, and a knowledge gap between farmers and technology. The major ideas behind AI in agriculture are its adaptability, excellence, accuracy, and economy [72]. In order to increase crop yields and use less water, fertilizer, and pesticides, AI systems will be able to anticipate which crop to grow in a given year and when the ideal times to sow and harvest are in a certain area. By utilizing AI technology, it is possible to lessen the impact on natural ecosystems and improve worker safety, which will help to keep food prices low and guarantee that food production will keep up with the growing population [73, 74]. AI technology can be used in a variety of ways to fight cybercrime. There are ideas for using neural networks in Denial of Service (DoS) detection, computer worm detection, spam detection, Zombie detection, malware classification, and forensic investigations. Newer versions of anti-virus software have also been developed using AI techniques like data mining, neural networks, and heuristics [75]. Natural disasters have increased in frequency and severity, resulting in catastrophic damage and severe economic loss [76]. Every day, huge amounts of data, including actual data and simulated data, are produced. Disaster management can be supported by using either type of data. Large amounts of actual data are now available due to the development of information and communication technologies including social media, telecommunications data, and remote sensing. Real data are occasionally hard to find. Many computational models [77, 78] are created to produce simulation data for evaluating the disaster-induced impact and identifying vulnerable structures. Enough big data, collected fast, and processed in large quantities are required to enable efficient disaster management.

It is becoming more and more common to employ AI to quickly extract relevant and accurate information from the large amount of data being analysed to enable successful decision-making in disaster management [79]. Enhanced individualized financial advice, fraud detection, and algorithmic trading are all made possible by AI-driven algorithms in the financial sector. By extracting hidden patterns from data to enhance the accuracy of financial judgements, AI is speeding up the development of financial services. But in addition to frequently demanded properties like model correctness, financial services also need reliable AI with qualities that haven't been fully realized [80]. In business sectors, virtual assistants improve customer service, chatbots, and expedite communications. The AI-based software chatbots stimulate human conversation and it is designed to serve as the virtual assistant's primary entertainment function. Business organizations are also using chatbots more frequently since they may cut down on the price of customer care while simultaneously supporting numerous customers [81].

Artificial intelligence assists healthcare professionals in reducing documentation time by digitally preserving patient data and creating a database that can be utilized for regular medical care, diagnosis, and treatment. In the present scenario, doctors and surgeons become more inventive due to the development of AI. These intelligent machines behave like humans and quickly pick up on the language used to capture medical data, text, photos, bioinformatics, and financial transactions. For flawless decision-making, these machines are capable of understanding human language [82]. By giving the patient the necessary information, it makes possible for an accurate surgery. With the use of AI technology, it is possible to identify patients, gather sufficient amounts of high-quality patient data, and utilize that information to forecast patient outcomes, shorten hospital stays, and reduce risk during joint replacements while also increasing the likelihood that patients will recover [83]. In scanning technologies like X-rays, computed tomography, magnetic resonance imaging, and three-dimensional scanners, AI is a crucial factor. These can be used to help in patient decision-making. AI also recommends a healthy diet and eating behaviours. It effectively handles patient scheduling and sends appointment reminders [84]. AI can address a variety of medical issues, such as resolving various levels of complexity while carrying out intricate operations with higher quality and results. The several other applications of AI in the healthcare sector are to predict upcoming diseases, precise and effective diagnosis, gather information during surgery that will help to better upcoming operations, increase pathological results, maintain clinical records, proper training for medical students, and be helpful for complicated and new treatments [85].

All things taken into account, like predictive modelling, resource allocation, genome analysis and monitoring, AI is crucial for controlling infectious diseases since it makes it easier for us to detect, prevent, and control epidemics. It allows for a data-driven approach to manage these health issues and support conventional public initiatives (Figure **7.2**).

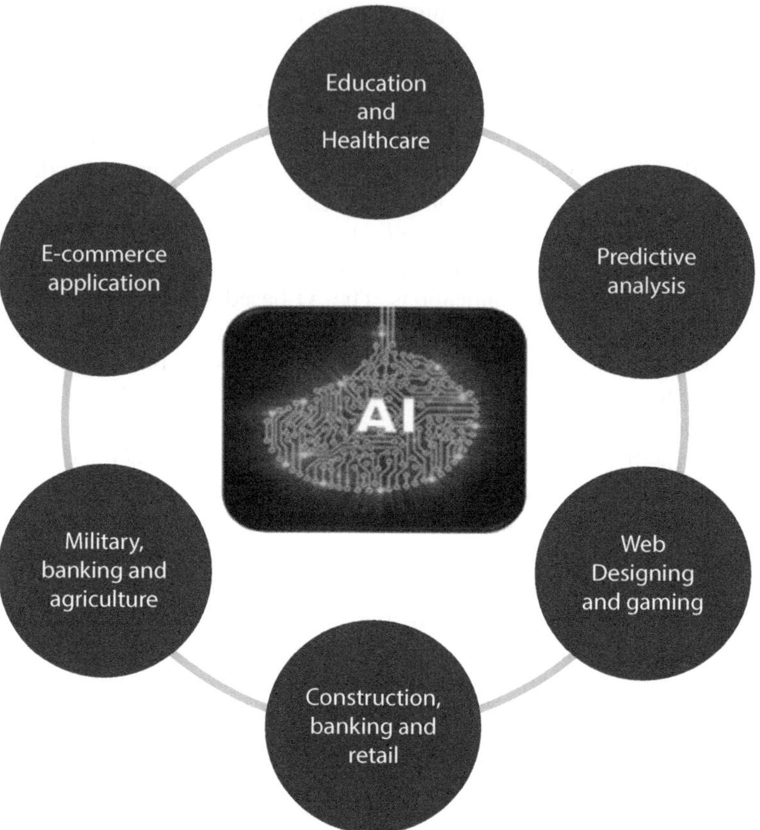

FIGURE 7.2 Applications of artificial intelligence (AI).

7.4.1 MACHINE LEARNING

One of the most transformational, revolutionary, and emerging technologies of the 21st century was machine learning. It is a subset of artificial intelligence (AI) that gives computer systems the ability to learn from data, spot patterns, and make wise judgements without having to be explicitly programmed. Machine learning has become increasingly useful over the years in a variety of fields, including healthcare, finance, transportation, and entertainment. The idea of creating intelligent machines was in between 1940 and 1950, when machine learning began [86]. However, the phrase "machine learning" wasn't even coined until the 1960s. ML algorithms and techniques made great progress in the 1980s and 1990s as a result of improvements in computing power and the accessibility of massive datasets [87]. With the emergence of deep learning in the 2000s, a branch of artificial neural networks with several layers capable of learning hierarchical representations, machine learning experienced a paradigm change. Since then, deep learning has revolutionized a number of fields, including speech recognition, natural language processing, and computer vision [88]. The important features of ML algorithm are the algorithm is trained on labelled data in supervised learning, where input data are linked with appropriate target labels [89]. In order to make predictions on new, unknown data, the algorithm must learn a mapping between inputs and outputs. In unsupervised learning, the algorithm is trained on unlabelled data and remains to discover patterns or structures on its own. Common unsupervised learning tasks include dimensionality reduction and clustering. In behavioural psychology, an agent learns to act in a way that maximizes a cumulative reward; this is the basis of reinforcement learning. Trial and error are involved, and the agent receives feedback in the form of rewards or punishments [90]. The well-known ML algorithms include Support Vector Machines, Neural Networks, and Random Forest. It has a substantial impact on finance, transportation, natural language processing, healthcare sectors, and image and video analysis. The application of ML in healthcare has significant advantages for both medical professionals and patients. Some of the extremely extensively used applications in healthcare sectors are automating healthcare invoicing, offering medical decision support, and developing regulations for medical treatment. There are numerous instances of how ML and healthcare models are used in medicine. The wide range of ML applications in general healthcare that are currently being used includes improved radiotherapy, individualized treatment, crowdsourced data collection, smart health records, ML-based behavioural modification, clinical trials, and research [91]. To anticipate serious side effects for patients receiving radiation therapy for head and neck cancers, the first machine learning approach has been developed [92]. Deep learning-based ML system in healthcare analyses radiology reports, scans, and conventional radiography to identify complex patterns automatically in radiology and help radiologists make wise decisions [93, 94]. There are numerous instances of ML techniques and algorithms being utilized to develop clinical decision support systems that aid physicians. One instance is the classification of the mortality risk of patients with the disease COVID-19 using an ensemble model made up of four independent models, namely a neural network, a gradient-boosted decision tree, a support vector machine, and logistic regression [95]. There are numerous additional examples of clinical decision support systems that help with the treatment of periodontal disease, early detection of circular RNAs, the identification of shock situations, and aiding with back pain self-referral decisions [96]. In order to obtain the higher accurate feature, which is a crucial learning module, the technique of automatic classification of COVID-19 can be applied by comparing general deep learning-based feature extraction frameworks. Among a group of deep convolutional neural networks (CNN), Dense Net, Res Net were chosen. After that, the classification was accomplished by feeding the collected features through a few machine learning classifiers to identify them as a COVID-19 or other cases of diseases [97]. Modern machine learning algorithms can evaluate and integrate vast amounts of data pertaining to COVID-19 patients to offer the best understanding of the viral spread pattern, boost diagnostic precision, enhance novel, efficient therapeutic approaches, and even identify people who are at risk of the disease based on genetic and physiological characteristics [98]. In order to effectively address the infodemic at the grassroots level among the general public, health applications must use machine learning to give the correct information while continuously understanding misinformation patterns [99].

7.4.2 DIFFERENT AI AND ML TECHNOLOGIES USED IN THE SMART HEALTH SYSTEMS

AI is a group of technologies rather than a single one. Although the specific work and processes that these technologies assist vary greatly, the majority of them have immediate significance to the healthcare sector. The following provides an overview of a few specific AI technologies that are very significant to the healthcare industry.

7.4.2.1 Natural Language Processing

Natural language processing (NLP) is most commonly used in the healthcare industry for the generation, interpretation, and categorization of published research and clinical documentation. NLP systems can perform conversational AI, create reports, evaluate unstructured clinical notes on patients, and translate patient interactions [100]. Applications in speech recognition, text analysis, translation, and other language-related fields are included in the field of NLP [101]. Semantic and statistical NLP are the two main methods for approaching it. Recent improvements in recognition accuracy have been attributed to statistical NLP, which is based on machine learning, specifically deep learning neural network [102].

7.4.2.2 Robotic Process Automation

Using information systems, this technology performs structured digital tasks for administrative purposes as if they were being performed by a human user adhering to a script or set of guidelines. These technologies are less expensive, simpler to programme, and behave transparently in comparison to other types of AI [103]. Robotic process automation uses computer programmes running on servers instead of actual robots. It acts as a semi-intelligent user of the information systems through a combination of workflow, business rules, and "presentation layer" integration [104]. This technology performs routine tasks in the healthcare industry, such as prior atomization, billing, and patient record updates. In conjunction with other technologies such as image recognition, they can be employed to retrieve information from e.g. faxed photographs for incorporation into transactional systems [105].

7.4.2.3 Rule-Based Expert System

For expert systems, to create a set of rules in a certain knowledge domain, knowledge engineers and human experts are needed [106]. They are simple to understand and function well up to a level. But they frequently implode when there are a lot of rules – often thousands or more and when those rules start to contradict one another. In addition, rules can be complex and time-consuming to modify if the knowledge domain changes. More methods in healthcare that rely on data and machine learning algorithms are gradually replacing them. In the 1980s, expert systems that relied on sets of "if–then" rules dominated AI technology and were widely employed in the previous and later decades for commercial purposes [107]. They have been widely used in the healthcare industry for "clinical decision support" purposes for a few decades, and their use is still widespread today. Nowadays, a lot of sectors that offer electronic health record systems include a set of guidelines.

7.5 CHALLENGES AND OPPORTUNITIS OF AI AND ML APPROACHES

The challenges facing AI in healthcare must be addressed as more and more healthcare organizations engage in using this technology for a variety of purposes. There are numerous ethical and regulatory issues that may not apply in other contexts. The most significant challenges are obtaining physician approval and trust, integrating AI with current information technology systems, data privacy and security, patient safety and accuracy, training algorithms to identify trends in medical data, and making sure regulatory guidelines are followed [108]. AI systems acquire a lot of personal health data, which might be misused if not handled appropriately. For this reason, data privacy is very crucial [109]. Furthermore, it is imperative to implement appropriate security protocols to safeguard confidential patient information against malevolent use. By using machine learning, we can link current data for the predictions of potential diseases. Better forecasts require novel methods that maximize data information while utilizing the best ML model, improve clinical results and tackle major healthcare issues with continuous data inflow. Advanced analytics and automation, together with reliable anomaly detection in diagnostics and disease screening, are just two examples of the many areas where ML may improve decision-making. Increasing administrative efficiency and reducing waste, fraud, and abuse in the healthcare industry are other factors [110]. The data that AI systems receive instruction may contain biases, which may end up with unfair results. It is a huge challenge to ensure fairness and minimize bias [111]. Considering that AI systems analyse enormous volumes of personal data, preserving privacy and avoiding abuse are top priorities. And, increasing job automation may result in major job displacement, necessitating programmes to reskill and upskill workers [112], which are the major challenges of AI approaches. The pharmaceutical industry and researchers consider that drug development should take less time and be less expensive. Molecular docking has been widely used to filtre the most desired drug candidates. Machine learning can introduce new methods for scoring a complex in molecular docking methods either by improving an existing scoring function or developing a new scoring function using the structure of a complex as input. In addition, ML is occasionally applied to the virtual screening process and binding prediction tasks. The ML model can be developed once the data set has been selected and the data representation has been determined [113]. Though both AI and ML have demonstrated enormous potential in the fight against infectious diseases, both ML and AI techniques also address a number of obstacles like data privacy, interpretability, generalization, and security risks. Data scientists, medical practitioners, and ethical experts must work together to address these issues to ensure that AI and ML technologies can effectively treat infectious diseases while minimizing any potential negative effects.

7.6 CONCLUSION AND FUTURE PERSPECTIVE

Machine learning has a substantial impact on the development of smart healthcare systems. Here are some possible viewpoints. In order to provide precise diagnoses and find trends, machine learning algorithms can scan vast amounts of patient data, genetic data and medical records, and test results. Healthcare can become more successful and efficient when AI-powered systems can recommend individualized treatment solutions based on unique patient features. Real-time analysis of patient data by machine learning algorithms can be used to forecast the propensity for specific diseases or consequences. Healthcare professionals may be able to intervene earlier and more successfully prevent or manage problems with its aid. For instance, using genetic data and lifestyle factors, AI algorithms can forecast the likelihood of strokes or heart attacks. Vital signs and other health indicators can be remotely monitored constantly by sensors and devices driven by AI. This makes it possible for medical professionals to immediately identify any changes or irregularities and take appropriate action. In addition to enabling remote consultations and giving patients individualized healthcare advice, telehealth platforms powered by AI can also lessen the need for in-person visits and increase access to healthcare. It can find prospective medication candidates and forecast their efficacy and safety by analyzing enormous datasets of biological and chemical data. This has the potential to significantly speed up the process of discovering novel drugs and developing new therapeutics for a variety of ailments. To create individualized treatment regimens, machine learning algorithms can examine patient data, including genetics, lifestyle choices, and medical history. This can assist healthcare professionals in customizing therapies to meet the unique needs of each patient, enhancing outcomes and minimizing negative effects. By automating administrative duties, optimizing workflows, and enhancing resource allocation, AI-powered technologies can improve hospital operations. This can lower expenses, increase effectiveness, and free up healthcare workers to concentrate on patient care. Patients can receive individualized health information, have their queries answered, and receive advice on how to manage their diseases via these chatbots and virtual assistants. As a result, patients may be more motivated to participate actively in their treatment and have better overall health results. Ethics related to data privacy, security, and bias become more crucial as machine learning and AI are integrated more deeply into healthcare systems. Building trust and guaranteeing the success of intelligent healthcare systems will rely heavily on ensuring that patient data are protected and utilized properly. Overall, machine learning and AI in smart healthcare systems have a bright future in terms of enhancing patient outcomes, boosting productivity, and revolutionizing the way healthcare is provided. To make sure that these technologies are applied in a responsible and advantageous way, it is crucial to address the difficulties and ethical issues.

ACKNOWLEDGEMENTS

M. Moharana, F. Khan, S. K. Pattanayak are thankful to the Department of Chemistry, National Institute of Technology, Raipur, for providing laboratory facilities and support.

REFERENCES

1. Minopoulos, G. M., Memos, V. A., Stergiou, C. L., Stergiou, K. D., Plageras, A. P., Koidou, M. P., & Psannis, K. E. (2022). Exploitation of emerging technologies and advanced networks for a smart healthcare system. *Applied Sciences*, 12(12), 5859.
2. Morse, S. S. (2001). Factors in the Emergence of Infectious Diseases. Plagues and Politics: Infectious Disease and International Policy. In *Plagues and Politics. Global Issues Series*, Price-Smith, A.T. (ed.). London: Palgrave Macmillan, (pp. 8–26). https://doi.org/10.1057/9780230524248_2
3. Wu, T., Perrings, C., Kinzig, A., Collins, J. P., Minteer, B. A., & Daszak, P. (2017). Economic growth, urbanization, globalization, and the risks of emerging infectious diseases in China: A review. *Ambio – A Journal of the Human Environment*, 46(1), 18–29.
4. Safavi, S., & Shukur, Z. (2014). Conceptual privacy framework for health information on wearable device. *PLoS One*, 9(12), e114306.
5. Safadi, H., Chan, D., Dawes, M., Roper, M., & Faraj, S. (2015). Open-source health information technology: A case study of electronic medical records. *Health Policy and Technology*, 4(1), 14–28.
6. Kallinikos, J., & Tempini, N. (2014). Patient data as medical facts: Social media practices as a foundation for medical knowledge creation. *Information Systems Research*, 25(4), 817–833.
7. Surya, L. (2018). How government can use AI and ML to identify spreading infectious diseases. *International Journal of Creative Research Thoughts (IJCRT)*, 6(1), 899–902. https://ssrn.com/abstract=3785649
8. Taiwo, O., & Ezugwu, A. E. (2020). Smart healthcare support for remote patient monitoring during Covid-19 quarantine. *Informatics in Medicine Unlocked*, 20, 100428.
9. Mbunge, E. (2020). Integrating emerging technologies into COVID-19 contact tracing: Opportunities, challenges and pitfalls. *Diabetes and Metabolic Syndrome: Clinical Research and Reviews*, 14(6), 1631–1636.
10. Shuo, T., Wenbo, Y.,Jehane, M. L. G.,Peng , W.,Wei, H., & Zhewe, Y. (2019) Smart healthcare: making medical care more intelligent. *Global Health Journal*,3(3), 62–65. https://doi.org/10.1016/j.glohj.2019.07.001.
11. Pereira, L., Mutesa, L., Tindana, P., & Ramsay, M. (2021). African genetic diversity and adaptation inform a precision medicine agenda. *Nature Reviews. Genetics*, 22(5), 284–306.
12. Manupati, V. K., Schoenherr, T., Subramanian, N., Ramkumar, M., Soni, B., & Panigrahi, S. (2021). A multi-echelon dynamic cold chain for managing vaccine distribution. *Transportation Research: Part E: Logistics and Transportation Review*, 156, 102542.
13. Álvarez-Machancoses, Ó., & Fernández-Martínez, J. L. (2019). Using artificial intelligence methods to speed up drug discovery. *Expert Opinion on Drug Discovery*, 14(8), 769–777.
14. Kapoor, A., Guha, S., Das, M. K., Goswami, K. C., & Yadav, R. (2020). Digital healthcare: The only solution for better healthcare during COVID-19 pandemic? *Indian Heart Journal*, 72(2), 61–64.

15. Oueida, S., Aloqaily, M., & Ionescu, S. (2019). A smart healthcare reward model for resource allocation in smart city. *Multimedia Tools and Applications*, 78(17), 24573–24594.

16. Agrebi, S., & Larbi, A. (2020). Use of artificial intelligence in infectious diseases. In *Artificial Intelligence in Precision Health*, Debmalya Bar (ed.), (pp. 415–438). Academic Press. https://doi.org/10.1016/B978-0-12-817133-2.00018-5.

17. Fauci, A. S. (2001). Infectious diseases: Considerations for the 21st century. *Clinical Infectious Diseases*, 32(5), 675–685.

18. Leung, K., Jit, M., Lau, E. H., & Wu, J. T. (2017). Social contact patterns relevant to the spread of respiratory infectious diseases in Hong Kong. *Scientific Reports*, 7(1), 7974.

19. Dhand, R., & Li, J. (2020). Coughs and sneezes: Their role in transmission of respiratory viral infections, including SARS-CoV-2. *American Journal of Respiratory and Critical Care Medicine*, 202(5), 651–659.

20. Hu, D. J., Kane, M. A., & Heymann, D. L. (1991). Transmission of HIV, hepatitis B virus, and other bloodborne pathogens in health care settings: A review of risk factors and guidelines for prevention. World Health Organization. *Bulletin of the World Health Organization*, 69(5), 623.

21. Centers for Disease Control and Prevention. (2017). *HIV and Viral Hepatitis. South Carolina State Documents Depository*. Centers for Disease Control and Prevention.

22. Baneth, G. (2014). Tick-borne infections of animals and humans: A common ground. *International Journal for Parasitology*, 44(9), 591–596.

23. Rubin, R. H. (1993). Infectious disease complications of renal transplantation. *Kidney International*, 44(1), 221–236.

24. Kramer-Schadt, S., Fernández, N., Eisinger, D., Grimm, V., & Thulke, H. H. (2009). Individual variations in infectiousness explain long-term disease persistence in wildlife populations. *Oikos*, 118(2), 199–208.

25. Gottlieb, S. L., Low, N., Newman, L. M., Bolan, G., Kamb, M., & Broutet, N. (2014). Toward global prevention of sexually transmitted infections (STIs): The need for STI vaccines. *Vaccine*, 32(14), 1527–1535.

26. Auld, G., Bernstein, S., Cashore, B., & Levin, K. (2021). Managing pandemics as super wicked problems: Lessons from, and for, COVID-19 and the climate crisis. *Policy Sciences*, 54(4), 707–728.

27. Li, Q., Li, M., Lv, L., Guo, C., & Lu, K. (2017). A new prediction model of infectious diseases with vaccination strategies based on evolutionary game theory. *Chaos, Solitons, and Fractals*, 104, 51–60.

28. Rao, A. K., Petersen, B. W., Whitehill, F., Razeq, J. H., Isaacs, S. N., Merchlinsky, M. J., … Bell, B. P. (2022). Use of JYNNEOS (smallpox and monkeypox vaccine, live, non-replicating) for preexposure vaccination of persons at risk for occupational exposure to orthopoxviruses: Recommendations of the Advisory Committee on Immunization Practices—United States, 2022. *Morbidity and Mortality Weekly Report*, 71(22), 734.

29. De Melker, H. E., Van den Hof, S., Berbers, G. A. M., & Conyn-van Spaendonck, M. A. E. (2003). Evaluation of the national immunisation programme in the Netherlands: Immunity to diphtheria, tetanus, poliomyelitis, measles, mumps, rubella and Haemophilus influenzae type b. *Vaccine*, 21(7–8), 716–720.

30. Acter, T., Uddin, N., Das, J., Akhter, A., Choudhury, T. R., & Kim, S. (2020). Evolution of severe acute respiratory syndrome coronavirus 2 (SARS-CoV-2) as coronavirus disease 2019 (COVID-19) pandemic: A global health emergency. *Science of the Total Environment*, 730, 138996.

31. Tso, F. Y., Lidenge, S. J., Peña, P. B., Clegg, A. A., Ngowi, J. R., Mwaiselage, J., … Wood, C. (2021). High prevalence of pre-existing serological cross-reactivity against severe acute respiratory syndrome coronavirus-2 (SARS-CoV-2) in sub-Saharan Africa. *International Journal of Infectious Diseases*, 102, 577–583.

32. Harapan, B. N., & Yoo, H. J. (2021). Neurological symptoms, manifestations, and complications associated with severe acute respiratory syndrome coronavirus 2 (SARS-CoV-2) and coronavirus disease 19 (COVID-19). *Journal of Neurology*, 268(9), 3059–3071.

33. Chan, J. F. W., Siu, G. K. H., Yuan, S., Ip, J. D., Cai, J. P., Chu, A. W. H., ... To, K. K. W. (2022). Probable animal-to-human transmission of severe acute respiratory syndrome coronavirus 2 (SARS-CoV-2) Delta variant AY. 127 causing a pet shop-related coronavirus disease 2019 (COVID-19) outbreak in Hong Kong. *Clinical Infectious Diseases*, 75(1), e76–e81.

34. Lloyd-Smith, J. O., George, D., Pepin, K. M., Pitzer, V. E., Pulliam, J. R., Dobson, A. P., ... Grenfell, B. T. (2009). Epidemic dynamics at the human-animal interface. science, 326(5958), 1362–1367.

35. Jain, S., Nehra, M., Kumar, R., Dilbaghi, N., Hu, T., Kumar, S., ... Li, C. Z. (2021). Internet of medical things (IoMT)-integrated biosensors for point-of-care testing of infectious diseases. *Biosensors and Bioelectronics*, 179, 113074.

36. Glass, T. A., & Schoch-Spana, M. (2002). Bioterrorism and the people: How to vaccinate a city against panic. *Clinical Infectious Diseases*, 34(2), 217–223.

37. Bissonnette, L., & Bergeron, M. G. (2012). Infectious disease management through point-of-care personalized medicine molecular diagnostic technologies. *Journal of Personalized Medicine*, 2(2), 50–70.

38. Hahn, A., Podbielski, A., Meyer, T., Zautner, A. E., Loderstädt, U., Schwarz, N. G., ... Frickmann, H. (2020). On detection thresholds–a review on diagnostic approaches in the infectious disease laboratory and the interpretation of their results. *Acta Tropica*, 205, 105377.

39. Srivastava, S., Singh, P. K., Vatsalya, V., & Karch, R. C. (2018). Developments in the diagnostic techniques of infectious diseases: Rural and urban prospective. *Advances in Infectious Diseases*, 8(3), 121.

40. Lee, J. H., Seo, H. S., Kwon, J. H., Kim, H. T., Kwon, K. C., Sim, S. J., ... Lee, J. (2015). Multiplex diagnosis of viral infectious diseases (AIDS, hepatitis C, and hepatitis A) based on point of care lateral flow assay using engineered proteinticles. *Biosensors and Bioelectronics*, 69, 213–225.

41. Crowther, J. (2008). Enzyme Linked Immunosorbent Assay (ELISA). Molecular Biomethods Handbook. In *Molecular Biomethods Handbook. Springer Protocols Handbooks*, Walker, J. M. and Rapley, R. (eds.), (pp. 657–682). Humana Press. https://doi.org/10.1007/978-1-60327-375-6_37

42. Tian, T., Shu, B., Jiang, Y., Ye, M., Liu, L., Guo, Z., ... Zhou, X. (2020). An ultralocalized Cas13a assay enables universal and nucleic acid amplification-free single-molecule RNA diagnostics. *ACS Nano*, 15(1), 1167–1178.

43. Krishnan, S. (2022). Colorimetric visual sensors for point-of-needs testing. *Sensors and Actuators Reports*, 4, 100078.

44. Bissonnette, L., & Bergeron, M. G. (2010). Diagnosing infections—Current and anticipated technologies for point-of-care diagnostics and home-based testing. *Clinical Microbiology and Infection*, 16(8), 1044–1053.

45. Younger, M., Morrow-Almeida, H. R., Vindigni, S. M., & Dannenberg, A. L. (2008). The built environment, climate change, and health: Opportunities for co-benefits. *American Journal of Preventive Medicine*, 35(5), 517–526.

46. Alshehri, F., & Muhammad, G. (2020). A comprehensive survey of the Internet of Things (IoT) and AI-based smart healthcare. *IEEE Access*, 9, 3660–3678.

47. Fernandez, F., & Pallis, G. C. (2014, November). Opportunities and challenges of the Internet of Things for healthcare: Systems engineering perspective. *2014 4th International Conference on Wireless Mobile Communication and Healthcare-Transforming Healthcare through Innovations in Mobile and Wireless Technologies (MOBIHEALTH)*. IEEE, pp. 263–266.

48. De Pessemier, T., & Martens, L. (2018). Heart rate monitoring, activity recognition, and recommendation for e-coaching. *Multimedia Tools and Applications*, 77(18), 23317–23334.

49. Mohammed, M. N., Syamsudin, H., Al-Zubaidi, S., AKS, R. R., & Yusuf, E. (2020). Novel COVID-19 detection and diagnosis system using IOT based smart helmet. *International Journal of Psychosocial Rehabilitation*, 24(7), 2296–2303.

50. Nazir, S., Ali, Y., Ullah, N., & García-Magariño, I. (2019). Internet of things for healthcare using effects of mobile computing: A systematic literature review. *Wireless Communications and Mobile Computing*, 2019, 1–20.

51. Sood, S. K., & Mahajan, I. (2017). Wearable IoT sensor-based healthcare system for identifying and controlling Chikungunya virus. *Computers in Industry*, 91, 33–44.

52. Bajwa, J., Munir, U., Nori, A., & Williams, B. (2021). Artificial intelligence in healthcare: Transforming the practice of medicine. *Future Healthcare Journal*, 8(2), e188.

53. Johnson, K. B., Wei, W. Q., Weeraratne, D., Frisse, M. E., Misulis, K., Rhee, K., … Snowdon, J. L. (2021). Precision medicine, AI, and the future of personalized health care. *Clinical and Translational Science*, 14(1), 86–93.

54. Naveed, A. (2023). Transforming clinical trials with informatics and AI/ML: A data-driven approach. *International Journal of Computer Science and Technology*, 7(1), 485–503.

55. Kausar, A., & Ahmad, M. A. (2023). Artificial intelligence—Applications across industries (healthcare, pharma, education). In *Era of Artificial Intelligence*, Rik, D., Madhumi, M., and Chandrani, S. (eds.), (pp. 15–31). Chapman and Hall/CRC.

56. Ray, K. S. (2021). Quest for I (Intelligence) in AI (Artificial Intelligence): A non-elusive attempt. In *Artificial Intelligence-Latest Advances, New Paradigms and Novel Applications*. IntechOpen. doi: 10.5772/intechopen.96324

57. Vinichenko, M.V., Melnichuk, A.V., & Karácsony, P. (2020). Technologies of improving the university efficiency by using artificial intelligence: Motivational aspect. *Entrepreneurship and Sustainability Issues*, 7(4), 2696.

58. Ekmekci, P. E. & Arda, B. (2020). History of artificial intelligence. In *Artificial Intelligence and Bioethics* (pp. 1–15). Springer, Cham: Springer Briefs in Ethics. https://doi.org/10.1007/978-3-030-52448-7_1

59. Menzies, T. (2003). 21st-century AI: Proud, not smug. *IEEE Intelligent Systems*, 18(3), 18–24.

60. Khan, F. H., Pasha, M. A., & Masud, S. (2021). Advancements in microprocessor architecture for ubiquitous AI—An overview on history, evolution, and upcoming challenges in AI implementation. *Micromachines*, 12(6), 665.

61. Hirschberg, J., & Manning, C. D. (2015). Advances in natural language processing. *Science*, 349(6245), 261–266.

62. Lavallin, A., & Downs, J. A. (2021). Machine learning in geography–Past, present, and future. *Geography Compass*, 15(5), e12563.

63. Hardwick, T., & Ahmed, N. (2020). Digitising chemical synthesis in automated and robotic flow. *Chemical Science*, 11(44), 11973–11988.

64. Pereira, G., & Moreschi, B. (2021). Artificial intelligence and institutional critique 2.0: Unexpected ways of seeing with computer vision. *AI and Society*, 36(4), 1201–1223.

65. Ongsulee, P. (2017, November). Artificial intelligence, machine learning and deep learning. 2017 15th International Conference on ICT and Knowledge Engineering (ICT&KE). IEEE, pp. 1–6.

66. Dongbo, M., Miniaoui, S., Fen, L., Althubiti, S. A., & Alsenani, T. R. (2023). Intelligent chatbot interaction system capable for sentimental analysis using hybrid machine learning algorithms. *Information Processing and Management*, 60(5), 103440.

67. Dipsis, N., & Stathis, K. (2020). A RESTful middleware for AI controlled sensors, actuators and smart devices. *Journal of Ambient Intelligence and Humanized Computing*, 11(7), 2963–2986.

68. Korteling, J. H., van de Boer-Visschedijk, G. C., Blankendaal, R. A., Boonekamp, R. C., & Eikelboom, A. R. (2021). Human-versus artificial intelligence. *Frontiers in Artificial Intelligence*, 4, 622364.

69. Das, K., & Behera, R. N. (2017). A survey on machine learning: Concept, algorithms and applications. *International Journal of Innovative Research in Computer and Communication Engineering*, 5(2), 1301–1309.

70. Rao, S., Verma, A. K., & Bhatia, T. (2021). A review on social spam detection: Challenges, open issues, and future directions. *Expert Systems with Applications*, 186, 115742.

71. Karim, A., Azam, S., Shanmugam, B., Kannoorpatti, K., & Alazab, M. (2019). A comprehensive survey for intelligent spam email detection. *IEEE Access*, 7, 168261–168295.

72. Tian, H., Wang, T., Liu, Y., Qiao, X., & Li, Y. (2020). Computer vision technology in agricultural automation—A review. *Information Processing in Agriculture*, 7(1), 1–19.

73. Vathsala, A. V., Lakshmi, H. N., Yedukondalu, G., Rao, C. R. S., Kotha, M., & Changala, R. (2023). Optimization of irrigation and herbicides using artificial intelligence in agriculture. *International Journal of Intelligent Systems and Applications in Engineering*, 11(3), 503–518.

74. Eli-Chukwu, N. C. (2019). Applications of artificial intelligence in agriculture: A review. *Engineering, Technology and Applied Science Research*, 9(4).

75. Dilek, S., Çakır, H., & Aydın, M. (2015). Applications of artificial intelligence techniques to combating cyber crimes: A review. *arXiv Preprint ArXiv:1502.03552*.

76. Coronese, M., Lamperti, F., Keller, K., Chiaromonte, F., & Roventini, A. (2019). Evidence for sharp increase in the economic damages of extreme natural disasters. *Proceedings of the National Academy of Sciences of the United States of America*, 116(43), 21450–21455.

77. Ellingwood, B. R., Cutler, H., Gardoni, P., Peacock, W. G., van de Lindt, J. W., & Wang, N. (2016). The Centerville virtual community: A fully integrated decision model of interacting physical and social infrastructure systems. *Sustainable and Resilient Infrastructure*, 1(3–4), 95–107.

78. Sun, W., Bocchini, P., & Davison, B. D. (2019). Comparing decision models for disaster restoration of interdependent infrastructures under uncertainty. Proceedings 13th International Conference on Applications of Statistics and Probability in Civil Engineering (ICASP13), pp. 26–30.

79. Sun, W., Bocchini, P., & Davison, B. D. (2020). Applications of artificial intelligence for disaster management. *Natural Hazards*, 103(3), 2631–2689.

80. Zhou, J., Chen, C., Li, L., Zhang, Z., & Zheng, X. (2022). FinBrain 2.0: When finance meets trustworthy AI. *Frontiers of Information Technology and Electronic Engineering*, 23(12), 1747–1764.

81. Suhel, S. F., Shukla, V. K., Vyas, S., & Mishra, V. P. (2020, June). Conversation to automation in banking through chatbot using artificial machine intelligence language. 8th International Conference on Reliability, Infocom Technologies and Optimization (Trends and Future Directions) (ICRITO). IEEE, pp. 611–618.

82. Misawa, M., Kudo, S. E., Mori, Y., Cho, T., Kataoka, S., Yamauchi, A., ... Mori, K. (2018). Artificial intelligence-assisted polyp detection for colonoscopy: Initial experience. *Gastroenterology*, 154(8), 2027–2029.

83. Haleem, A., Javaid, M., & Vaishya, R. (2019). Industry 4.0 and its applications in orthopaedics. *Journal of Clinical Orthopaedics and Trauma*, 10(3), 615–616.

84. Haleem, A., Javaid, M., & Khan, I. H. (2019). Current status and applications of Artificial Intelligence (AI) in medical field: An overview. *Current Medicine Research and Practice*, 9(6), 231–237.

85. Lee, E. J., Kim, Y. H., Kim, N., & Kang, D. W. (2017). Deep into the brain: Artificial intelligence in stroke imaging. *Journal of Stroke*, 19(3), 277.

86. Mintz, Y. & Brodie, R. (2019). Introduction to artificial intelligence in medicine. *Minimally Invasive Therapy & Allied Technologies*, 28(2), 73–81.

87. Kocheturov, A., Pardalos, P. M., & Karakitsiou, A. (2019). Massive datasets and machine learning for computational biomedicine: Trends and challenges. *Annals of Operations Research*, 276(1–2), 5–34.

88. Ongsulee, P. (2017, November). Artificial intelligence, machine learning and deep learning. 2017 15th International Conference on ICT and Knowledge Engineering (ICT&KE). IEEE, pp. 1–6.

89. Nasteski, V. (2017). An overview of the supervised machine learning methods. *Horizons. B*, 4, 51–62.

90. Matsuo, Y., LeCun, Y., Sahani, M., Precup, D., Silver, D., Sugiyama, M., ... Morimoto, J. (2022). Deep learning, reinforcement learning, and world models. *Neural Networks*, 152, 267–275.

91. Kalaiselvi, K., & Deepika, M. (2020). Machine learning for healthcare diagnostics. In *Machine Learning with Health Care Perspective. Learning and Analytics in Intelligent Systems*, Jain, V. and Chatterjee, J. (eds), (pp. 91–105). Springer, Cham. https://doi.org/10.1007/978-3-030-40850-3_5

92. Bak, B., Skrobala, A., Adamska, A., & Malicki, J. (2022). What information can we gain from performing adaptive radiotherapy of head and neck cancer patients from the past 10 years? *Cancer/Radiothérapie*, 26(3), 502–516.

93. Mehta, M., Passi, K., Chatterjee, I., & Patel, R. (Eds.). (2021). *Knowledge Modelling and Big Data Analytics in Healthcare: Advances and Applications*. CRC Press.

94. Leibig, C., Brehmer, M., Bunk, S., Byng, D., Pinker, K., & Umutlu, L. (2022). Combining the strengths of radiologists and AI for breast cancer screening: A retrospective analysis. *The Lancet Digital Health*, 4(7), e507–e519.

95. Gao, Y., Cai, G. Y., Fang, W., Li, H. Y., Wang, S. Y., Chen, L., ... Gao, Q. L. (2020). Machine learning based early warning system enables accurate mortality risk prediction for COVID-19. *Nature Communications*, 11(1), 5033.

96. Gulshan, V., Peng, L., Coram, M., Stumpe, M. C., Wu, D., Narayanaswamy, A., ... Webster, D. R. (2016). Development and validation of a deep learning algorithm for detection of diabetic retinopathy in retinal fundus photographs. *JAMA*, 316(22), 2402–2410.

97. Bishop, C. M., & Nasrabadi, N. M. (2006). *Pattern Recognition and Machine Learning* (Vol. 4, No. 4, p. 738). Springer.

98. Khanday, A. M. U. D., Rabani, S. T., Khan, Q. R., Rouf, N., Mohi, U., & Din, M. (2020). Machine learning based approaches for detecting COVID-19 using clinical text data. *International Journal of Information Technology*, 12(3), 731–739.

99. Pandey, R., Gautam, V., Pal, R., Bandhey, H., Dhingra, L. S., Misra, V., ... Sethi, T. (2022). A machine learning application for raising wash awareness in the times of Covid-19 pandemic. *Scientific Reports*, 12(1), 810.

100. Demner-Fushman, D., Chapman, W. W., & McDonald, C. J. (2009). What can natural language processing do for clinical decision support? *Journal of Biomedical Informatics*, 42(5), 760–772.
101. Bharadiya, J. (2023). A comprehensive survey of deep learning techniques natural language processing. *European Journal of Technology*, 7(1), 58–66.
102. Alshemali, B., & Kalita, J. (2020). Improving the reliability of deep neural networks in NLP: A review. *Knowledge-Based Systems*, 191, 105210.
103. Syed, R., Suriadi, S., Adams, M., Bandara, W., Leemans, S. J., Ouyang, C., ... Reijers, H. A. (2020). Robotic process automation: Contemporary themes and challenges. *Computers in Industry*, 115, 103162.
104. Talukdar, J., Singh, T. P., & Barman, B. (2023). Artificial intelligence in healthcare. In *Artificial Intelligence in Healthcare Industry. Advanced Technologies and Societal Change* (pp. 127–143). Springer Nature Singapore. https://doi.org/10.1007/978-981-99-3157-6_7
105. Davenport, T. & Kalakota, R. (2019). The potential for artificial intelligence in healthcare. *Future Healthcare Journal*, 6(2), 94.
106. Gennari, J. H., Musen, M. A., Fergerson, R. W., Grosso, W. E., Crubézy, M., Eriksson, H., ... Tu, S. W. (2003). The evolution of Protégé: An environment for knowledge-based systems development. *International Journal of Human-Computer Studies*, 58(1), 89–123.
107. Rychener, M. D. (1985). Expert systems for engineering design. *Expert Systems*, 2(1), 30–44.
108. Ellahham, S., Ellahham, N., & Simsekler, M. C. E. (2020). Application of artificial intelligence in the health care safety context: Opportunities and challenges. *American Journal of Medical Quality*, 35(4), 341–348.
109. Thapa, C., & Camtepe, S. (2021). Precision health data: Requirements, challenges and existing techniques for data security and privacy. *Computers in Biology and Medicine*, 129, 104130.
110. Nayyar, A., Gadhavi, L., & Zaman, N. (2021). Machine learning in healthcare: Review, opportunities and challenges. *Machine Learning and the Internet of Medical Things in Healthcare*, Krishna Kant S., Mohamed, E., Akansha, S., and Ahmed, A. E. (eds.), 23–45. Academic Press.
111. Tolan, S. (2019). Fair and unbiased algorithmic decision making: Current state and future challenges. *arXiv Preprint ArXiv:1901.04730*.
112. Pradhan, I. P., & Saxena, P. (2023). Reskilling workforce for the Artificial Intelligence age: Challenges and the way forward. In *The Adoption and Effect of Artificial Intelligence on Human Resources Management, Part B* (pp. 181–197). Emerald Publishing Limited.
113. Crampon, K., Giorkallos, A., Deldossi, M., Baud, S., & Steffenel, L. A. (2022). Machine-learning methods for ligand–protein molecular docking. *Drug Discovery Today*, 27(1), 151–164.

8 Facemask and Hand Gloves Detection Using Hybrid Deep Learning Model

Akash Das, Dwaipayan Mistry, Raj Kamal,
Sabyasachi Ganguly, and Sanjay Chakraborty

8.1 INTRODUCTION

In the battle against the spread of infectious diseases, personal protective equipment (PPE) has emerged as a critical line of defense. Facemasks and hand gloves have become integral components of preventive measures, particularly in the context of air-borne diseases such as COVID-19 [23, 24]. The widespread adoption of these safety measures has highlighted the need for efficient and reliable systems to detect whether individuals are wearing facemasks and hand gloves in various settings [10, 28].

In recent years, computer vision and deep learning techniques have revolutionized the field of object detection and recognition. These technologies have shown great potential for automating the detection of facemasks and hand gloves in images and videos, thereby aiding in the enforcement of PPE compliance. Current research in this area has focused on developing models that can accurately identify the presence or absence of facemasks and hand gloves, utilizing advanced deep learning algorithms such as YOLOv8 (You Only Look Once) and Region-based Convolutional Neural Network (RCNN). YOLOv8 is a popular object-detection algorithm known for its real-time performance and ability to detect multiple objects in an image. On the other hand, RCNN (Region-based Convolutional Neural Network) is a powerful technique for object detection and classification. By combining the strengths of both YOLOv8 and RCNN within a hybrid model, we can leverage YOLOv8's efficient object-detection capabilities and RCNN's accurate classification abilities, thereby improving the overall performance of the model. The rise of air-borne diseases has underscored the importance of taking proactive measures to mitigate their spread. Wearing facemasks and hand gloves has proven to be an effective strategy in reducing the transmission of infectious agents and minimizing the associated health risks. Therefore, it is crucial to develop robust systems that can automatically detect

DOI: 10.1201/9781003464884-12

whether individuals are adhering to these preventive measures in various environments. The motivation behind this research is to compare different models for facemasks and hand glove detection and to propose a hybrid form that can enhance the accuracy and efficiency of these detection systems. By conducting a thorough evaluation and comparison of existing approaches, we can identify their strengths and weaknesses. Building upon these insights, the hybrid model can be designed to leverage the complementary strengths of YOLOv8 and RCNN, ultimately yielding a system that achieves state-of-the-art performance in detecting facemasks and hand gloves.

The objective of this research is twofold: first, to assess the effectiveness of current models for facemasks and hand glove detection, and second, to develop a new hybrid method that surpasses the limitations of individual models and provides improved detection accuracy and real-time performance. The proposed hybrid model aims to deliver a robust and efficient solution that can accurately detect and monitor compliance with PPE usage guidelines in various scenarios. By developing an advanced and reliable system for facemasks and hand glove detection, we aim to contribute to public health efforts and reduce the impact of air-borne diseases. The subsequent sections of this chapter will delve into the methodology, experimental results, and discussions, providing a comprehensive overview of the development and performance of the hybrid deep learning model for facemasks and hand glove detection. Through this research, we strive to enhance the effectiveness of PPE compliance monitoring system.

The use of personal protective equipment, such as facemasks and hand gloves, has become an essential aspect of this effort. In recent years, computer vision and deep learning techniques have been applied to various tasks. In the context of COVID-19, there has been increasing interest in using these techniques for the detection of facemasks and hand gloves in images and videos. Current research in this area has focused on developing models that can accurately detect the presence of facemasks and hand gloves in images. YOLOv8 and RCNN are two popular deep learning algorithms that have been used for this task. These models have shown promising results, achieving high accuracy in detecting facemasks and hand gloves in various settings. The model consists of YOLOv8 and RCNN; the YOLO is a great technique for object detection which helps to detect multiple objects and with the combination of RCNN, the classification gives a better result. The rise of diseases mainly air-borne diseases can cause dangerous health problems[9]. The usage of these masks with the addition of hand gloves may reduce the spread of the disease. The motivation to stop the spread made us venture into this research to compare different models and create a hybrid deep learning model to detect them so that it can stop the spread and reduce diseases.

8.1.1 Problem Definition

The COVID-19 pandemic has highlighted the critical role of personal protective equipment (PPE) in preventing the spread of infectious diseases, particularly facemasks and hand gloves [2,3]. However, ensuring compliance with PPE guidelines in public spaces or crowded environments presents significant challenges. Manual monitoring of individuals for wearing facemasks and hand gloves is time-consuming, resource-intensive, and prone to errors. Therefore, there is a need for an automated system that can accurately detect whether individuals are wearing facemasks and hand gloves to enhance disease prevention efforts [25–27].

The main problem addressed in this research is the development of a robust and efficient system for facemask and hand glove detection using computer vision and deep learning techniques. The system should be capable of processing real-time video or image data and accurately identifying whether individuals are wearing facemasks and hand gloves. This automated approach will enable proactive monitoring and enforcement of PPE compliance, reducing the risk of disease transmission and ensuring the safety of individuals in various settings, such as public transportation, healthcare facilities, and crowded public spaces. Several challenges need to be addressed to achieve accurate and reliable detection. These include variations in lighting conditions, occlusions, diverse facial appearances, different types of masks and gloves, and the presence of other objects that may resemble masks or gloves. Furthermore, the system should be able to handle real-world complexities, such as individuals wearing masks improperly or removing them temporarily. Overcoming these challenges requires the development of a sophisticated model that can handle variations and adapt to different scenarios while maintaining high detection accuracy.

The proposed solution aims to address these challenges by developing a hybrid model that combines the strengths of computer vision techniques and deep learning algorithms. The model leverages a pre-trained convolutional neural network (CNN) as a feature extractor to capture meaningful representations from input images or video frames. These features are fed into a classification module to determine the presence or absence of facemasks and hand gloves. The hybrid model is trained and evaluated using a diverse dataset [13–15], encompassing various scenarios and demographics, to ensure its adaptability and robustness in real-world conditions.

The rest of the chapter is organized as follows. Section 8.2 discusses a set of existing research works using supervised learning techniques for the detection of facemask and hand gloves during any kind of pandemic situation. Section 8.3 describes the background, preparation of dataset, and the used methodology for this work. Section 8.4 shows a detailed analysis of results after rigorous training through our proposed hybrid model and provides a prediction output based on some important parameters analysis. Section 8.5 discusses the conclusions of this chapter and future works in this domain for interested readers and researchers.

8.2　RELATED WORKS

In recent years, the detection of facemasks and hand gloves in images and videos has become a popular research topic due to the pandemic situation [22]. Many researchers have developed various deep learning models and algorithms to detect facemasks and hand gloves in images and videos. In this section, we have given a review of some works in this area. One very common approach to detect facemasks is using the convolutional neural networks (CNN) [19]. A recent study by Wang et al. (2021)

[4] proposed a YOLO-based model for detecting facemasks and hand gloves in images. The model achieved high accuracy in detecting facemasks and hand gloves, and the authors claim that their model can be used in real-world scenarios. Another popular deep learning model for object detection is Faster RCNN (Region-based Convolutional Neural Network). In a research work [1], a Faster RCNN-based technique is proposed for the detection of facemasks and hand gloves in images and videos. The authors claim that their model achieved high accuracy and can be used in real-time scenarios. In a recent study by Liu et al. (2021) [6], a hybrid model is proposed that combines the strengths of both YOLOv5[3,7] and Faster RCNN for the detection of facemasks and hand gloves in images and videos. The proposed model achieved high accuracy in detecting facemasks and hand gloves and outperformed existing models in terms of speed and accuracy. Another study by Xiong et al. (2021) proposed a deep learning-based model for the detection of facemasks and hand gloves in videos. The proposed model used a spatiotemporal attention mechanism and achieved high accuracy in detecting facemasks and hand gloves in videos. In summary, various deep learning models and algorithms have been proposed for the detection of facemasks and hand gloves in images and videos. The proposed models have shown promising results in terms of accuracy and speed, and some of them have been evaluated in real-world scenarios. Our study builds upon these previous works by proposing a hybrid model using YOLOv8 and RCNN for the detection of facemasks and hand gloves in images and videos.

Using numerous face picture datasets, a new deep-learning-based approach is proposed in this study [16] for detecting and recognizing masked faces, as well as for identifying the face and deciding whether or not it is appropriately masked. A convolutional neural network (CNN) with cross-validation and early halting is used to train the suggested system. A binary classification model is initially developed to distinguish between faces that are and are not covered in masks. The masked face photos are then classified into three labels, namely correctly, incorrectly, and non-masked faces, using a multi-class model that had been developed.

An article [17] detects the trends of COVID-19 using machine learning techniques in Pakistan. This work introduces a computer-aided design (CAD) face mask identification system [18]. The proposed design system is based on the nose, mouth, and face detections in the gathered image. This work's main goal is to create a software-based system that mitigates the transmission of respiratory illnesses and regulates face mask use in hospitals that treat respiratory infections by using mask detection and mask color detection. The suggested approach was created for a hospital with three departments for respiratory disorders and three mask colors, with each mask color being applied for each department. The local binary pattern histogram (LBPH) algorithm-based cascaded object detector employed by the mask recognition system was followed by a method based on artificial intelligence for color detection using images of face masks in the RGB color space. Convolutional neural network (CNN) technology is finally used to classify data [18].

This work [20] has developed a novel model to detect and recognize faces and persons for authentication by using scale invariant features (SIFT) for the full segmented face and local binary texture features (DLBP) in the area of the eyes in the covered face. The image is segmented using the fuzzy C mean. An extensive amount of training is done on these combined features using convolution neural network (CNN) technology [20].

The SARS-CoV-2 virus is very dangerous, contaminated and spread faster. According to a study [21], HCWs' hands occasionally contained SARSCoV-2 RNA after providing direct and indirect treatment to early COVID-19 patients. The facemask detector dataset is used in a research study [29] to train the model and provide ground truth labels for training and assessment. Using this dataset, the researchers apply transfer learning techniques to fine-tune the YOLOv8 model [12], making it capable of reliably classifying circumstances related to facemask wearing. An article [30] suggests a real-time glove identification system that makes use of video surveillance. To improve detection average precision, the method makes use of an attention mechanism and transfer learning. The following are the main concepts of our algorithm: the combine attention partial network (CAPN) is a convolutional neural network-based system that can detect whether gloves are on or off. It can also be used to: (1) extract deeper feature information and improve recognition accuracy; (2) combine channel attention and spatial attention modules; and (3) use transfer learning to transfer human hand features in various states to gloves in order to improve the small sample dataset of gloves. CCA-YOLO [31] is presented based on YOLOv5 to realize the rip and scratch defect detection in nitrile medical gloves, with the goal of addressing the problem of low efficiency. The YOLOv5 network backbone now has a small-target detection layer thanks to CCA-YOLO, which also suggested a novel channel coordinate attention technique [31]. A study [8] uses YOLOv4 to identify glove use among laboratory workers.

8.3 BACKGROUND AND METHODOLOGY

8.3.1 BACKGROUND

This section mainly deals with the two-object detection models from images that work as base models in our hybrid model approach. The YOLO and RCNN models are discussed below.

8.3.1.1 You Only Look Once (YOLO)

The YOLO is a method that provides real-time object detection using convolutional neural networks (CNNs) [5]. This algorithm (which operates in real time) can find and identify different items in images. The YOLO object identification process inspired by regression problem provides the class probabilities of the discovered photos. Due to its improved performance over the aforementioned object detection algorithms in a single run, the YOLO algorithm has grown in popularity [11]. Tiny YOLO and YOLOv3 are two popular variations. YOLOv8 has been used in this work. The first version of YOLO, version 8, is launched on January 10, 2023. The YOLO algorithm employs the following three methods:

- **Residual blocks**: First, the image is divided into many grids. Each grid has a size of S × S. Items that enter a grid cell will be detectable by all of the cells. When an object's center appears within a grid cell, for example, that grid cell will be responsible for recognizing the object.

- **Regression by bounding box**: The YOLO uses a single bounding box regression to ascertain an object's height, width, center, and class. The following characteristics are present in each bounding box in the image: width (M_w), Height (M_h), 'c' stands for class, which includes elements like person, car, traffic signal, etc. and (b_x, b_y) represents bounding box center ($[M_w, M_h, c, (b_x, b_y),$ Score]) .
- **Intersection over union (IOU)**: It describes box overlapping. If the planned bounding box and the actual box match, IOU gives '1.' This method gets rid of bounding boxes that aren't the same as the real box.

8.3.1.2 Region-Based Convolutional Neural Networks (RCNN)

In 2014, Ross Girshick, Jeff Donahue, Trevor Darrell, and Jitendra Malik unveiled RCNN. In RCNN, we feed the image through selective search, choose the first 2,000 region proposals from the result, and run classification on those instead of running classification on a massive number of regions. In this manner, we just need to classify the top 2,000 regions rather than a large number of them. As a result, this approach is quicker than earlier methods of object detection. Rather than working on a huge number of areas, the RCNN approach recommends a number of boxes in the image and determines whether any of these boxes contain any objects. These boxes, also known as regions, are extracted from an image by RCNN using selective search. Various scales, colors, textures, and enclosures are the main four areas that make up an object. These patterns are recognized by selective search in the image, and several regions are suggested as a result. An overview of the operation of selective search is provided below:

1. First image is used as the input.
2. After that, it generates initial sub-segments, allowing us to have various segments of this image.
3. The approach then joins the comparable parts to create a bigger zone (based on color, texture, size, and shape compatibility).d. Final locations of objects are then produced by these regions.

An outline of the procedures taken by RCNN to detect objects is shown below:

- A pre-trained convolutional neural network is what we start with.
- The model is then retrained. Depending on how many classes need to be identified, we train the network's final layer.
- Obtaining the region of interest for each image is the third step. Then, we restructure each of these regions to meet the CNN input size.
- After obtaining the regions, we train the SVM to categorize the background and objects. One binary SVM is trained for each class.
- In order to create narrower bounding boxes for each recognized object in the image, we lastly train a linear regression model.

We have thus far witnessed the value of RCNN in object detection. However, this method has its own drawbacks. Due to the following procedures, training an RCNN model is expensive and time-consuming:

1. 2,000 areas are extracted from each image using a selective search.
2. Use CNN to extract features from each image region. If there are N photos, then there will be N*2,000 CNN features.
3. Three models make up the complete RCNN object detection process:

- CNN to extract features.
- Object classification using a linear SVM classifier.
- Regression model to make the bounding boxes more precise.

The sum of all these operations makes RCNN extremely slow. The model is essentially difficult to create when faced with a massive dataset because it takes a little bit of time to produce detection for each new image.

8.3.2 PREPARATION OF DATASET

The dataset plays a crucial role in training models for the detection of facemasks and hand gloves. In this section, we describe the preparation of our dataset, which encompasses a large and diverse collection of images to ensure the development of a robust and accurate model. The dataset comprises two main categories: real-world datasets and simulated datasets [13–15]. By including data from both sources, we aim to create a comprehensive dataset that captures a wide range of scenarios and variations commonly encountered in practical settings.

a) **Real-world Dataset:** 5,620 images for training, 1,280 images for validation, and 300 images for testing. The real-world dataset consists of a substantial number of images collected from various sources, including public spaces, healthcare facilities, and other relevant environments. The dataset has been carefully curated to encompass different demographics, lighting conditions, and diverse settings to ensure its representativeness of real-world scenarios. For the training phase, we have included a total of 5,620 images, providing a rich variety of examples for the model to learn from. To assess the performance and generalization ability of the trained model, we have set aside 1,280 images for validation. Additionally, we have reserved a separate set of 300 images specifically for testing the model's accuracy and robustness (Figure 8.1).

b) **Simulated Dataset**: 3,500 images for training, 1,000 images for validation, and 200 for testing. To complement the real-world dataset, we have generated a simulated dataset consisting of synthetically created images. These images are generated using computer graphics techniques to simulate

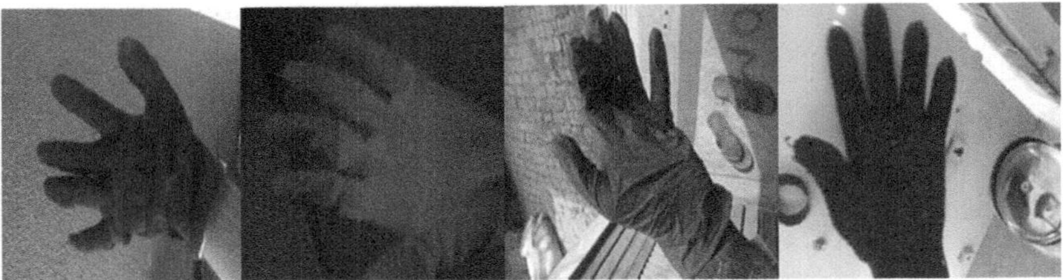

FIGURE 8.1   Real-world dataset.

different scenarios and variations. This approach allows us to augment the dataset and introduce controlled variations to evaluate the model's performance under specific conditions. The simulated dataset consists of 3,500 images for training, providing a diverse range of simulated scenarios and variations. To ensure the generalization capability of the model, we have allocated 1,000 images for validation purposes. Additionally, we have reserved 200 images for testing, specifically designed to evaluate the model's ability to handle simulated scenarios. All the images in the experimented dataset have RGB resolution (Figures 8.2 and 8.3).

8.3.3   Experimented Models

Hand gloves and facemasks detection has become critical task in today's world due to the ongoing COVID-19 pandemic. Object detection models like YOLOv8 and RCNN have proven to be effective in detecting objects in images and videos. In this proposed model, we will combine both YOLOv8 and RCNN to detect hand gloves and facemasks in images and videos.

The proposed model will have two stages of object detection: first, we will use YOLOv8 to detect hand gloves and facemasks in the image or video frames. Then, we will use RCNN to further analyze and classify the detected objects. Modern object identification models like the YOLOv8 model are renowned for their excellent accuracy and quick detection times. It predicts the bounding boxes and class probabilities for each cell in a grid created from the input image. YOLOv8 is a superior version of YOLO than its predecessors since it makes use of a stronger backbone network and improved training methods.

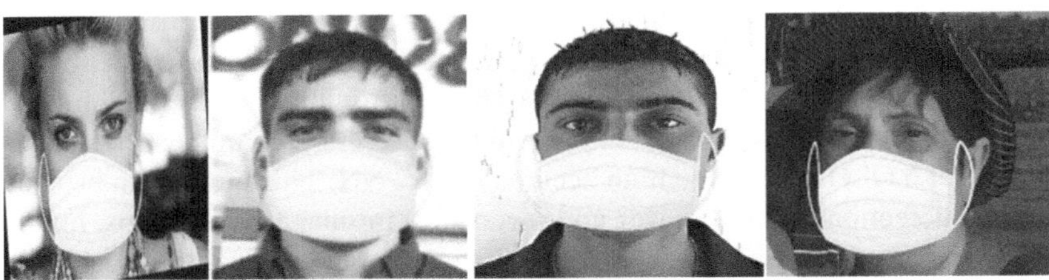

FIGURE 8.2   Simulated dataset.

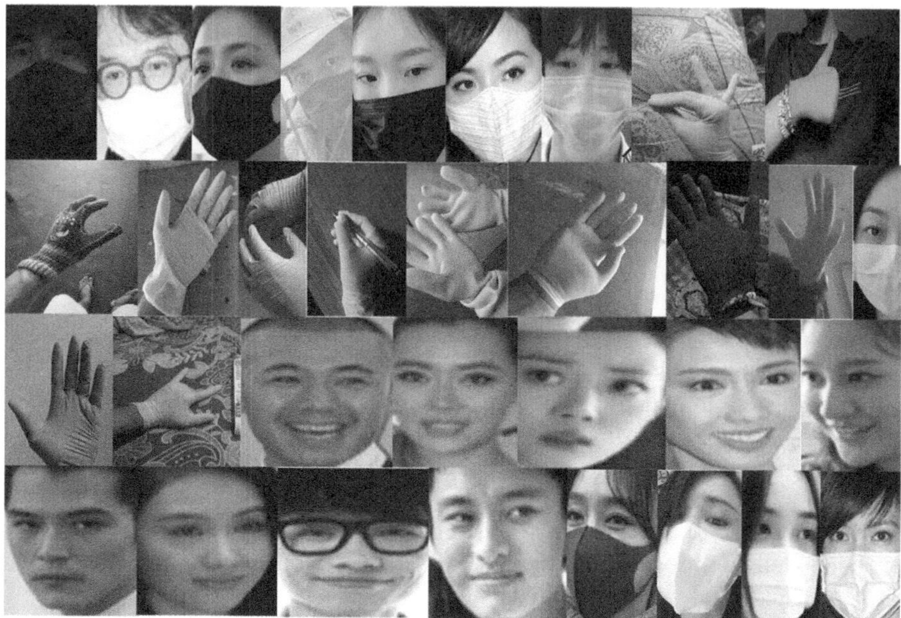

FIGURE 8.3   Real-world masked and non-masked dataset.

In our proposed model, we will train YOLOv8 on a dataset of images and videos that contain people wearing hand gloves and facemasks. The model will learn to detect the bounding boxes for hand gloves and facemasks in the input images. After YOLOv8 has detected the objects, we will use RCNN to further analyze and classify them. Region-based convolutional neural networks, or RCNNs for short, are a common class of object identification models that categorize items in an image by first using a CNN to generate region recommendations for those objects. Although RCNN has a reputation for being highly accurate, YOLOv8 is faster. In our proposed model, we will use RCNN to analyze the regions of the image where YOLOv8 has detected hand gloves and facemasks. RCNN will classify the objects into different categories, such as medical gloves or industrial gloves, and surgical masks or N95 masks. Finally, we will combine the results of YOLOv8 and RCNN to produce the final output. The output will be a set of bounding boxes for hand gloves and facemasks, along with their respective classes. This output can be used to alert individuals who are not wearing hand gloves or facemasks, or it can be used for statistical purposes to analyze compliance with public health guidelines. The proposed model for hand gloves and facemasks detection combines the speed and accuracy of YOLOv8 with the high accuracy of RCNN. This model can be used for real-time detection of hand gloves and facemasks in images and videos, making it useful for monitoring compliance with public health guidelines during the COVID-19 pandemic.

8.3.3.1 Working with You Only Look Once (YOLO)

The process to detect facemasks and hand gloves using YOLOv8 involves collecting a dataset of images and videos that contain people wearing hand gloves and facemasks and annotating the dataset by labeling the hand gloves and facemasks in each image or video frame with bounding boxes. The dataset is then split into training and validation sets, and the YOLOv8 model is trained on the training set using the annotated bounding boxes as ground truth. The model's performance is evaluated on the validation set, and hyperparameters are adjusted as necessary. Once the model is trained, it can be tested on new images or videos to detect hand gloves and facemasks. The results are visualized by drawing bounding boxes around the detected objects and displaying the corresponding class probabilities. The YOLOv8 model achieves high accuracy and fast detection speed by dividing the input image into a grid of cells and predicting the bounding boxes and class probabilities for each cell. The model can be trained to accurately identify hand gloves and facemasks in fresh photos and videos by using a dataset of images and videos with people wearing them (Figure 8.4).

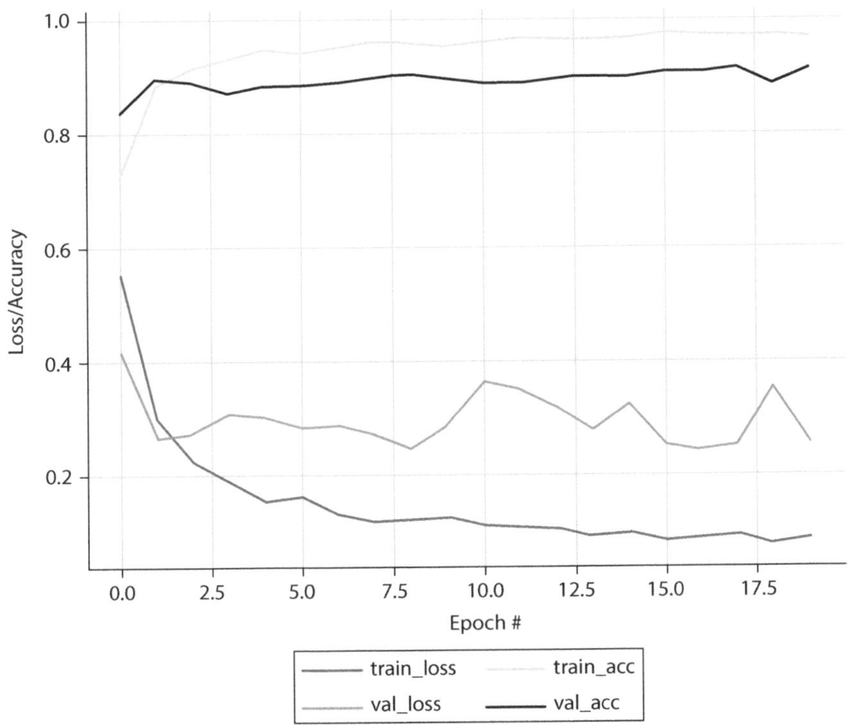

FIGURE 8.4 Relationship among training, validation loss, and accuracy.

8.3.3.2 Working with Region-Based Convolutional Neural Networks (RCNN)

Detecting facemasks and hand gloves using RCNN (Region-based Convolutional Neural Network) involves several steps. First, we gather a dataset comprising images with and without facemasks and hand gloves. Then, we mark the regions of interest (ROIs) in these images to indicate the presence of facemasks and hand gloves. This annotated dataset will be used to train our RCNN model.

Next, we select an RCNN-based model suitable for object detection, such as Faster RCNN or Mask RCNN. These models have been proven to be effective in accurately detecting objects. We train the selected model using the annotated dataset, allowing it to learn the distinctive features and patterns associated with facemasks and hand gloves.

If we have a large enough dataset, we can consider fine-tuning a pre-trained model. Fine-tuning can save training time and potentially enhance performance. After training the model, we evaluate its performance on a separate validation or test set. This step helps us assess the model's ability to accurately detect facemasks and hand gloves. During inference, we apply the trained model to new, unseen images. The model detects regions containing facemasks and hand gloves, outputting bounding boxes or masks to indicate their presence. To refine the detections and remove false positives, we can apply post-processing techniques such as non-maximum suppression or filtering based on the size and shape of the detected regions. Finally, we integrate the trained model into our desired application or system, enabling real-time or batch processing of facemasks and hand glove detection (Figure 8.5).

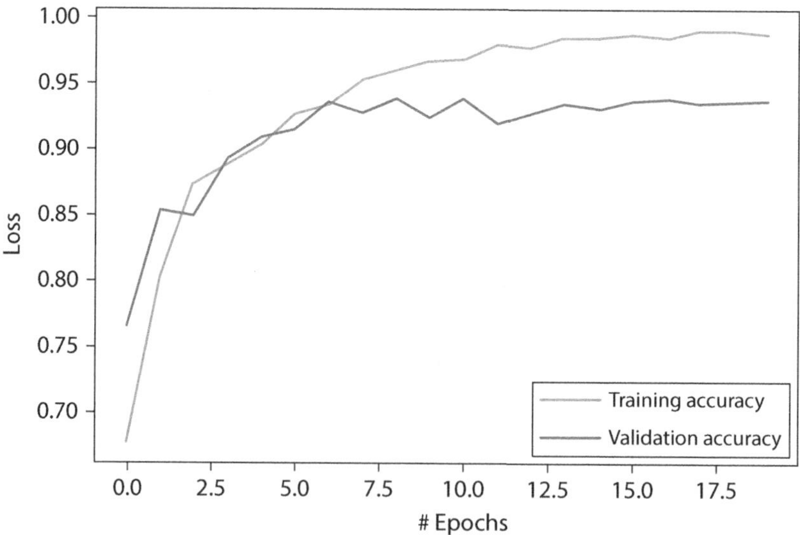

FIGURE 8.5 Accuracy of RCNN model.

8.3.3.3 Proposed Hybrid Model

Detecting facemasks and hand gloves using region-based convolutional neural network (RCNN) and you only look once (YOLOv8) involves a comprehensive process. First, we gather a dataset consisting of images with and without facemasks and hand gloves. We annotate the images by marking the regions of interest (ROIs) where these objects are present (Figure 8.6).

This annotated dataset will be used for training the models. We select both RCNN and YOLOv8 models for object detection. RCNN is known for its accuracy, while YOLOv8 offers real-time detection capabilities. We train the RCNN model using the annotated dataset, enabling it to learn the distinctive features and patterns associated with facemasks and hand gloves. Similarly, we train the YOLOv8 model using the same dataset, focusing on its ability to detect objects quickly. During inference, we apply both models to new, unseen images. The RCNN model detects facemasks and hand gloves by outputting bounding boxes or masks, while the YOLOv8 model provides real-time detection with bounding boxes. To refine the detections and remove false positives, we can apply post-processing techniques such as non-maximum suppression or filtering based on the size and shape of the detected regions. We integrate both trained models into our desired application or system, enabling us to detect facemasks and hand gloves efficiently and in real time.

8.3.3.4 Proposed Hybrid Algorithm

Input:
Gather dataset with annotated ROIs.

Output:
Real-time detection of facemasks and hand gloves.

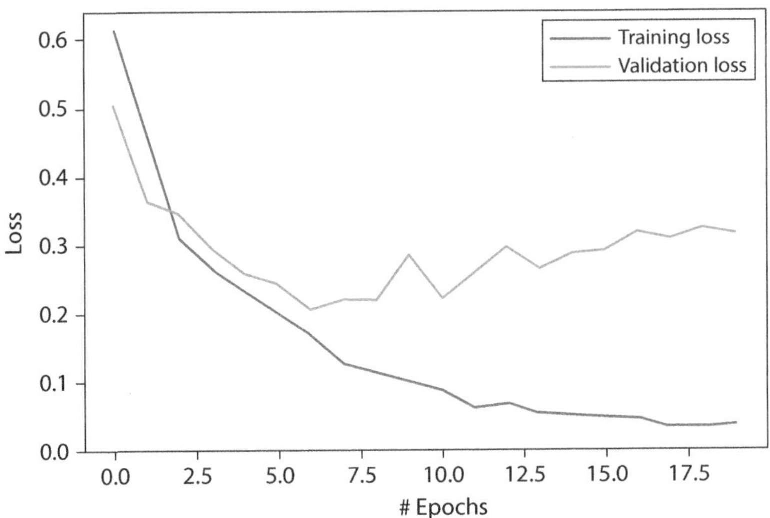

FIGURE 8.6 Loss of RCNN model.

Procedure:

a) Train RCNN model on the input image set. Input unseen image into RCNN model.
b) Evaluate RCNN model and RCNN model detects facemasks and hand gloves (bounding boxes or masks).
c) Train YOLOv8 model. Input unseen image into YOLOv8 model.
d) YOLOv8 model detects facemasks and hand gloves (bounding boxes).

Post-processing:

a) Refine detections (non-maximum suppression, filtering based on size and shape).
b) Integrate RCNN and YOLOv8 models into application/system.

End

Figure 8.7 represents the pictorial diagram of the overall working process.

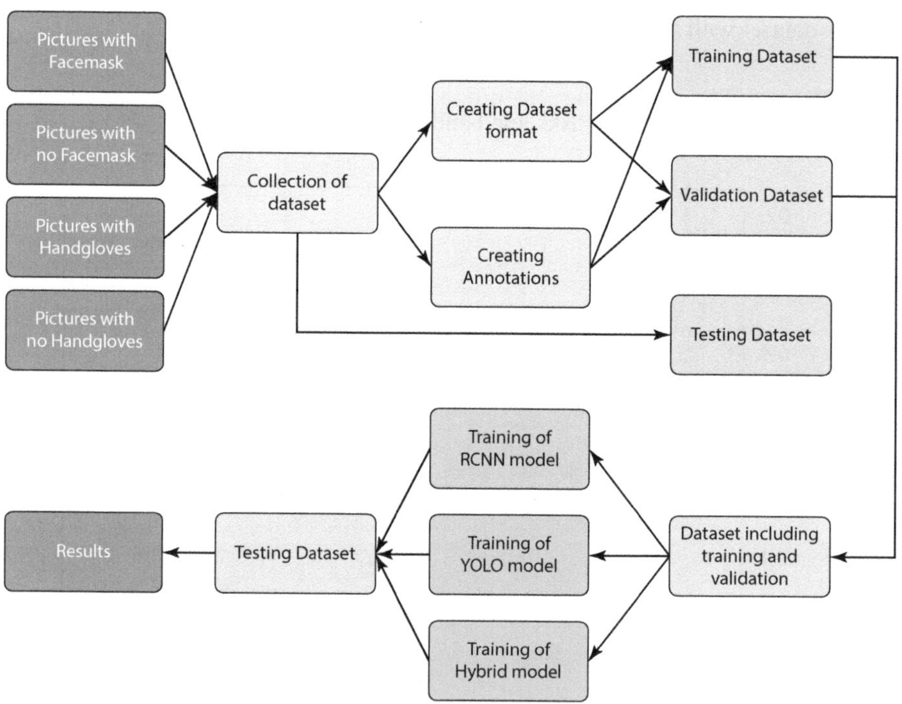

FIGURE 8.7   Overall flowchart of the working process

8.4   RESULT ANALYSIS

This section discusses and analyses the results of facemasks and hand gloves detections with respect to the different measurement parameters. Figure 8.8 and Figure 8.9 represent the relationship between training and validation loss and F1 curve with confidence scores for facemask detection, respectively. Figure 8.10 represents the relationship between training and validation loss for hand gloves detection. Figure 8.11 shows the relationship between precision and recall for both the cases.(Tables 8.1 and 8.2).

In this study, we present a detailed analysis of the performance of a hybrid model that combines YOLOv8 and RCNN for the detection of facemasks and hand gloves. The model aims to accurately identify instances of individuals wearing facemasks and hand gloves in images or video frames. The evaluation metrics used to assess the model's performance include accuracy, F1 score curve, and precision confidence. The hybrid model achieved a remarkable accuracy of 98% in detecting facemasks and hand gloves. This high accuracy demonstrates the effectiveness of the model in accurately identifying and localizing these personal protective equipment items. The model's ability to distinguish between masked and unmasked individuals and individuals wearing hand gloves contributes to its practical utility in various applications, such as public health monitoring, safety compliance enforcement, and crowd surveillance. A comparison among YOLOv8, RCNN, and our proposed hybrid model is

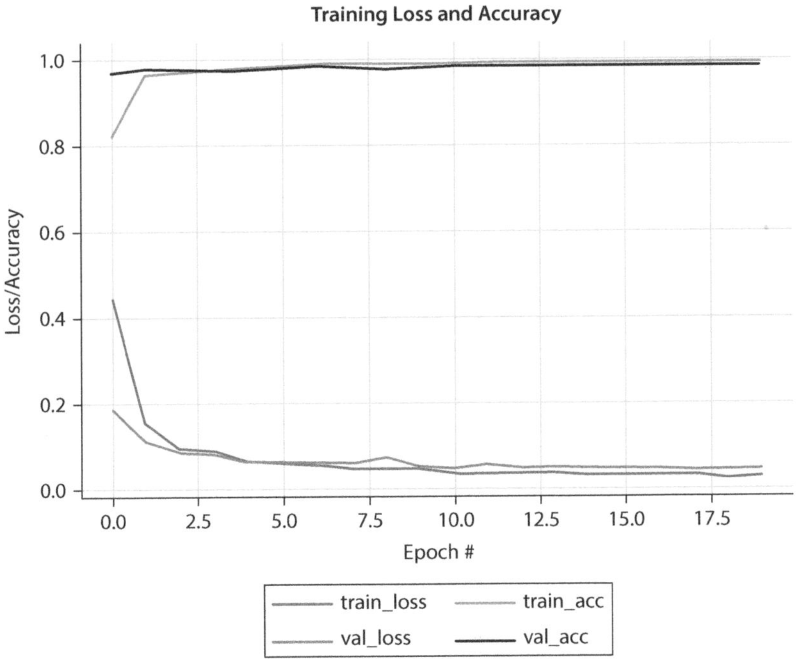

FIGURE 8.8   Training and validation loss with accuracy for facemasks detection.

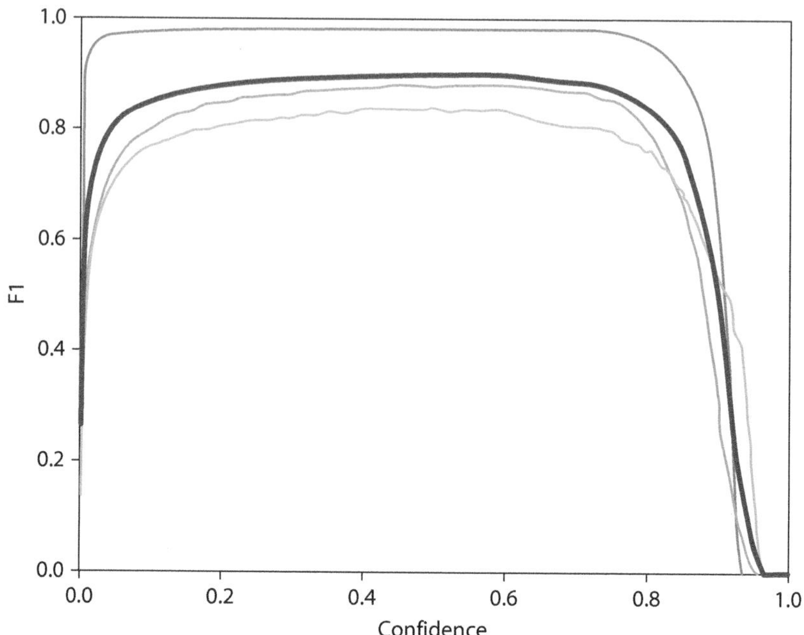

FIGURE 8.9 F1 curve with respect to confidence scores for facemasks.

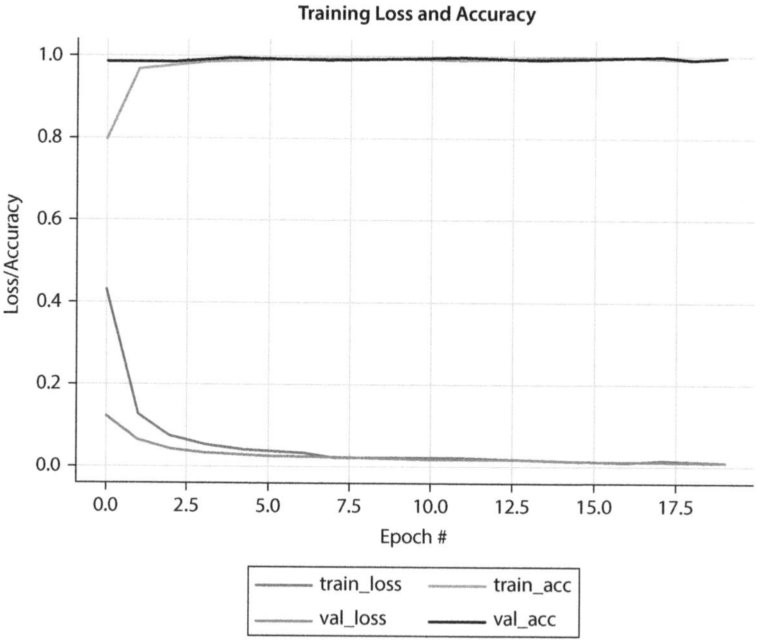

FIGURE 8.10 Training and validation loss with accuracy for handgloves detection.

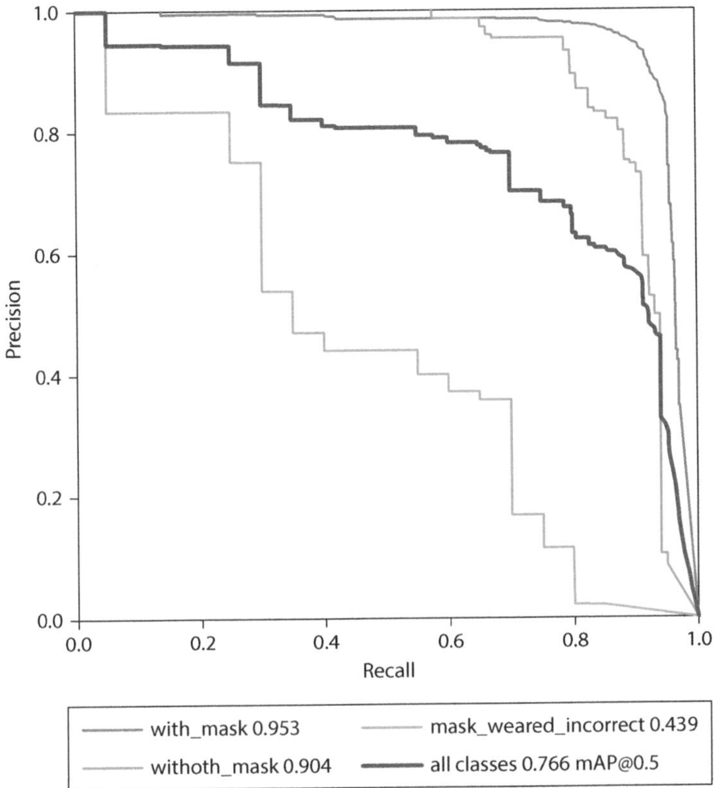

FIGURE 8.11   Relation between precision and recall.

TABLE 8.1

Resultant Table of Hybrid Model for Facemasks Detection

Model	Training Accuracy	Training Loss	Validation Accuracy	Validation Loss	F1
Hybrid Model	99%	0.16	98.6%	0.18	0.93

shown in Table 8.3 and Figure 8.12. From, the comparison results, it is clearly seen that our proposed hybrid model outperforms the YOLOv8 and RCNN models.

At various confidence thresholds, the F1 score curve showed a smooth trade-off between precision and recall. This curve allows for selecting an optimal threshold based on the specific requirements of the application. In this case, the optimal threshold is determined to be 0.95, where the F1 score is the highest. This threshold

TABLE 8.2
Resultant Table of Hybrid Model for Handgloves Detection

Model	Training Accuracy	Training Loss	Validation Accuracy	Validation Loss	Fl
Hybrid Model	98.7%	0.12	95.2%	0.14	0.95

TABLE 8.3
Comparison among Hybrid Model, YOLOv8, and RCNN

Purpose of Task	Models	Training Accuracy (%)	Validation Accuracy (%)
Face Masks Detection	YOLOv8	97.6	95.3
	RCNN	95.4	91.07
	Hybrid	**99**	**98.6**
Handgloves Detection	YOLOv8	95.9	94.2
	RCNN	93.41	90.7
	Hybrid	**98.7**	**95.2**

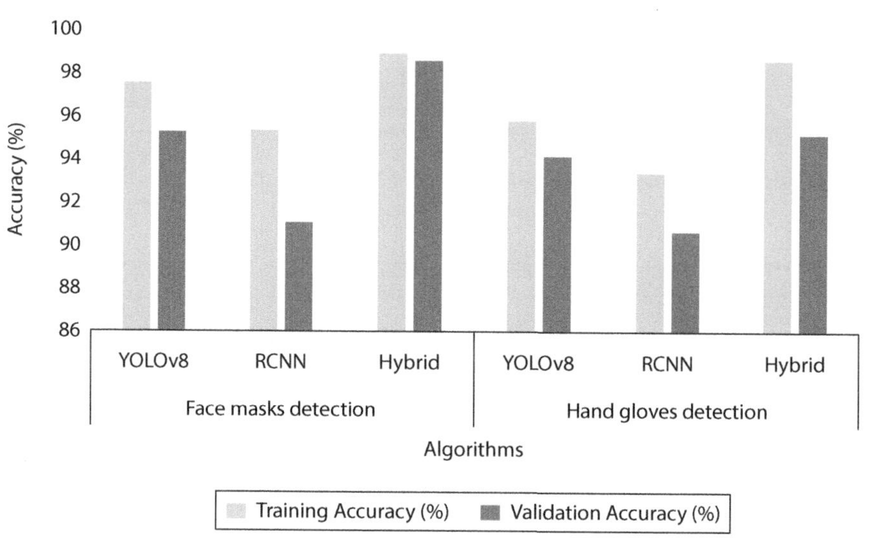

FIGURE 8.12 Accuracy comparison among hybrid model, YOLOv8, and RCNN.

strikes a balance between precision (correct identification of individuals wearing facemasks and hand gloves) and recall (capturing all instances of facemasks and hand gloves), making it suitable for various real-world scenarios. The precision confidence of the hybrid model is measured at 0.95, indicating a high level of certainty

Results

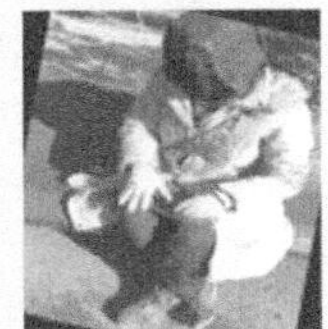

Fig 6. Original image

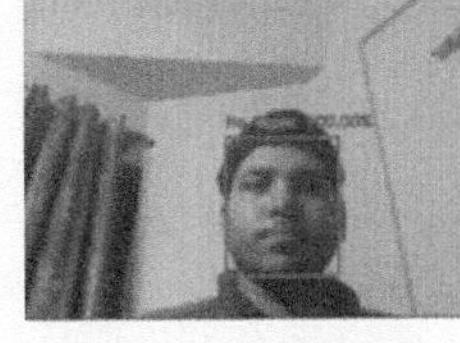

Fig 8. No mask Facemask detected

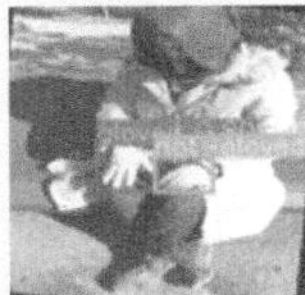

Fig 7. Gloved and not- gloved detected

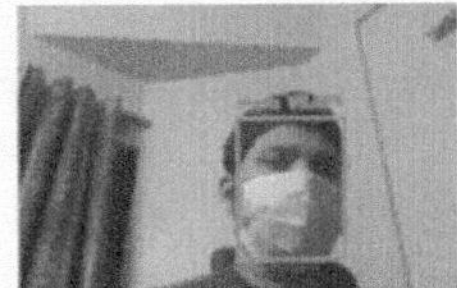

Fig 9. Mask detected

FIGURE 8.13   Handgloves and facemask detection testing on real-time sample images.

in its predictions. This implies that the model had a 95% confidence in correctly identifying instances of facemasks and hand gloves. High precision confidence is crucial, particularly in critical scenarios where accurate detection is required, such as in healthcare facilities, airports, or crowded public places. Figure 8.13 represents the testing results on some sample images of the proposed hybrid model for both hand gloves and facemask detection.

In Figure 8.13, a sample testing of the proposed hybrid model is executed and represented on real-life images to identify facemask and hand gloves. The tested results are on the real-life images. The images are the authors themselves where we have executed and tested our hybrid algorithm to check whether it is actively working with mask/gloves and without mask/gloves.

8.5   CONCLUSIONS AND FUTURE WORK

The detection of facemasks and hand gloves using computer vision and deep learning techniques has emerged as a valuable tool in the fight against infectious diseases, with relevance during the pandemic situation. This chapter has explored the current state of research in this area, highlighting the use of models such as YOLOv8, RCNN, and hybrid approaches for accurate detection in images and videos. The findings from related works showcased the progress made in detecting facemasks and hand gloves, demonstrating high accuracy and promising results in various real-world and simulated scenarios. The use of deep learning models, such as YOLOv8 and RCNN, has proven to be effective in achieving accurate and efficient detection, leveraging the strengths of both object detection and classification. The preparation of a robust dataset played a pivotal role in training the detection models. By combining real-world and simulated datasets, encompassing diverse scenarios and variations, the dataset enabled the models to learn from a wide range of examples. The careful annotation of the dataset provided ground truth information for training, validation, and testing, ensuring the reliability and accuracy of the models. Looking ahead, there are several exciting avenues for future exploration in this field. Improving the accuracy and robustness of existing models remains a priority, focusing on addressing challenges such as occlusions, diverse facial appearances, and variations in lighting conditions. Real-time deployment and integration with surveillance systems and IoT devices can enhance the practical applicability of these detection systems in high-traffic areas and healthcare facilities. The integration of multimodal approaches, such as thermal imaging or depth sensing, holds promise for improving the accuracy and reliability of detection systems, especially in scenarios where visual cues alone may be insufficient. Transfer learning techniques can be employed to leverage pre-trained models and adapt them to new environments, reducing the need for extensive labeled datasets for every unique scenario. Ethical considerations and privacy concerns should be at the forefront of future research endeavors. Developing privacy-preserving techniques and addressing ethical implications will foster trust and ensure responsible deployment of these systems. Additionally, exploring techniques for assessing the proper usage of facemasks, such as analyzing their positioning and fit, can further enhance the effectiveness of detection systems. In conclusion, the use of computer vision and deep learning techniques for the detection of facemasks and hand gloves has shown significant potential in combating the spread of infectious diseases. The advancements made in this field, coupled with future research and development, hold promise for improving the accuracy, real-time deployment, and integration of these detection systems, ultimately contributing to public health and safety in various settings. By continuously innovating and addressing emerging challenges, we can create more reliable, efficient, and scalable solutions to mitigate the impact of infectious diseases.

One area of future development is enhancing the accuracy and robustness of existing models and algorithms. While current models have achieved high accuracy in detecting facemasks and hand gloves, there is still room for improvement. Future research can focus on refining these models to better handle challenging scenarios, such as occlusions, diverse facial appearances, and variations in lighting conditions. By addressing these issues, detection systems can become even more reliable and effective. Real-time deployment is another important aspect that can be further explored. Ensuring that facemasks and hand glove detection systems can operate in real time is crucial for their practical implementation. Future efforts can concentrate on optimizing models and algorithms for real-time performance, reducing latency, and enabling the deployment of these systems in high-traffic areas, healthcare facilities, and other contexts where immediate monitoring and enforcement of PPE compliance are necessary. Incorporating multimodal approaches can also enhance the accuracy and reliability of detection systems. Future research can explore the integration of computer vision with other technologies, such as thermal imaging, depth sensing, or audio analysis. By combining multiple sensing modalities, detection systems can overcome limitations associated with visual cues alone and improve accuracy, especially in challenging scenarios where facemasks or hand gloves might not be clearly visible. Transfer learning and generalization are important considerations for the practical applicability of detection systems. Future work can investigate transfer learning techniques to leverage pre-trained models on large-scale datasets and adapt them to new environments or specific domains. This approach would reduce the dependency on collecting extensive labeled datasets for every unique scenario, making the detection systems more scalable and adaptable. As facemasks and hand glove detection systems become more prevalent, it is essential to address privacy concerns and ethical considerations. Future research can focus on developing privacy-preserving techniques, such as anonymization or edge-computing approaches, to ensure the protection of individuals' privacy while still maintaining effective detection capabilities. Ethical considerations, such as consent and data usage, should also be carefully addressed to build trust and ensure responsible deployment of these systems. Integration with existing surveillance systems and IoT devices is another area of future development. By integrating facemasks and hand glove detection systems with surveillance cameras and IoT devices, their functionality and impact can be enhanced. This integration can enable real-time alerts, automate enforcement mechanisms, and contribute to overall public safety efforts. Furthermore, future research can explore techniques to not only detect the presence of facemasks but also assess the proper usage of masks. This can involve advanced image analysis and pattern recognition techniques to analyze the positioning and fit of masks on individuals' faces. Ensuring that masks cover the nose and mouth adequately is essential for their effectiveness in preventing the spread of infectious diseases.

REFERENCES

1. Lee, A., Jiang, B., Zeng, I., & Aibin, M. (2022, October). Ocean Medical Iste Detection for CPU-Based Underwater Remotely Operated Vehicles (ROVs). 2022 IEEE 13th Annual Ubiquitous Computing, Electronics & Mobile Communication Conference (UEMCON). IEEE, pp. 385–389.
2. Buragohain, A., Mali, B., Saha, S., & Singh, P. K. (2022). A Deep Transfer Learning Based Approach to Detect COVID-19 Iste. *Internet Technology Letters*, 5(3), e327.
3. Pham, T. N., Nguyen, V. H., & Huh, J. H. (2023). Integration of Improved YOLOv5 for Facemasks Detector and Auto-labeling to Generate Dataset for Fighting against COVID-19. *The Journal of Supercomputing*, 79, 8966–8992.
4. Wang, C. Y., Bochkovskiy, A., & Liao, H. Y. M. (2022). YOLOv7: Trainable Bag-of-Freebies Sets New State-of-the-Art for Real-Time Object Detectors. *arXiv Preprint ArXiv:2207.02696*.
5. Wang, X., Zhao, Q., Jiang, P., Zheng, Y., Yuan, L., & Yuan, P. (2022). LDS-YOLO: A Lightweight Small Object Detection Method for Dead Trees from Shelter Forest. *Computers and Electronics in Agriculture*, 198, 107035.
6. Liu, W., Shan, S., Chen, H., Wang, R., Sun, J., & Zhou, Z. (2022). X-ray Weld Defect Detection Based on AF-RCNN. *Welding in the World*, 66(6), 1165–1177.

7. Tang, J., Liu, S., Zhao, D., Tang, L., Zou, W., & Zheng, B. (2023). PCB-YOLO: An Improved Detection Algorithm of PCB Surface Defects Based on YOLOv5. *Sustainability*, 15(7), 5963.

8. Al Bari, A. K., Rachmawati, E., & Kosala, G. (2023). Glove Detection System on Laboratory Members Using Yolov4. *Journal of Information System Research (JOSH)*, 4(4), 1270–1276.

9. Singh, M. P., Prinja, S., Rajsekar, K., Gedam, P., Aggarwal, V., Sachin, O., ... Bhargava, B. (2022). Cost of Surgical Care at Public Sector District Hospitals in India: Implications for Universal Health Coverage and Publicly Financed Health Insurance Schemes. *PharmacoEconomics – Open*, 6(5), 745–756.

10. Docto, J. P., Labininay, A. I., & Villaverde, J. F. (2022, September). Third Eye Hand Glove Object Detection for Visually Impaired Using You Only Look Once (YOLO) v4-Tiny Algorithm. 2022 IEEE International Conference on Artificial Intelligence in Engineering and Technology (IICAIET). IEEE, pp. 1–6.

11. Yunefri, Y., Sutejo, S., Fadrial, Y. E., Anggraini, K., Ramadhani, M., & Hardianto, R. (2022). Implementation of Object Detection With You Only Look Once Algorithm in Limited Face-to-Face Times in Pandemic. *Journal of Applied Engineering and Technological Science (JAETS)*, 4(1), 400–404.

12. Gugssa, M., Gurbuz, A., Wang, J., Ma, J., & Bourgouin, J. (2021). PPE-Glove Detection for Construction Safety Enhancement Based on Transfer Learning. In *Computing in Civil Engineering*. Reston, VA: ASCE Library, (pp. 58–65).

13. https://www.kaggle.com/datasets/aditya276/face-mask-dataset-yolo-format (accessed: 10 October 2023).

14. https://www.kaggle.com/datasets/dataclusterlabs/palm-and-gloves-dataset (accessed: 8 October 2023).

15. https://universe.roboflow.com/search?q=hand%20gloves (accessed: 11 October 2023).

16. Al-Dmour, H., Tareef, A., Alkalbani, A. M., Hammouri, A., & Alrahmani, B. (2023). Masked Face Detection and Recognition System Based on Deep Learning Algorithms. *Journal of Advances in Information Technology*, 14(2), 224–232.

17. Hassan, H. (2023). Assessing the COVID-19 Trends in Pakistan Using Predictive Machine Learning Techniques: An Empirical Study. *Graduate Journal of Pakistan Review (GJPR)*, 3(1), 1–120.

18. Mohamed, A., & Khairi, A. (2023). CAD System Based on Facemasks Recognition for Respiratory Infections Diseases Hospital. *Journal of Image Processing and Intelligent Remote Sensing (JIPIRS)*, 3(01), 40–48. ISSN 2815–0953.

19. Madhurya, C., & Goutham, N. (2022, February). Facemask Detection Using Convolutional Neural Networks (CNN). 2022 2nd International Conference on Artificial Intelligence and Signal Processing (AISP). IEEE, pp. 1–6.

20. Aljarallah, N. F., & Uliyan, D. M. (2022). Masked Face Recognition via a Combined SIFT and DLBP Features Trained in CNN Model. *IJCSNS*, 22(6), 319.

21. Legeay, C., Peron, W., Le Bihan, C., Pivert, A., & Lefeuvre, C. (2022). SARS-CoV-2 Detection on Healthcare Workers' Hands Caring for COVID-19 Patients. *Journal of Hospital Infection*, 126, 78–80.

22. Mohammed Ali, F. A., & Al-Tamimi, M. S. (2022). Facemasks Detection Methods and Techniques: A Review. *International Journal of Nonlinear Analysis and Applications*, 13(1), 3811–3823.

23. Fong, S. J., Dey, N., Chaki, J., Fong, S. J., Dey, N., & Chaki, J. (2021). An Introduction to COVID-19. In *Artificial Intelligence for Coronavirus Outbreak*. Springer Briefs in Applied Sciences and Technology, Springer, (pp. 1–22).

24. Chakraborty, S., & Dey, L. (2022). The Implementation of AI and AI-Empowered Imaging System to Fight Against COVID-19—A Review. *Smart Healthcare System Design: Security and Privacy Aspects*, 1, 301–311.
25. Mondal, A., Mallick, A., Das, S., Mondal, A., & Chakraborty, S. (2022). A COVID-19 Infection Rate Detection Technique Using Bayes Probability. In *Emerging Technologies in Data Mining and Information Security: Proceedings of IEMIS 2022*, Paramartha Dutta,Satyajit Chakrabarti, Abhishek Bhattacharya, Soumi Dutta, and Celia Shahnaz (eds.), (Vol. 2, pp. 575–584). Springer Nature Singapore
26. Shinde, G. R., Kalamkar, A. B., Mahalle, P. N., & Dey, N. (2020). *Data Analytics for Pandemics: A COVID-19 Case Study*. CRC Press.
27. Dey, L., Chakraborty, S., & Mukhopadhyay, A. (2020). Machine Learning Techniques for Sequence-Based Prediction of Viral–Host Interactions between SARS-CoV-2 and Human Proteins. *Biomedical Journal*, 43(5), 438–450.
28. Mishra, A., Paul, P., Mondal, K., & Chakraborty, S. (2023). A Study on Facemask Detection and Maintaining Safe Distance Using AI and ML to Prevent COVID-19. International Conference on Robotics, Control and Computer. Vision (ICRCCV), Vol. 1009, Springer LNEE.
29. Tamang, S., Sen, B., Pradhan, A., Sharma, K., & Singh, V. K. (2023). Enhancing COVID-19 Safety: Exploring YOLOv8 Object Detection for Accurate Face Mask Classification. *International Journal of Intelligent Systems and Applications in Engineering*, 11(2), 892–897.
30. Yu, F., Zhu, J., Chen, Y., Liu, S., & Jiang, M. (2023). CAPN: A Combine Attention Partial Network for Glove Detection. *PeerJ Computer Science*, 9, e1558.
31. Jin, H., Du, R., Qiao, L., Cao, L., Yao, J., & Zhang, S. (2023). CCA-YOLO: An Improved Glove Defect Detection Algorithm Based on YOLOv5. *Applied Sciences*, 13(18), 10173.

Part V

Machine Learning in Medical Diagnosis and Treatment Planning

9 Utilization of Machine Learning and Deep Learning Classifiers in Predicting Users' Performance in Augmented Reality Surgical Environments
A Comparative Analysis

Hamza Ghandorh

9.1 INTRODUCTION

The potential of machine learning (ML) methods to improve patient outcomes and improve teaching is drawing interest in the field of surgical education. ML methods are strong in pattern recognition, big data analysis, and creating specific training modules. These methods can analyze many kinds of data, which help with training evaluation and skill assessment. In surgical training, ML may replicate surgical scenarios, pinpoint areas for improvement, and offer immediate feedback. Yet, issues, such as data privacy, and workflow integration must be resolved. Despite these obstacles, ML methods are a viable strategy for patient care and surgical education.

ML techniques known as deep learning (DL) methods are becoming increasingly prevalent in surgical education because of their capacity to extract intricate representations from massive amounts of data. Through data analysis, DL methods in surgical training seek to enhance knowledge, expertise, and patient care. These methods can help with surgery planning, find patterns and correlations, and create augmented and virtual reality (AR/VR) simulators. Large labeled datasets and incorporating DL into current workflows are two obstacles that must be overcome, though.

DOI: 10.1201/9781003464884-14

Medical researchers have employed several cutting-edge technologies, such as augmented reality (AR) or virtual reality (VR) simulators, which are utilized to train surgeons in complex procedures, providing a realistic, risk-free environment for practice and performance improvement and ultimately enhancing patient outcomes [1]. These simulators have two main advantages: (1) to replicate purposeful training and (2) to provide precise, objective, and prompt feedback. On the one hand, neurosurgical procedures, for example, require hard and soft skills, including medical knowledge, judgment, and dexterity. Surgeons' training curricula should include these skills, focusing on targeted tasks to build mastery in effective ways [1]. On the other hand, the utilization of simulation technologies offers an objective means of assessing a range of surgical activities. For example, surgeons-in-training or novice surgeons could be evaluated using objective metrics such as hand–eye coordination, surgical technique, and decision-making skills. These assessments could then be analyzed to identify common errors or trends among trainees, enabling targeted interventions and improvements in surgical performance [1]. The development of ML and DL classifiers would enhance the healthcare decision-making process by enabling the analysis of relevant data to forecast the success of trainees[1] in many medical domains. The incorporation of ML and DL classifiers and AR technology has the potential to bring about a transformative impact on various aspects of the healthcare industry.

In this chapter, we hypothesize that both ML and DL classifiers could accurately predict trainees' performance during their interactions within AR surgical simulation environments. This work will act as an extension of our work [2] that aimed to predict the performance of surgical trainees in an AR surgical simulation environment using ML classifiers.

This chapter is organized as follows: Section 9.2 introduces some concepts related to the chapter's scope and current related work. Section 9.3 briefly describes the evaluation techniques used to predict trainees' performance in AR surgical environments. Section 9.4 depicts the outcomes of the comparative analysis between the applied ML and DL classifiers and Fitts' law. Sections 9.5 and 9.6 give a discussion and conclusion of this chapter, respectively.

9.2 BACKGROUND AND RELATED WORK

This section provides a brief introduction to AR and VR surgical simulation and a review of their application to assess users' performance in the healthcare domain. Azuma [3] described AR technology as the process of incorporating or merging three-dimensional (3D) virtual information upon the actual environment into the users' perception. AR does not completely replace the user's reality; rather, it enhances the user's existing experience. The role of AR is to not only retrieve and present pertinent information to our immediate focus but also enhance one or more of our senses, including visual, aural, olfactory, gustatory, and tactile.

AR enables users to develop a more profound comprehension of their surroundings, which is achieved through the collection and cultivation of knowledge, leading to an improved understanding and enhancement of their performance [4]. An AR system integrates both physical and virtual environments, enabling users to interact with real-time interactive modes, while ensuring the accurate alignment of 3D objects and sceneries. Every AR system consists of three essential components: a 3D scene generator, a display or multimodal device, and tracking and sensing equipment [3]. The integration of 3D objects into real-world surroundings, namely for surgical navigation and trainee evaluation, has become a focal point for clinical, academic, and industrial laboratories due to the emergence of medical augmented reality (MAR) display technologies. MAR technologies can provide real-time patient information for surgeons during surgeries. By using these technologies, trainees experience better precision and efficiency during simulated procedures in a virtual environment. NeuroTouch, a typical example of MAR display technology, enables accurate navigation within brain structures, mimics actual surgical operations, and allows for the assessment of trainees' performance, thereby improving surgical precision and training outcomes [5].

Within AR and VR surgical simulations, a few works considered the integration of ML and DL classifiers to predict users' performance for training purposes [6–11]. Ledwos et al. identified a set of the most pertinent criteria for assessing the educational advancement of surgeons within a virtual environment that simulates neurosurgical procedures [6]. They utilized the k-nearest neighbors (k-NN) classifier to examine a set of performance indicators obtained from a dataset of surgeons' performance at various points in their skill development. k-NN successfully identified several crucial variables that exhibited noteworthy variations as surgeons advanced in their learning trajectory, namely, accuracy, precision, task completion time, and movement fluidity.

Siyar et al. created a system capable of effectively evaluating and categorizing the proficiency levels of neurosurgeons by analyzing their performance in a simulated tumor-removal process [7]. The researchers utilized several ML classifiers, including the support vector machine (SVM) and k-NN, to examine and classify performance data and to assess and classify the proficiency levels of the surgeons. The results indicated that the SVM method was successful in accurately distinguishing between various proficiency levels among the subjects with a significant level of accuracy (90%). Alkadri et al. examined the use of a multilayer perceptron artificial neural network (ANN) for assessing the efficacy of a VR surgical procedure [8].

To determine the performance of the ANN, the researchers conducted a comparative analysis between the assessments made by the ANN and those made by human experts. The findings demonstrated that there was a significant correlation accuracy (80%) between the evaluations conducted by the ANN and the assessments made by the experts. Reich et al. created a system that accurately evaluates and delivers feedback on the proficiency levels of trainees in the context of competency-based training [9]. Using the ANN classifier, the system could accurately evaluate and offer constructive feedback on the proficiency levels of trainees across multiple domains and disciplines. The researchers discovered that ANN proved to be effective in accurately evaluating the trainees' accuracy (83.3%). Karlik et al. evaluated surgical proficiency through the utilization of hybrid deep neural network algorithms within the context of VR simulation, using convolutional neural networks and recurrent neural networks (RNNs) [10]. They examined and interpreted data related to surgical performance based on the collected data from expert surgeons. The findings of the study indicated that the hybrid deep neural network algorithms were successful in accurately differentiating between expert and beginner surgeons by analyzing their performance indicators. The algorithms demonstrated a notable level of accuracy in evaluating surgical expertise, thereby highlighting their potential as a dependable assessment tool. Winkler-Schwartz et al. conducted a systematic review and maintained a comprehensive framework for reporting and analyzing research papers that involve the utilization of VR surgical simulation and ML classifiers [11]. The researchers reported that a total of 12 studies published between 2003 and 2018 were examined to evaluate the application of ML and DL classifiers in the classification of expertise within the context of VR surgical simulation. The researchers primarily emphasized that SVM, decision tree (DT), hidden Markov models, Naive Bayes, and other ML classifiers were chosen to be applied.

9.3 METHODOLOGY

This section describes the approach employed to predict users' performance in an AR simulation environment. The objective of this chapter is to examine the impact of different ML and DL classifiers on predicting users' performance using an AR surgical simulation dataset.

9.3.1 AR SURGICAL DATASET

The dataset was curated as the outcome of an AR surgical simulation training study [2], where a total of 14 novice subjects were enlisted as trainees and a series of 378 trials were conducted on the target throughout 27 scenarios, with the order of scenarios being randomized. The objective of the study was to assess the performance of participants in 3D virtual activities that involved targeting designed to simulate a neurosurgical activity.

The study was conducted utilizing an AR simulator system [12] that utilized virtual 3D anatomical models of the human brain and a surgical probe. A user manipulated a virtual probe tool with the intention of precisely inserting it into the most suitable entrance site of a predetermined target to achieve a precise penetration. Every trial provided insight into the performance of each subject in relation to activity-related variables, enabling subsequent assessment within the same conditions. The dataset comprised both task-related and event-related attributes from an AR surgical study for trainees. A sample of the dataset and its features is listed in Figure 9.1.

9.3.2 FITTS' LAW ASSESSMENT TECHNIQUE

Paul Fitts [13, 14] explained the correlation between (1) the level of difficulty associated with a pointing task, (2) the distance between the user and the target, and (3) the size of the target itself. This correlation is referred to as Fitts' law. It is a foundational concept within the domains of human–computer interaction and human movement

TimeStamp (YYYY/MM/DD HH:MM:SS:FFFF)	User Trial Number	Event Type	Caustive Object	Caustive Object Position X	Caustive Object Position Y	Caustive Object Position Z	Caustive Object Rotation X	Caustive Object Rotation Y	Caustive Object Position Z	Receptive Object Name	Incidence Angle	Receptive Object Width	Sesion Elapsed Time
2016/06/21 17:17:52:2410	27	Objects At Single Line	Endscopy_Head	4.29	48.13	4.51	0.73	0.16	-0.20	Skull	157.18	-576.51	
2016/06/21 17:17:52:3118	27	Objects At Single Line	Endscopy_Head	4.29	48.04	4.52	0.73	0.16	-0.20	Skull	157.38	-576.51	
2016/06/21 17:17:52:4261	27	Objects At Single Line	Endscopy_Head	4.24	48.02	4.59	0.73	0.17	-0.21	Skull	155.53	-576.51	
2016/06/21 17:17:52:5450	27	Objects At Single Line	Endscopy_Head	4.20	47.94	4.60	0.73	0.17	-0.21	Skull	155.25	-576.51	
2016/06/21 17:17:52:6450	27	Objects At Single Line	Endscopy_Head	4.20	47.74	4.56	0.73	0.16	-0.20	Skull	156.36	-576.51	
2016/06/21 17:17:52:7685	27	Objects At Single Line	Endscopy_Head	4.16	47.66	4.56	0.73	0.16	-0.21	Skull	155.58	-576.51	
2016/06/21 17:17:52:8573	27	Objects At Single Line	Endscopy_Head	4.13	47.62	4.56	0.73	0.17	-0.21	Skull	154.50	-576.51	
2016/06/21 17:17:52:9893	27	Objects At Single Line	Endscopy_Head	4.25	47.48	4.46	0.74	0.16	-0.20	Skull	157.45	-576.51	
2016/06/21 17:17:53:1081	27	Objects At Single Line	Endscopy_Head	4.42	47.57	4.32	0.74	0.16	-0.20	Skull	158.90	-576.51	
2016/06/21 17:17:53:2402	27	Objects At Single Line	Endscopy_Head	4.75	48.20	3.97	0.73	0.18	-0.20	Skull	160.52	-576.51	
2016/06/21 17:17:53:3352	27	Objects At Single Line	Endscopy_Head	4.95	48.65	3.73	0.72	0.19	-0.20	Skull	161.55	-576.51	
2016/06/21 17:17:53:4581	27	Objects At Single Line	Endscopy_Head	5.04	49.08	3.47	0.72	0.19	-0.21	Skull	160.93	-576.51	
2016/06/21 17:17:53:5526	27	Objects At Single Line	Endscopy_Head	5.06	49.37	3.38	0.72	0.19	-0.20	Skull	161.93	-576.51	
2016/06/21 17:17:53:6809	27	Objects At Single Line	Endscopy_Head	4.91	49.67	3.18	0.72	0.19	-0.20	Skull	159.47	-576.51	
2016/06/21 17:17:53:7572	27	Objects At Single Line	Endscopy_Head	4.91	50.20	3.10	0.72	0.17	-0.19	Lateral Ventricles	161.17	-247.77	
2016/06/21 17:17:53:8846	27	Objects At Single Line	Endscopy_Head	4.86	51.15	3.03	0.71	0.18	-0.19	Lateral Ventricles	160.15	-247.77	
2016/06/21 17:17:53:9574	27	Objects At Single Line	Endscopy_Head	4.85	51.43	2.99	0.71	0.18	-0.19	Lateral Ventricles	159.39	-247.77	
2016/06/21 17:17:54:0817	27	Objects At Single Line	Endscopy_Head	4.76	52.47	2.99	0.70	0.19	-0.19	Lateral Ventricles	159.28	-247.77	
2016/06/21 17:17:54:2176	27	Objects At Single Line	Endscopy_Head	4.80	52.79	2.97	0.70	0.18	-0.18	Lateral Ventricles	159.51	-247.77	
2016/06/21 17:17:55:4391	27	Interaction Detected	Endscopy_Head	4.68	53.99	3.62	0.69	0.20	-0.19	Ellipse27_R2_P2_S2	88.16	0.05	00:00:43.15
2016/06/21 17:17:57:7446	Session ended												

FIGURE 9.1 A sample of the augmented reality surgical dataset and its attributes (position, rotation, size) vectors, including virtual 3D anatomical brain structures, surgical task-related features, and event-related features.

science. It aims to estimate the duration needed for accurate target selection and movement using a pointing device, such as a mouse or finger. In addition, it specifies that the duration of movement exhibits a direct correlation with the distance to the designated goal while displaying an inverse correlation with the breadth of the target. It is measured by the index of performance (IP) in bits per second. The mathematical representation of Fitts' law [13, eq. (1)]:

$$IP = \frac{\log_2\left(\frac{A}{W}+1\right)}{MT} = \frac{ID}{MT} \; , \qquad\qquad (\text{eq. } 1)$$

where ID is how accurately and fast the participants completed the tasks, MT denotes the duration of the movement, A indicates the distance between the initial position and the intended goal, W signifies the width of the target, and the coefficients a and b are generated from empirical observations.

9.3.3   MACHINE LEARNING CLASSIFIERS

The ML classifiers refer to a set of algorithms that are autonomously used to acquire patterns and subsequently generate predictions or conclusions by analyzing input data. They constitute integral elements of numerous applications spanning diverse disciplines that encompass image recognition, natural language processing, medical diagnostics, and fraud detection. Every classifier possesses distinct strengths and weaknesses, rendering these classifiers appropriate for varying problem types and datasets [15].

9.3.3.1   Nearest Centroid

The nearest centroid (NC) classifier is a simple and effective algorithm commonly used for the purpose of classification. It aims to assign a given test sample to the class that possesses a centroid with the closest proximity to the sample inside the feature space [16]. A centroid is a representation of the average values of the feature vectors derived from the training samples belonging to each class.

9.3.3.2   k-Nearest Neighbors

The k-NN classifier is a simple, nonparametric algorithm that is utilized for performing classification. It aims to allocate a test sample to a specific class or forecast its value through the process of majority voting or averaging its k-nearest neighbors in the feature space. The number of nearest neighbors to consider while making predictions in a k-NN classifier is determined by the value of k. The assignment of a test sample is determined by selecting the class that appears most frequently among its k-nearest neighbors [16].

9.3.3.3   Support Vector Machine

The SVM is a supervised learning classifier that is utilized for the purposes of classification problems. It aims to identify an ideal hyperplane inside the space of features that effectively divides different classes while also increasing the margin between those classes. A hyperplane is determined to divide the classes with the biggest margins. The samples closest in proximity to the decision boundary, commonly referred to as the support vectors, play a critical role in determining the hyperplane [17].

9.3.3.4   Linear Support Vector Machine

The linear support vector machine (LSVM) classifier identifies a suitable hyperplane inside the space of features that effectively divides into many classes while also maximizing the margin between them. The primary goal is to optimize the margin between the hyperplane and the support vectors, which are the samples that are in closest proximity to the decision boundary. The LSVM classifier offers a quick and easy solution for binary classification tasks, making it particularly helpful when working with linearly separable data [18].

9.3.3.5   Decision Tree

A DT is a widely utilized machine learning method that uses a model resembling a tree structure, which represents decisions and their corresponding outcomes. The training data is recursively partitioned according to the features' values to generate nodes and branches that reflect decision rules. DT functions by recursively dividing the feature space into smaller subsets, utilizing the values of various features as criteria for division. DT choose the most optimal feature to partition the data at each internal node, utilizing parameters such as entropy or Gini impurity [19]. The Gini index [20, eq. (2)] and entropy criteria [20, eq. (3)] are calculated as follows:

$$Gini_{index} = 1 - \sum_j p_j^2, \qquad\qquad (eq.\ 2)$$

where $0 \le Gini_{index} \le 1$ and p_j is the probability of class j and

$$entropy = -\sum_j p_j * log_2 p_j, \qquad\qquad (eq.\ 3)$$

where p_j is the probability of class j.

9.3.3.6   Random Forest

The random forest (RF) classifier aggregates the results of numerous decision tree classifiers to make accurate predictions. It uses an ensemble approach to combine individual tree predictions, thus reducing overfitting and improving generalization performance while also identifying influential variables. At every node in the tree, a subset of features is chosen randomly for the purpose of splitting, which serves to mitigate overfitting and enhance the heterogeneity of the trees [21].

9.3.4   Deep Learning Classifiers

The DL classifiers are a specific category of machine learning methods that employ deep neural networks for the purpose of acquiring intricate representations and generating predictions. DL classifiers have gathered substantial attention and demonstrated notable achievements in diverse domains, including computer vision, natural language processing, and speech recognition. DL classifiers hold the distinctive attribute of being capable of autonomously acquiring hierarchical representations from unprocessed input data. The utilization of hierarchical representation learning facilitates the ability of DL classifiers to effectively capture complex patterns and interdependencies within a given dataset [22].

9.3.4.1   Long Short-term Memory

The long short-term memory (LSTM) is a specific architecture of an RNN that has been developed to effectively mitigate the issue of vanishing gradients and model long-range relationships across sequential input. The LSTM networks employ memory cells that possess the capability to store and update information for a duration, thereby enabling them to discerningly keep or discard information contingent upon the input. The fundamental components of every memory cell encompass an input gate, a forget gate, and an output gate. The goal of these gates is to regulate the transmission of data into, out of, and within the memory cell [23]. The architecture of LSTM comprises a set of equations [24, eq. (4), eq. (5), eq. (6)] that regulate the information transmission within the network. The primary equations that govern the behavior of LSTM cells i.e. the forget gate f_t, the input gate i_t, and the output gate o_t, can be expressed as follows:

$$i_t = \sigma\left(W_i * \left[H_{t-1} - x_t\right] + b_i\right) \tag{eq. 4}$$

$$f_t = \sigma\left(W_f * \left[H_{t-1} - x_t\right] + b_f\right) \tag{eq. 5}$$

$$o_t = \sigma\left(W_0 * \left[H_{t-1} - x_t\right] + b_0\right) \tag{eq. 4}$$

where x_t is an input to the current timestamp t, W is the weight associated with the input, H_{t-1} is the hidden state of the previous timestamp t, and b is a bias value for the gate.

9.3.4.2   Artificial Neural Network

The ANN is a computational model that draws inspiration from the form and functionality of a biological neural network. It is composed of interconnected nodes, referred to as artificial neurons, which are arranged in layers. The main element of an ANN is an artificial neuron or a perceptron. Every individual neuron inside a neural network receives input signals, which are subsequently subjected to mathematical modification, ultimately resulting in the generation of an output signal. The synaptic connections between neurons are characterized by numerical values known as weights, which quantitatively determine the magnitude of the impact exerted by one neuron on another. The ANNs are structured in a hierarchical manner, comprising several levels i.e. an input layer, one or more hidden layers, and an output layer. The input layer is responsible for receiving the input data, whereas the output layer is responsible for generating the final prediction or judgment. The concealed layers of a neural network are responsible for doing intermediary computations and acquiring representations of the incoming data [22]. The cost of an ANN is determined by an activation function [25 , eq. (7)] as follows:

$$\hat{y} = w[0]*x[0] + w[1]*x[1] + \cdots + w[p]*x[p] + b,\qquad \text{(eq. 5)}$$

where $\hat{y}$ is the weighted sum of the input features $x[0]$ to $x[p]$ and the weighted sum of the learned coefficients $w[0]$ to $w[p]$. Each neuron in the network has a bias value b that can be learned, and the activating function is moved around with the help of b.

9.3.5 PERFORMANCE MEASURES

According to the existing literature, Malhotra and Jain [26] suggested that there are two evaluation criteria that can be utilized to assess the similarity of actual and predicted values: the mean magnitude of relative error (MMRE)[2] [26, eq. (8)] and the average pairwise relative distance (PRED)[3] [26, eq. (9)]. Both criteria are used to determine the similarity of ML and DL classifiers (NC, k-NN, SVM, LSVM, RF, DT, LSTM, and ANN) predictions and then compare them against Fitts' law. These metrics are calculated as follows:

$$MMRE = \frac{1}{n}\sum_{i=1}^{n}\frac{|P_i - A_i|}{|A_i|},\qquad \text{(eq. 6)}$$

where P_i is the predicted value for datapoint i, A_i is the actual value for datapoint i, and n is the total number of data points.

$$PRED(A) = \frac{d}{n},\qquad \text{(eq. 7)}$$

where d is the value of MRE where a data point n is less than or equal to A.

9.4 RESULTS

This section demonstrates the outcomes of our comparative analysis between the actual users' performance measured by Fitts' law and ML and DL classifiers within an AR surgical simulation environment. The users' performance features, namely, the target width (W), the distance between the target and the user (A), the user's effort (ID), and the trails' time (MT) were utilized as inputs to the NC, k-NN, SVM, LSVM, RF, DT, LSTM, and ANN classifiers and the value of the IP. Prior work [2] examined the potential for predicting users' performance by comparing a few ML classifiers, namely, NC, k-NN, SVM, and DT, with the conventional human performance evaluation approach (Fitts' law) in an AR surgical environment. In this chapter, additional ML and DL classifiers were included, namely, LSVM, RF, LSTM, and ANN, to examine the potential for predicting users' performance in AR surgical simulation environments.

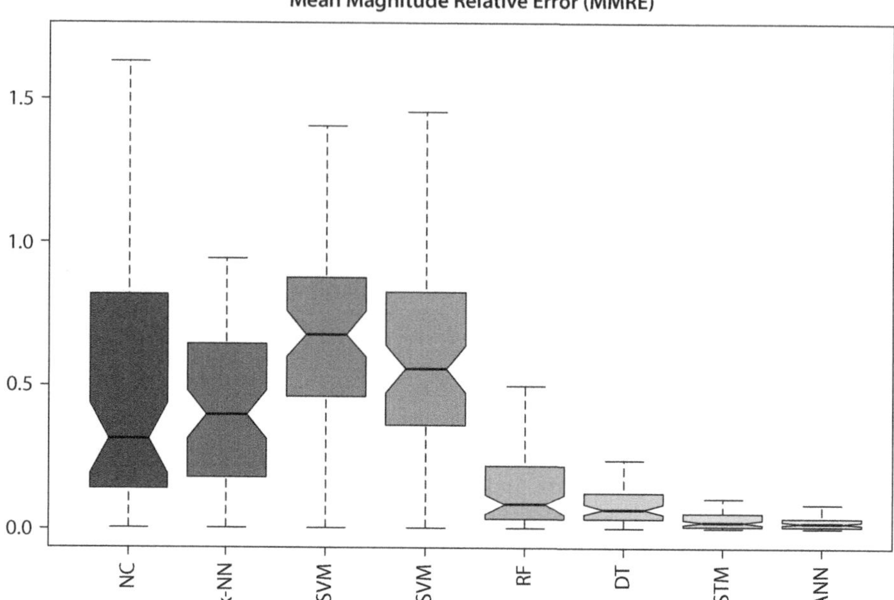

FIGURE 9.2 Mean magnitude relative error of a variety of the applied machine learning and deep learning classifiers.

Figure 9.2 and Table 9.1 indicate the values of the MMRE for the ML and DL classifiers used. Comparing values of minimum MMRE and maximum PRED(A) for the RF, DT, LSTM, and ANN classifiers shows that they maintain better performance than NC, k-NN, SVM, and LSVM classifiers. When we compare them against actual users' performance, NC, k-NN, SVM, and LSVM yielded MMRE values (0.791, 0.430, 0.655, 0.733 with a relatively high error, which means that these

TABLE 9.1

Mean Magnitude Relative Error and Maximum Pairwise Relative Distance (A) of the Machine Learning and Deep Learning Classifiers

no.	Classifier	MMRE	PRED (25)	PRED (50)	PRED (75)
1	NC	0.791	0.447	0.632	0.711
2	k-NN	0.430	0.329	0.618	0.816
3	SVM	0.655	0.145	0.289	0.579
4	LSVM	0.733	0.171	0.408	0.684
5	RF	0.234	0.776	0.868	0.947
6	DT	0.105	0.829	0.921	0.947
7	LSTM	0.049	0.974	0.987	1.000
8	ANN	0.040	0.974	0.987	1.000

classifiers are bad predictors of the trainees' performance. In addition, the RF and DT methods yielded MMRE values (0.234 and 0.105, respectively) with a relatively low error, which means that these classifiers are good predictors of the trainees' performance. Moreover, LSTM and ANN yielded MMRE values (0.049 and 0.040, respectively) with a very low error, which means that these classifiers are the best predictors of trainees' performance.

Figures 9.3, 9.4, 9.5, 9.6, and 9.7 depict the actual performance measured by Fitts' law against the NC and k-NN classifiers, Fitts' law against the SVM and LSVM classifiers, Fitts' law against the RF and DT classifiers, Fitts' law against the LSTM classifier, and Fitts' law against the ANN classifier, respectively. We compared the predicted performance using the ML and DL classifiers (i.e. dotted in blue and green lines) against actual users' performance (i.e. solid red line). The closer the blue and green dotted lines are to the red line, the more accurate the classifier is at predicting the users' performance. From Figure 9.3, we compared the results from the NC and k-NN classifiers against the actual users' performance and found that both classifiers were not effective predictors of the actual users' performance, as indicated by the huge error margins.

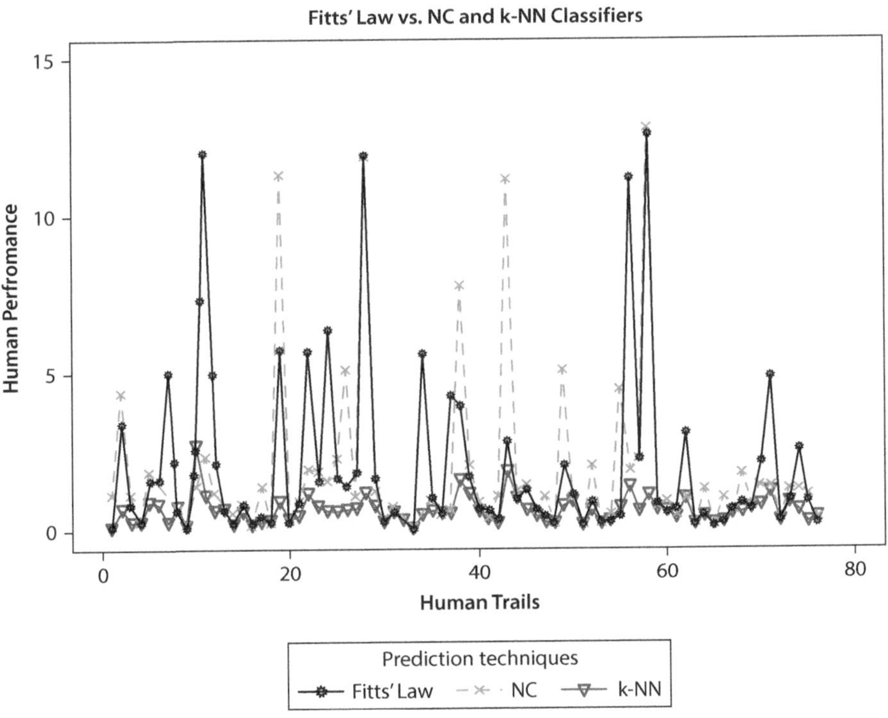

FIGURE 9.3 Actual and predicted performance using Fitts' law and the nearest centroid and k-nearest neighbors classifiers.

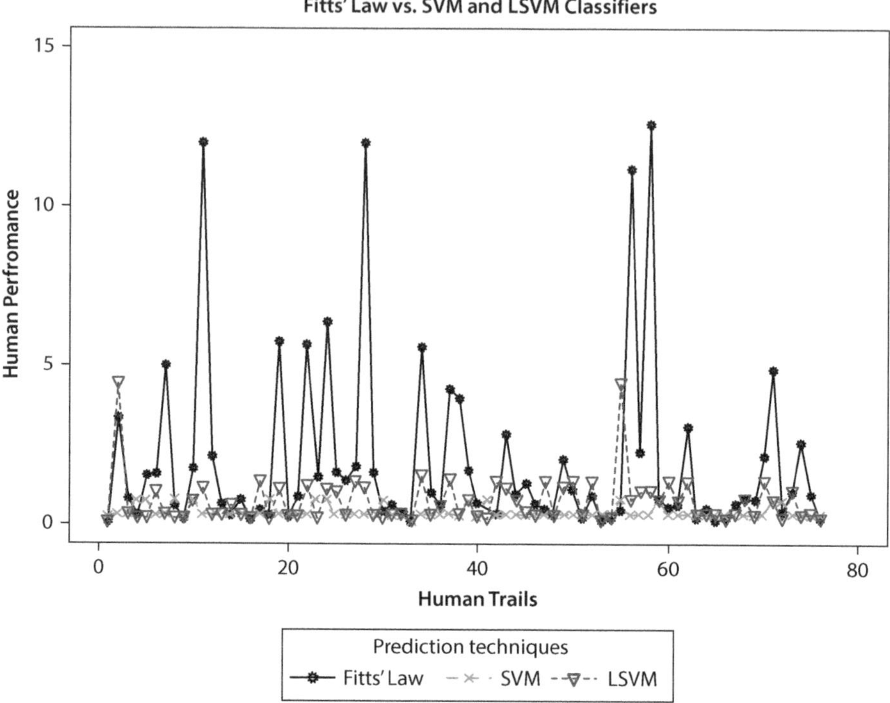

FIGURE 9.4 Actual and predicted performance using Fitts' law and the support vector machine and linear support vector machine classifiers.

From Figure 9.4, we compared the results from the SVM and LSVM classifiers against the actual users' performance and also found that both classifiers were not effective predictors of the actual users' performance, as they had huge error margins.

From Figure 9.5, we compared the results from the RF and DT classifiers against the actual users' performance and found that the RF classifier was a reasonably effective predictor of the actual users' performance, with low error margins, while the DT classifier was a good predictor of the actual users' performance, with acceptable error margins.

We compared the LSTM and the ANN classifiers against the actual users' performance and found that the LSTM and ANN classifiers were excellent predictors of the actual users' performance, with almost zero error margins.

9.5 DISCUSSION

The integration of the AR, ML, and DL classifiers should bring about a significant transformation in healthcare decision-making processes, as these classifiers facilitate the analysis of data and the prediction of performance outcomes. By analyzing datasets derived from AR technologies employed in past surgical procedures,

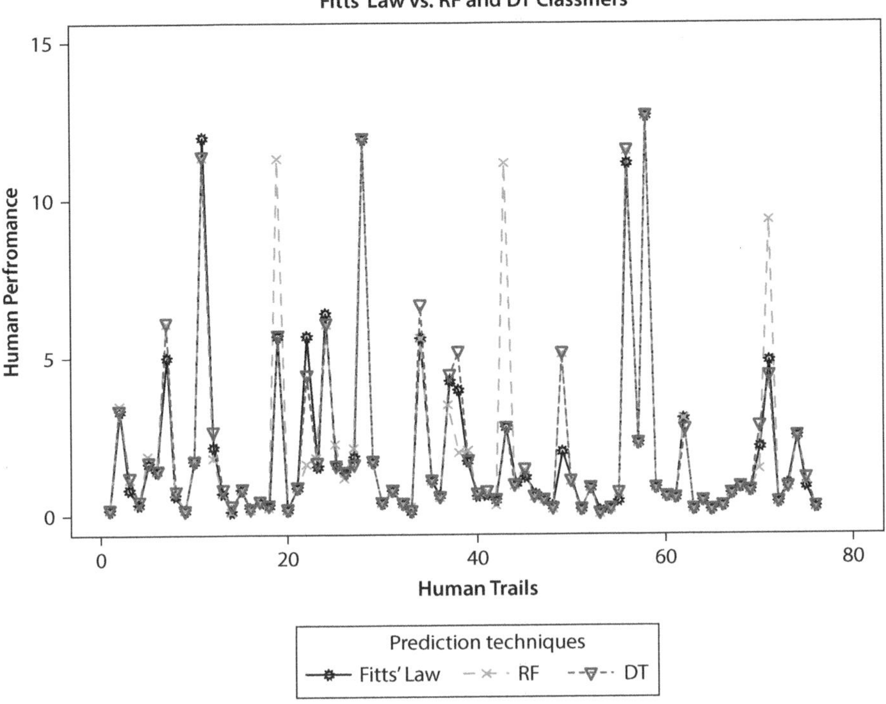

FIGURE 9.5 Actual and predicted performance using Fitts' law and the random forest and decision tree classifiers.

valuable insights may be gleaned, enabling the identification of patterns and trends. Consequently, this knowledge can be utilized to provide personalized recommendations while taking into account the associated advantages and disadvantages.

Fitts' law is a theoretical concept that is primarily used in primitive pointing tasks with discrete targets and equal difficulty. However, it may not be applicable in complex situations with diverse targets and complex interactions. It also overlooks cognitive variables and does not consider factors such as attention, task complexity, and user experience, which could limit its applicability in practical situations. Moreover, Fitts' law may not be optimal for large or distant targets, as it can take longer to accurately aim from a distance. Small close targets can be quickly selected without significant challenges in pointing accuracy. Thus, complex tasks, cognitive variables, or targets size might negatively affect Fitts' law and lead to inaccurate assessment results.

It is important to keep in mind that ML and DL classifiers have their own limitations that might affect the evaluation outcomes. The NC method is sensitive to outliers in datasets, as it assumes a uniform data spread and orientation within each class. While using the k-NN method, the presence of certain features with wider ranges can exert an excessive impact on distance estimations, leading to outcomes that are

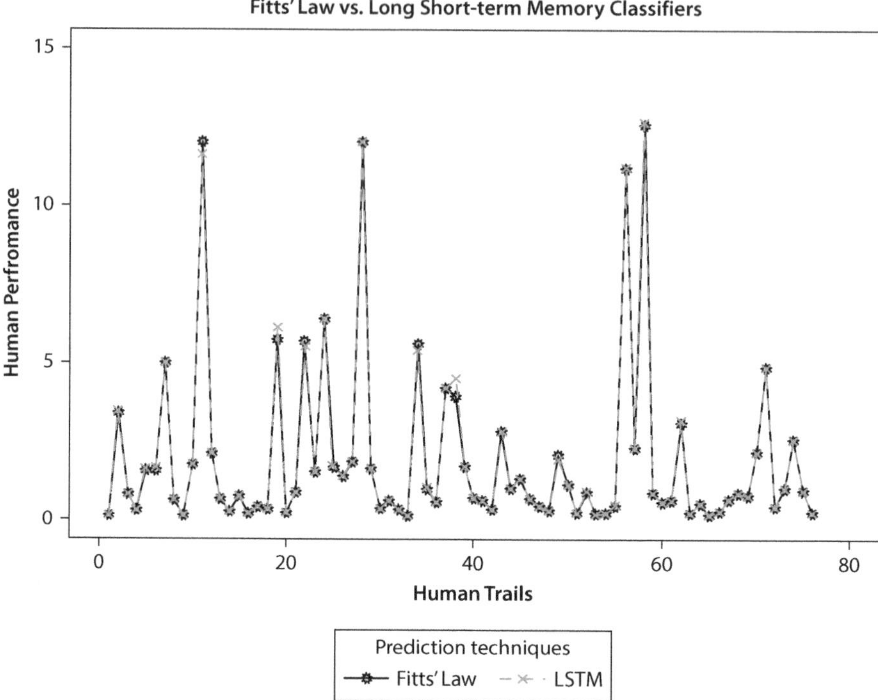

FIGURE 9.6 Actual and predicted performance using Fitts' law and the long short-term memory classifier.

skewed. In addition, k-NN assigns equal importance to all features, which can have a negative impact on its performance when irrelevant or noisy features are present. The SVM method is susceptible to the effects of parameter tuning, which can lead to an increased likelihood of overfitting. The LSVM classifier exhibits vulnerability to outliers and noisy data instances, leading to notable effects on the positioning and orientation of the decision boundary. Consequently, this might lead to unsatisfactory outcomes in the classification process.

The DT method is sensitive to small changes in training data, with even minor modifications causing a significantly different decision tree structure. The DT can also overfit when grown to maximum depth or with noisy or outlier data. While using the RF method, it is difficult to comprehend decision-making procedures and feature importance because they aggregate many tree forecasts. As such, it can be difficult to interpret the connections and interactions between characteristics. The complex architecture of the LSTMs, which includes numerous memory cells and gates, can make it difficult to track information flow and process particular input patterns. It may take a long time for the LSTM computations to update and propagate information through these connections, which slows down training and inference times. For large complex networks in particular, the ANN training is computationally

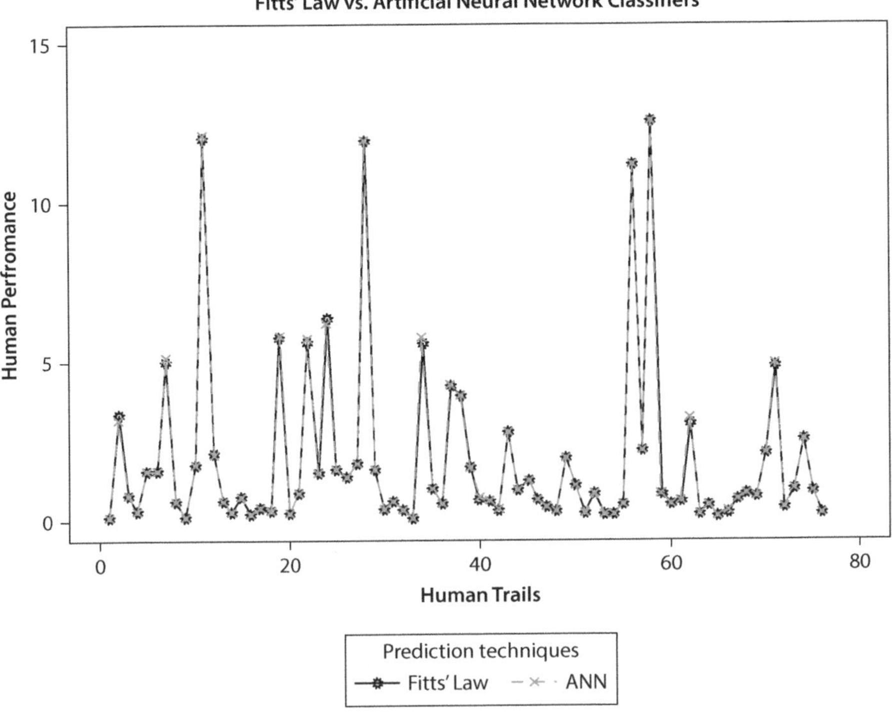

FIGURE 9.7 Actual and predicted performance using Fitts' law and the artificial neural network classifier.

demanding and time-consuming, necessitating a substantial amount of labeled data. The inner workings of the ANNs are also difficult to understand and interpret due to their complexity and nonlinearity.

9.6 CONCLUSION AND FUTURE WORK

The objective of this chapter was to compare multiple classifiers i.e. NC, k-NN, SVM, LSVM, RF, DT, LSTM, and ANN, predictive potential of subjects' performance with the conventional human performance evaluation approach (Fitts' law) in the AR surgical environments. The NC method is an easy instance-based method of learning that classifies instances in feature space using centroids; however, because it depends on mean vectors, it may incorrectly classify instances as a result of outliers. The k-NN method handles both linear and nonlinear decision boundaries. The k-NN is a nonparametric, instance-based learning method that classifies instances based on similarity. For the best results, it needs to be scaled appropriately because it is sensitive to feature scale. The best hyperplanes for separating data points are found using the SVM and LSVM algorithms; the LSVM is specifically designed for linearly separable data. Large datasets are their strong action, but parameter selection is difficult and affects performance. The DT is a visual representation of decision-making, resembling flowcharts. They provide a clear, understandable representation of decision-making, but can overfit when deep, potentially capturing irrelevant patterns and affecting generalization capabilities. The RF shows resilience in noisy datasets by combining several DTs to produce predictions. However, because of its ensemble nature, the RF is less interpretable, making it challenging to derive clear decision rules or explain the rationale underlying the prediction. Because the LSTM can recognize long-range correlations in input sequences, the recurrent neural network LSTM performs exceptionally well in sequential data analysis. However, regularization procedures are necessary because the LSTM is prone to overfitting. The ANN, inspired by biological neural networks, is a computational model with interconnected artificial neurons that can learn and predict based on input data. It's efficient on modern hardware, making it suitable for real-time applications and large datasets. However, its performance depends on the quality and quantity of training data.

This investigation used a dataset obtained from the AR simulation training conducted in a controlled study setting. The findings indicated that both the LSTM and the ANN classifiers were excellent predictors of the actual performance when using the same dataset features and trainees' trial attributes. Potential future research endeavors may involve the development of advanced predictive models that utilize a cluster of individual ML and DL classifiers, ensemble learning methods, or Adaboost methods to improve current predictors and locate new optimal predictors for any given AR surgical datasets.

NOTES

1. Trainees, novices, users, or subjects will be used interchangeably throughout the chapter.
2. MMRE measures the average magnitude of the relative errors between the anticipated values and the actual values.
3. PRED computes the relative distance between pairs of data points over two partitions.

REFERENCE

1. K. Abhari et al., "Training for Planning Tumour Resection: Augmented Reality and Human Factors," *IEEE Transactions on Bio-Medical Engineering*, vol. 62, no. 6, pp. 1466–1477, 2015. Available: https://ieeexplore.ieee.org/document/6998039/. [Accessed: Sep. 13, 2023]
2. H. Ghandorh, "Prediction of Users' Performance in Surgical Augmented Reality Simulation-Based Training Using Machine Learning Techniques," in *Digital Future of Healthcare*, edited by N. Dey et al. CRC Press, 2021, pp. 95–109.
3. R. T. Azuma, "A Survey of Augmented Reality," *Presence: Teleoperators and Virtual Environments*, vol. 6, no. 4, pp. 355–385, 1997. Available: https://direct.mit.edu/pvar/article/6/4/355-385/18336. [Accessed: Sep. 07, 2023]
4. N. Navab et al., "Medical Augmented Reality: Definition, Principle Components, Domain Modeling, and Design-Development-Validation Process," *Journal of Imaging*, vol. 9, no. 1, p. 4, Dec. 2022. Available: https://www.mdpi.com/2313-433X/9/1/4. [Accessed: Sep. 07, 2023]

5. S. Delorme, D. Laroche, R. DiRaddo, and R. F. Del Maestro, "NeuroTouch: A Physics-Based Virtual Simulator for Cranial Microneurosurgery Training," *Operative Neurosurgery*, vol. 71, pp. ons32–ons42, 2012. Available: https://journals.lww.com /01787389-201209001-00007. [Accessed: Sep. 10, 2023]

6. N. Ledwos et al., "Assessment of Learning Curves on a Simulated Neurosurgical Task Using Metrics Selected by Artificial Intelligence," *Journal of Neurologicalsurgery*, vol. 137, no. 4, pp. 1160–1171, Oct. 2022. Available: https://thejns.org/view/journals/j-neurosurg/137/4/article-p1160.xml. [Accessed: Sep. 10, 2023]

7. S. Siyar et al., "Machine Learning Distinguishes Neurosurgical Skill Levels in a Virtual Reality Tumor Resection Task," *Medical and Biological Engineering and Computing*, vol. 58, no. 6, pp. 1357–1367, 2020. Available: https://link.springer.com/10.1007/s11517 -020-02155-3. [Accessed: Sep. 10, 2023]

8. S. Alkadri et al., "Utilizing a Multilayer Perceptron Artificial Neural Network to Assess a Virtual Reality Surgical Procedure," *Computers in Biology and Medicine*, vol. 136, p. 104770, 2021. Available: https://linkinghub.elsevier.com/retrieve/pii/ S0010482521005643. [Accessed: Sep. 10, 2023]

9. A. Reich et al., "Artificial Neural Network Approach to Competency-Based Training Using a Virtual Reality Neurosurgical Simulation," *Operative Neurosurgery*, vol. 73. Publish Ahead of Print, May 2022. Available: https://journals.lww.com/10.1227/ons .0000000000000173. [Accessed: Sep. 10, 2023]

10. B. Karlik et al., "Assessment of Surgical Expertise in Virtual Reality Simulation by Hybrid Deep Neural Network Algorithms," *IJAE*, vol. 10, no. 3, pp. 47–59, Dec. 2021. Available: https://www.cscjournals.org/library/manuscriptinfo.php?mc=IJAE-206. [Accessed: Sep. 10, 2023]

11. A. Winkler-Schwartz et al., "Artificial Intelligence in Medical Education: Best Practices Using Machine Learning to Assess Surgical Expertise in Virtual Reality Simulation," *Journal of Surgical Education*, vol. 76, no. 6, pp. 1681–1690, 2019. Available: https:// linkinghub.elsevier.com/retrieve/pii/S1931720419301060. [Accessed: Sep. 10, 2023]

12. H. Ghandorh, J. Mackenzie, R. Eagleson, and S. De Ribaupierre, "Development of Augmented Reality Training Simulator Systems for Neurosurgery Using Model-Driven Software Engineering," 2017 IEEE 30th Canadian Conference on Electrical and Computer Engineering (CCECE). IEEE, Windsor, ON, 2017, pp. 1–6. Available: http://ieeexplore.ieee.org/document/7946843/. [Accessed: Sep. 06, 2023]

13. P. M. Fitts, "The Information Capacity of the Human Motor System in Controlling the Amplitude of Movement," *Journal of Experimental Psychology*, vol. 47, no. 6, pp. 381–391, 1954. Available: http://doi.apa.org/getdoi.cfm?doi=10.1037/h0055392. [Accessed: Sep. 06, 2023]

14. S. MacKenzie, "Fitts' Law as a Research and Design Tool in Human-Computer Interaction," *Human–Computer Interaction*, vol. 7, no. 1, pp. 91–139, Mar. 1992. doi: 10.1207/s15327051hci0701_3. Available: http://www.tandfonline.com/doi/abs/10.1207/ s15327051hci0701_3. [Accessed: Nov. 05, 2023]

15. M. Christopher, "Pattern Recognition and Machine Learning," in *Information Science and Statistics*, 1st ed. New York, NY: Springer, 2016. Available: https://link.springer .com/book/9780387310732. [Accessed: Sep. 06, 2023]

16. R. O. Duda, P. E. Hart, and D. G. Stork, *Pattern Classification*, 2nd ed. New York: Wiley, 2001. Available: https://www.wiley.com/en-it/Pattern+Classification,+2nd +Edition-p-9780471056690. [Accessed: Sep. 05, 2023]

17. J. C. Burges, "A Tutorial on Support Vector Machines for Pattern Recognition," *Data Mining and Knowledge Discovery*, vol. 2, no. 2, pp. 121–167, 1998. Available: http:// link.springer.com/10.1023/A:1009715923555. [Accessed: Sep. 05, 2023]

18. B. E. Boser, I. M. Guyon, and V. N. Vapnik, "A training algorithm for optimal margin classifiers," Proceedings of the Fifth Annual Workshop on Computational Learning Theory. ACM, Pittsburgh PA, 1992, pp. 144–152. Available: https://dl.acm.org/doi/10.1145/130385.130401. [Accessed: Sep. 05, 2023]

19. T. Hastie, R. Tibshirani, and J. Friedman, *The Elements of Statistical Learning.* Springer Series in Statistics. New York, NY: Springer, 2009. Available: http://link.springer.com/10.1007/978-0-387-84858-7. [Accessed: Sep. 06, 2023]

20. S. Dash, "Decision Trees Explained — Entropy, Information Gain, Gini Index, CCP Pruning," *Medium*, Nov. 02, 2022. Available: https://towardsdatascience.com/decision-trees-explained-entropy-information-gain-gini-index-ccp-pruning-4d78070db36c. [Accessed: Oct. 31, 2023]

21. L. Breiman, "Random Forests," *Machine Learning*, vol. 45, no. 1, pp. 5–32, Oct. 2001. https://doi.org/10.1023/A:1010933404324. [Accessed: Sep. 06, 2023]

22. Y. Goodfellow, *Bengio, and A. Courville, Deep Learning.* Cambridge, MA: The MIT Press, 2016. Available: http://www.deeplearningbook.org

23. S. Hochreiter and J. Schmidhuber, "Long Short-Term Memory," *Neural Computation*, vol. 9, no. 8, pp. 1735–1780, Nov. 1997. Available: https://direct.mit.edu/neco/article/9/8/1735-1780/6109. [Accessed: Sep. 06, 2023]

24. P. Gudikandula, "Recurrent Neural Networks and LSTM Explained," *Medium*, Mar. 27, 2019. Available: https://purnasaigudikandula.medium.com/recurrent-neural-networks-and-lstm-explained-7f51c7f6bbb9. [Accessed: Oct. 31, 2023]

25. L. Panneerselvam, "Activation Functions and Their Derivatives - A Quick & Complete Guide," *Analytics Vidhya*, Apr. 14, 2021. Available: https://www.analyticsvidhya.com/blog/2021/04/activation-functions-and-their-derivatives-a-quick-complete-guide/. [Accessed: Oct. 31, 2023]

26. R. Malhotra and A. Jain, "Software Effort Prediction Using Statistical and Machine Learning Methods," *IJACSA*, vol. 2, no. 1, 2011. Available: http://thesai.org/Publications/ViewPaper?Volume=2&Issue=1&Code=IJACSA&SerialNo=22. [Accessed: Oct. 31, 2023]

Part VI

*Use and Regulation of
Digital Health Technologies
in Healthcare*

10 The Future of Medical Imaging

Ensuring Ethical and Legal Compliance

Soubhik Acharya and Priti Paul

10.1 INTRODUCTION

The science and art of medical imaging are among the most important and revolutionary threads in the complex web of contemporary healthcare. The history and technical evolution that have shaped the field of medical imaging into what it is today—a vibrant and dynamic domain—are explored in this chapter.

Medical imaging offers windows into the hidden landscape of the human body through a wide range of innovative methods and state-of-the-art technologies [1]. Every modality has its unique combination of benefits and limitations, ranging from the time-tested yet reliable X-rays to the delicate secrets unearthed by ultrasounds, the complexities of computed tomography (CT), magnetic resonance imaging (MRI), nuclear medicine, and the complicated movement of molecular imaging. Their combined goal is to enable accurate clinical diagnosis, design strategic treatments, and play a crucial role in directing interventional procedures, which in turn directs the course of surgical interventions and tracks the effectiveness of therapy [2]. This noninvasive visual journey into interior anatomy has not only transformed but also revolutionized the healthcare field, resulting in unparalleled levels of patient care and outcomes.

The history of medical imaging begins in 1895 when Wilhelm Conrad Roentgen by chance discovered X-rays, a discovery that permanently changed the face of medicine. In addition to opening the doors to radiography, Roentgen's unintentional discovery ushered in a new age of medical imaging. The following eras saw the introduction of ultrasound in the 1950s and MRI in the 1970s, which subtly but significantly changed the field of diagnostics and added a new dimension to the complex web of medical imaging.

The advancement of technology and a growing understanding of human anatomy and pathology have driven a never-ending movement of research and innovation in the evolution of medical imaging. It has been a transformation to move from the celluloid embrace of film-based imaging to a digital perspective. With the

DOI: 10.1201/9781003464884-16

TABLE 10.1

An Extensive Overview of the Medical Imaging Legal Landscape

Legal Challenge	Abstract	Description	Government Standards/Acts
Current Legal Framework for Medical Imaging	Security and Efficiency	Ensures the efficacy and safety of patients during imaging.	• **HIPAA(US):** Health Insurance Portability and Accountability Act. • **FDA (U.S.):** Food, Drug, and Cosmetic Act, Radiation Control for Health and Safety Act. • **ACR:** American College of Radiology Standards.
	Obligation	Address the legal ramifications of using medical imaging methods.	• **Stark Law (U.S.):** Physician self-referral regulations.
	Data security and Confidentiality	Maintains the privacy of patient data in imaging.	• **HIPAA (U.S.):** Guidelines for protecting patient health information.
	Online Safety	Safeguards digital patient health data in imaging.	• **HIPAA Security Rule (U.S.):** Ensures security of electronic PHI. • **NIST Cybersecurity Framework:** Provides standards, and guidelines to manage cybersecurity risks. • **ISO/IEC 27001:** Information security management.
	The Law of Intellectual Property	Protects the rights to innovation in medical imaging.	• **Patent Law:** Protects imaging technology inventions. • **Copyright Law:** Safeguards imaging-related creative works. • **Trade Secrets Protections:** Secures confidential imaging technology information.
Observance of Medical Imaging Rules	Rules for Quality Assurance	Implements protocols for reliable and accurate imaging.	• Procedures guaranteeing dependability and precision in imaging.
	Details Regarding the Equipment	Meets regulatory guidelines for safe and efficient imaging technologies.	• Rules set out by regulatory bodies that guarantee secure and effective imaging.

(*Continued*)

TABLE 10.1
(Continued)

Legal Challenge	Abstract	Description	Government Standards/Acts
	Radiation Safety Rules	Adhere to protocols to minimize radiation exposure in imaging.	• Procedures that reduce radiation exposure while preserving the accuracy of the diagnosis.
	Accreditation Schemes	Achieve quality standards through accreditation from recognized bodies.	• Joint Commission and ACR accreditations ensuring quality standards.
Problems with Liability and Malpractice	Litigation Obligations	Addresses complexities in legal obligations for accurate diagnosis.	• Legal responsibilities regarding the subjective interpretation of images.
	Hazards and Difficulties	Manage potential legal consequences due to misinterpretation.	• Possible legal repercussions from incorrectly interpreting imaging data.
	Expert Responsibility	Balancing professional responsibility and accurate diagnosis.	• Implications for imaging diagnosis caused by mistakes, carelessness, and misconduct.
Global Standardization, and Harmonization	Standards from of ISO and IEC	Establishes global guidelines for imaging safety and practices.	• Standards include data formats, equipment specifications, and safety.
	Attempts toward Global Harmonization	Harmonize practices for consistent quality across borders.	• Ensuring uniform standards and procedures across international borders.
	Advantages of Harmonization	Promotes standardized, accurate, and reliable global imaging practices.	• Ensuring trustworthy and accurate diagnostic procedures worldwide.

help of artificial intelligence and machine learning, modern digital paradigms have expanded the definition of diagnosis and created systems that minimize radiation exposure to patients while increasing efficiency and accuracy [3].

The advancement of technology is inextricably linked to the evolutionary pulse of medical imaging. The transition from analog to digital imaging was a turning point that completely changed the ways that images are acquired, stored, and interpreted.

The digital domain provides not only flexibility and improved picture processing but also competent archival functionalities that meld with the vast network of electronic health records (EHRs) and the rapidly developing fields of telemedicine [4]. But the most interesting part of this tale is how machine learning and artificial intelligence (AI) are coming together to become the leading forces behind a paradigm shift in picture analysis and visualization. The integration of AI with medical imaging improves the accuracy of diagnosis, facilitates anomaly identification, and speeds up picture processing [5]. This partnership ushers in a new era of unmatched precision and efficiency in healthcare by providing physicians with accurate, fast, and actionable information that has a significant influence on decision-making. The trajectory of technical development in medical imaging is an account that is still developing but promises much more significant breakthroughs. Portable and more affordable imaging equipment is on the horizon, ready to make healthcare accessible even in the world's most rural or impoverished regions.

10.2 UNDERSTANDING "MEDICAL IMAGING"

The term "medical imaging" is a group of methods that help with clinical analysis and intervention by producing visual representations of the interior organs and tissues of the body. Instruments that provide finely detailed pictures of organs, tissues, and body systems include MRIs, CT scans, X-rays, and ultrasounds. These technologies help medical professionals diagnose diseases, plan treatments, and advance research. A crucial component of contemporary healthcare, medical imaging transforms diagnosis and therapy. Noninvasive, in-depth insights into the body are provided by technologies such as CT, MRI, ultrasound, and X-rays [6]. Soft tissue may be seen with ultrasound, and complicated problems can be identified and treated more effectively using the cross-sectional images that CT scans give. Improved treatment efficacy and diagnostic accuracy brought forth by advances in medical imaging technology have completely changed the healthcare industry. However, careful comprehension and control are necessary for ethical and legal issues such as patient privacy, permission, the use of AI, equitable access, and responsible data usage [7]. Medical imaging accessibility and cost in healthcare settings present difficulties, particularly in areas with few resources. For integration to be successful and responsible, rules governing ethics and the law must be established. Healthcare practitioners, legislators, and researchers must comprehend the technological, clinical, ethical, and societal ramifications [8]. Our main goals are to protect patient rights, integrate medical imaging technology ethically and responsibly, and investigate feasible avenues for improving healthcare globally. This chapter explores the complex field of medical imaging, looking at therapeutic uses, ethical concerns, legal frameworks, and wider societal effects in addition to technical improvements.

10.3 EMERGING TRENDS IN MEDICAL IMAGING

Technological developments in medical imaging have initiated a revolutionary shift that is improving the accuracy of diagnosis and changing the face of healthcare. This section of the chapter offers a thorough examination of the complex web of developing trends, ranging from advancements in imaging technology to the blending of AI, the incorporation of big data, and the growing impact of robots.

10.3.1 ADVANCEMENTS IN IMAGING TECHNOLOGIES

Medical imaging technologies are the result of a never-ending search for innovation. The breadth and depth of diagnostics have greatly increased due to the advancement of current modalities and the introduction of novel approaches. The once-miraculous imaging precision tool computed tomography (CT) has evolved to become faster, more accurate, and radiation-free [9]. Visualizing soft tissues and dynamic physiological processes with exceptional clarity is made possible by sophisticated and adaptable magnetic resonance imaging (MRI) technology (Figure 10.1).

However, on the other hand, the multi-modal imaging frontier has become a significant landmark. The ability to diagnose diseases more thoroughly and nuancedly has been made possible by combining several imaging modalities, such as positron emission tomography–computerized tomography (PET–CT) and positron emission tomography–magnetic resonance imaging (PET–MRI) [10]. The combination of these technologies has improved the capacity to identify anomalies, view anatomical features, and track physiological processes in real time. Through the use of 3D and 4D imaging, new avenues have been opened up for the immersive study of physiological activity and anatomical structures. In addition, the combination of nanotechnology and imaging with molecular probes has brought in a new dimension that allows for the viewing and tracking of molecular and cellular activity. With the use of this

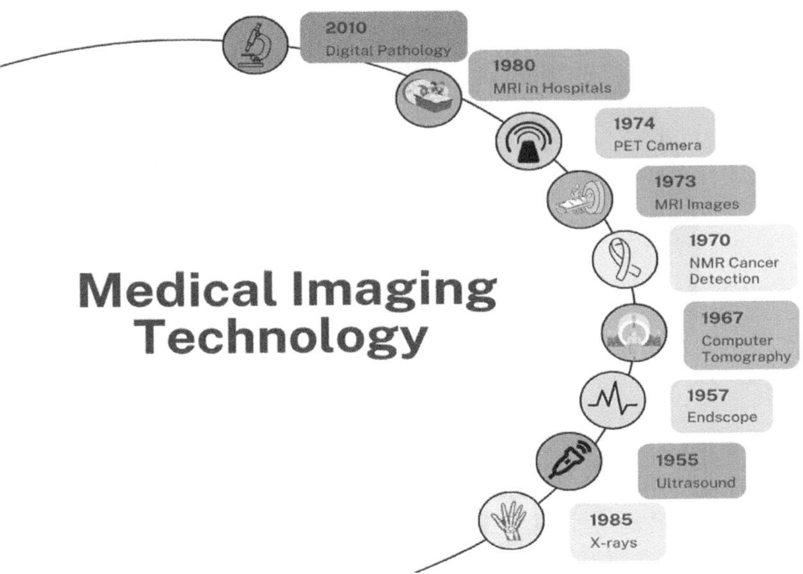

FIGURE 10.1 Evolution of Medical imaging technology

tiny lens, precision medicine is now possible, enabling early illness identification and individualized, customized therapies based on unique cellular characteristics [11].

10.3.2 Artificial Intelligence and Machine Learning in Medical Imaging

In the field of medical imaging, the fusion of machine learning (ML) and artificial intelligence (AI) is a game-changer, ushering in a new era of better efficiency and diagnostic precision. With the foundation laid in the development of machine learning, AI-driven algorithms have become vital resources for the healthcare industry [12]. These algorithms slow down the diagnostic process and reveal complex patterns that are sometimes invisible to the human eye by methodically sorting through large datasets. Their strongest points of catch are the ability to spot patterns, identify anomalies, and analyze images in great detail—all at a degree of precision and consistency that often exceeds human capacity (Figure 10.2).

Deep learning, a subset of machine learning, uses neural networks—more specifically, convolutional neural networks (CNNs)—to improve medical picture comprehension and interpretation. The neural networks of the human brain serve as the model for deep learning algorithms, which are very skilled at identifying minute details and patterns in complicated pictures. With a degree of accuracy and understanding that frequently surpasses human capabilities, CNNs that have been trained on large datasets do exceptionally well in pattern recognition [13]. Deep learning networks can automatically identify a hierarchy of characteristics inside pictures

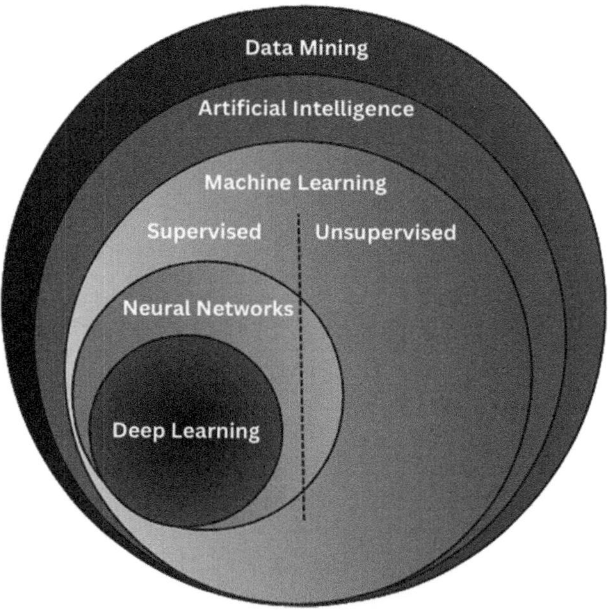

FIGURE 10.2   AI Revolution in medical imaging

because of their special architecture, especially the convolutional layers. The networks can identify characteristics of various sizes and abstractions because of this capacity, which provides unmatched precision in identifying complicated structures and abnormalities. Furthermore, deep learning algorithms are inherently flexible, constantly improving their comprehension and identification of patterns in visual data. They can detect minor differences and anomalies that may be difficult for humans to identify because of their extraordinary flexibility.

More than just accurate picture interpretation is possible with deep learning in medical imaging. With its ability to extract vital information from pictures, it may help with early illness identification and categorization, which leads to precise diagnoses as well as prognostic assessments and treatment planning [14].

Deep learning has revolutionized clinical interpretation standards by bringing exceptional precision to medical imaging systems and dramatically speeding up diagnostic procedures. The combination of deep learning with medical imaging also holds great promise for advancing personalized medicine by forecasting patient outcomes and customizing therapies based on individual profiles, therefore supporting preventative and predictive healthcare efforts [15]. A revolutionary future is being heralded by the fusion of AI, especially deep learning, with medical imaging. A new age in healthcare marked by increased accuracy, increased efficiency, and tailored patient care is promised by this integration, which is positioned to continuously improve and expand its capabilities. Medical imaging paradigms are being rewritten by these systems' ongoing progress, offering a future in which patient care will be profoundly transformed in addition to diagnostics being improved.

10.3.3 Integration of Big Data and Imaging

The fusion of big data analytics and medical imaging has brought about an amazing union that has yielded a wealth of new knowledge, increasing diagnostic precision to previously unheard-of levels and opening up new treatment options catered to the unique characteristics of each patient. This amalgamation combines large imaging datasets, electronic health records (EHRs), and genetic data to create a complex and complicated tapestry of data that is ready for in-depth analysis [16].

This convergence is primarily driven by the application of sophisticated pattern recognition algorithms and data mining techniques. These technologies are now essential for interpreting the complex links that exist between imaging results, the medical histories of patients, and the treatment outcomes that follow. In this combination, radiomics and imaging genetics stand out as pioneers, signifying a revolution in medical imaging analysis [17]. To identify minute features that forecast patient outcomes, treatment responses, and the course of illnesses, these areas carefully collect and evaluate quantitative data from medical pictures. These methods provide a better understanding of how illnesses appear and spread throughout the human body by interpreting and extrapolating a vast amount of data from photographs. The combination of this data is not just a reorganization of existing information; rather, it signifies a revolutionary advance in the precision of diagnoses and the arrival of proactive and predictive healthcare approaches. Through the process of deriving significant insights from imaging data, medical practitioners can anticipate possible outcomes, customize treatments to meet the needs of each patient, and even start preventive measures to slow the onset or spread of diseases [18] (Figure 10.3).

A bright future for healthcare is presented by the fusion of big data analytics with medical imaging through radiomics and imaging genomics. This is an important advancement toward a future of precision, personalized healthcare, and proactive disease management. It goes beyond simply studying images to include reading the stories they tell, projecting potential outcomes, and tailoring healthcare regimens to the individual needs of each patient.

10.3.4 Role of Robotics in Medical Imaging

The harmonious coexistence of robots and imaging technology has completely changed the way medical operations are carried out, improving accuracy and expanding healthcare's reach. The age of minimally invasive procedures has become the cornerstone of medical practice as a result of this integration. In this environment, surgical robots perform complex surgical procedures with unmatched precision when guided by real-time images. This presents a huge advancement in surgical accuracy since their operating skill reduces the possibility of human mistakes and greatly improves patient outcomes [19] (Figure 10.4).

The combination of robots and imaging technology has revolutionized the field of interventional radiology, taking it beyond standard surgery. With the aid of this fusion, medical experts may now maneuver through intricate anatomical structures with previously unheard-of accuracy [20]. Imaging and robots working together make complex interventions possible and pave the way for the emergence of remote treatments. With the assistance of this creative methodology, medical professionals

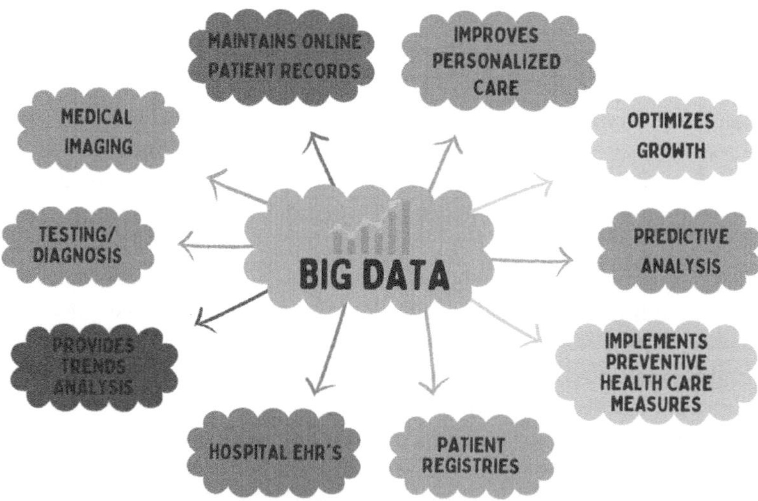

FIGURE 10.3 Big data fusion in medical imaging

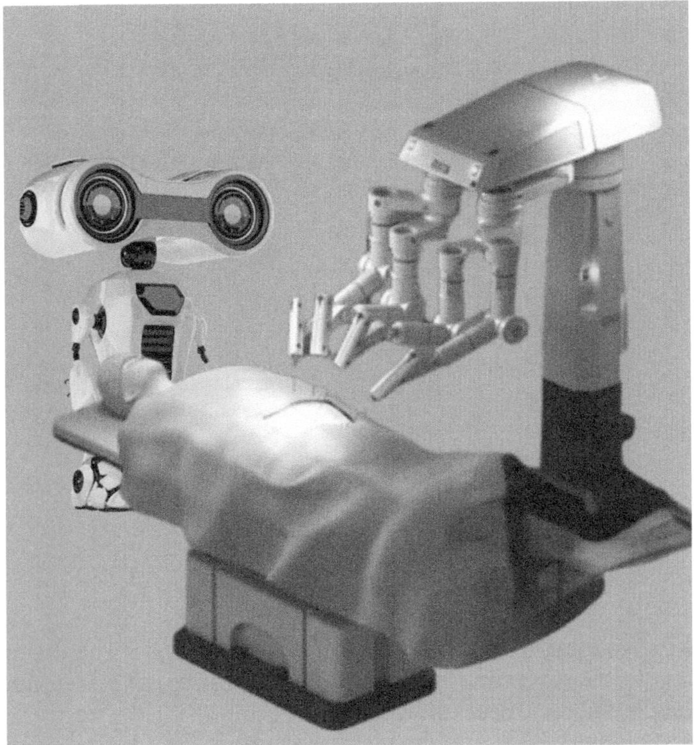

FIGURE 10.4 Robotics technology in advancing medical imaging

may embrace intercessions outside national borders, ensuring that specialized treatment can travel extraordinary distances and reach the most disconnected or underserved places. The combination of imaging and robotics technology could be a transformation that goes beyond the limits of routine healthcare delivery. It is almost more than fair-made strides and precision; it is almost making specialist care available to everybody, wherever within the globe [21]. This integration envisions a day when obstructions will disappear, precision will be valued over all else, and getting to master treatment will not be limited by topography.

10.4 ETHICAL CONSIDERATIONS IN MEDICAL IMAGING

The ethical implications of the field of therapeutic imaging are significant, including issues that are critical to understanding care, healthcare experts, and the general public (Figure 10.5).

10.4.1 PATIENT PRIVACY AND CONFIDENTIALITY

Medical imaging ethical issues are centered on the sacredness of patient privacy and confidentiality. Strict adherence to rules that protect patient information is necessary

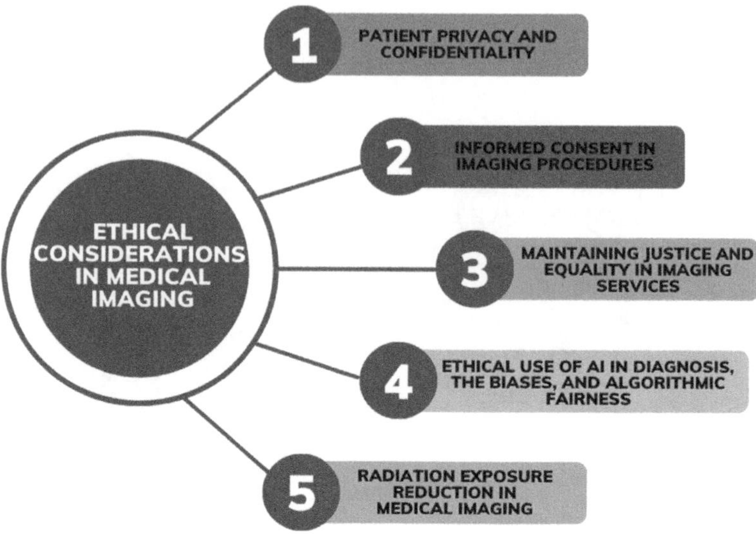

FIGURE 10.5   Ethical compass in medical imaging

for the taking, storing, and sharing of medical photographs. The digitalization of imaging data necessitates the implementation of strong data security protocols, encryption standards, and access restrictions. Assume the following scenario: a busy medical facility is switching to digital imaging technology. There are several advantages to switching from analog film-based records to digital imaging data in terms of easier access and quicker diagnosis. However, there are ethical problems with this move, especially in terms of information security.

Picture archiving and communication systems (PACS) are introduced by a hospital in this scenario to preserve and handle medical photographs. Healthcare professionals may quickly access patient information using the PACS, which expedites diagnosis and treatment choices. The PACS is designed to simplify picture storage and retrieval [22]. But there are difficulties in this digital world as well. Concerns regarding patient privacy and data security arise from the digitalization process. To secure understanding protection, it is basic to have solid information security instruments input. Strict access restrictions and encryption requirements are essential for protecting these digital archives from unwanted access. To safeguard the transmission and storage of critical imaging data, let's look at an example where strict encryption mechanisms are in place. Similar to how financial companies use strong security measures to protect confidential financial data, healthcare facilities also use strong security procedures to secure patient information [23]. It's also crucial to protect access to these documents. Only authorized individuals, such as attending physicians and specialists, can view certain patient data thanks to the implementation of a tiered access system. To ensure patient confidentiality and uphold the concept of least privilege, a cardiologist participating in the patient's treatment, for example, would have access to cardiac imaging data but not neuro-imaging information.

Patients and healthcare facilities can build a trustworthy connection because of the strict data security measures that protect the privacy and confidentiality of patient information. As a result, patients will feel more secure and certain within the healthcare framework, knowing that their private therapeutic data is protected from potential breaches and illegally obtained. Subsequently, securing persistent security within the advanced age of therapeutic imaging requires a solid and proactive approach to information security, rather than ensuring any other delicate individual data, in this manner, securing quiet secrecy in medical settings.

10.4.2 Informed Consent in Imaging Procedures

Imaging processes must uphold the autonomy of the patient and their freedom to make informed decisions. To empower patients to make knowledgeable decisions about their healthcare, informed consent entails the open sharing of procedure specifics, possible risks, benefits, and alternatives. When it comes to medical imaging, it is pivotal to ensure that patients fully understand the forms, risks, and potential outcomes before providing their consent for any imaging procedure [24]. Consider a situation where a patient has an appointment for an MRI scan to look into a possible neurological ailment. Before moving further, the patient feels that it is essential to comprehend the goal of the MRI, the process, and the possible results.

Assuring open communication about the MRI scan and the healthcare professional interacting with the patient diminishes the psychological barriers. It helps ensure transparency during information exchange, minimizing the chances of the patient being confused by the complexity of the process or unsure of his/her decisions related to healthcare. The complexities of the process are explained, including the type of imaging apparatus used, how long the scan will take, and whether sedation or contrast drugs are necessary. The patient is advised about the MRI machine's small size and the possibility of claustrophobia in certain people. The medical professional provides a comprehensive outline of the interest in magnetic resonance imaging (MRI), including how it may be utilized to diagnose neurological disorders. It also discusses potential hazards, such as the use of contrast chemicals and the infrequent allergic responses that can occur from them. To provide the patient with a complete picture and enable them to make an educated choice, they are also advised on potential alternative imaging techniques.

The patient is encouraged to actively participate in the diagnostic process and is equipped with this extensive knowledge. By providing the patient with the information they ought to make an informed well-being choice, this engagement builds belief and a sense of participation between the patient and their healthcare specialist. Patient participation in the choice-making process exemplifies the fundamentals of informed consent and highlights the significance of patient empowerment through thorough knowledge [25]. This situation not only highlights the moral necessity of informed permission for imaging treatments but also emphasizes how important open communication is to promote a patient-centered approach to healthcare.

10.4.3 Maintaining Justice and Equality in Imaging Services

Providing equal access to imaging services is a fundamental ethical principle in the medical field. Attention must be paid to differences in the availability of cutting-edge imaging services and technology across various socioeconomic classes and geographical areas. Initiatives to ensure that all societal strata, irrespective of their geographic location or socioeconomic status, have equitable access to state-of-the-art imaging services are necessary to address these inequities [26]. Imagine if access to cutting-edge imaging technology continues to differ between different locations. Modern hospitals and imaging facilities with the newest MRI equipment serve affluent residents of a bustling metropolis. Access to these cutting-edge imaging services is limited, though, in rural or underdeveloped locations.

Initiatives are presented to close the gap and advance fair access to resolve these discrepancies. In these isolated areas, mobile imaging units or satellite centers are erected to offer access to critical imaging services. This proactive measure guarantees equitable access to high-quality imaging services for inhabitants in these locations, irrespective of their geographic location or socioeconomic standing.

Furthermore, these units have policies in place to guarantee equitable resource distribution and combat prejudices. One example is the establishment of a policy whereby imaging visits are prioritized based on medical urgency as opposed to socioeconomic position. This guarantees equitable and prompt access to vital imaging services for all individuals, regardless of their background. An ethical commitment to healthcare is illustrated in this commitment to giving everybody impartial access to advanced imaging services. With impartial access to high-quality demonstrative apparatuses, everybody, notwithstanding financial status or geography, has an advantage. The objective of the health framework is to supply individuals with reasonable and impartial access to health services by diminishing inclination and empowering evenhanded allotment of assets.

10.4.4 Ethical Use of AI in Diagnosis, the Biases, and Algorithmic Fairness

An ethical framework must be carefully considered when integrating artificial intelligence (AI) into medical imaging. Artificial intelligence systems may be very useful in diagnosing and making decisions. Transparency about the operation of these systems is necessary for the ethical use of AI in this context, guaranteeing that the decisions and processes made by AI are transparent, responsible, and comprehensible [27]. Achieving an equilibrium between enhancing human proficiency and the moral obligation to prevent excessive dependence on artificial intelligence systems is crucial. AI-based algorithm integration opens up a crucial discussion on biases and fairness, especially in the field of medical imaging. Consider a situation in which radiologists use an artificial intelligence system to help them diagnose breast cancer from mammograms. As important as it is to ensure fairness and mitigate biases in these algorithms, they also have the potential to improve diagnostic accuracy.

Think about an artificial intelligence system that was mostly trained on datasets that had skewed representations of various demographic groupings. Due to possible biases in the system's decision-making caused by this imbalance, underrepresented groups may receive diagnoses that are not as accurate. For example, if the dataset is mostly made up of photographs of a single ethnic group, the AI may diagnose conditions for that group more accurately than for other ethnic groups since it has not had enough training data. It is necessary to take action which is needed to ensure algorithmic fairness to overcome these biases. To achieve equal representation, training datasets must be diverse and include multiple groups of subjects. To minimize the potential for biased decisions, it is important to maintain a balanced dataset that reflects patient diversity. This will help algorithms learn and generalize more successfully.

Regular assessment and auditing of AI algorithms is also crucial. Biases that may develop throughout the system's learning process can be found and corrected with the aid of ongoing monitoring. To address these biases and guarantee fair and accurate findings for all patient demographics, the AI models may need to be recalibrated or retrained [28]. For example, periodic evaluations may disclose disparities in diagnosis accuracy across various demographic groups. Reducing bias and improving equitable health outcomes for all patient groups is possible by committing to algorithmic equity in medical imaging. By aiming for equity in AI-based diagnostic systems, we can ensure that all patients, regardless of their demographics, receive an accurate and unbiased diagnosis, which will help create a more reliable and equitable healthcare system.

10.4.5   Radiation Exposure Reduction in Medical Imaging

To protect patients, it is crucial to reduce radiation exposure during medical imaging procedures. Patients receiving several imaging procedures using ionizing radiation should give particular thought to this ethical issue. Suppose, for illustration, that a patient in a medical environment requires routine imaging tests for diagnosis and monitoring.

As part of their treatment plan, the patient in this case needs routine CT scans. The medical facility uses techniques to lower radiation doses without sacrificing diagnostic precision since it is aware of the possible hazards connected to cumulative radiation exposure. The CT imaging makes use of sophisticated technical solutions, such as iterative reconstruction methods [29]. These innovative techniques maintain the high-quality pictures required for precise diagnosis while optimizing radiation doses. In addition, continual advancements in imaging technology are essential for reducing radiation exposure. To significantly lower radiation levels during imaging operations, for example, low-dose protocols in fluoroscopy or dose-reduction features integrated into digital radiography equipment are used [30]. Along with technology improvements, medical professionals and radiology technicians participate in ongoing education and training programs. With the help of these training programs, medical professionals will be better prepared to decide how to make the best use of imaging technology, resulting in more accurate diagnoses and less radiation exposure for patients. Placing patient safety at the center of imaging methods, the commitment to reduce radiation exposure is consistent with ethical healthcare standards. Healthcare institutions put the needs of their patients first by integrating cutting-edge technology and offering thorough training. This ensures that possible hazards related to radiation exposure are considerably avoided while diagnostic accuracy is maintained.

10.5 REGULATIONS AND THE LEGAL STRUCTURE

The regulatory environment around medical imaging is fundamental to keeping up an understanding of security, ethical practice, and regulatory compliance. This chapter segment goes into detail about a few lawful and regulatory variables that have formed the medical imaging industry. It covers universal measures, obligation concerns, compliance methods, and modern lawful systems (Figure 10.6).).

10.5.1 PRESENT MEDICAL IMAGING LEGAL ENVIRONMENT

The laws and rules that ensure understanding protection, information security, and moral behavior are all portions of the lawful system that apply to the field of medical imaging [31]. The Health Insurance Portability and Accountability Act (HIPAA), is at the front. The HIPAA establishes guidelines for maintaining patient privacy, restricting disclosure, and safeguarding private health information. Healthcare practitioners are required to uphold stringent protocols to safeguard patient data that is maintained in any format, including records of medical imaging. The Privacy Rule

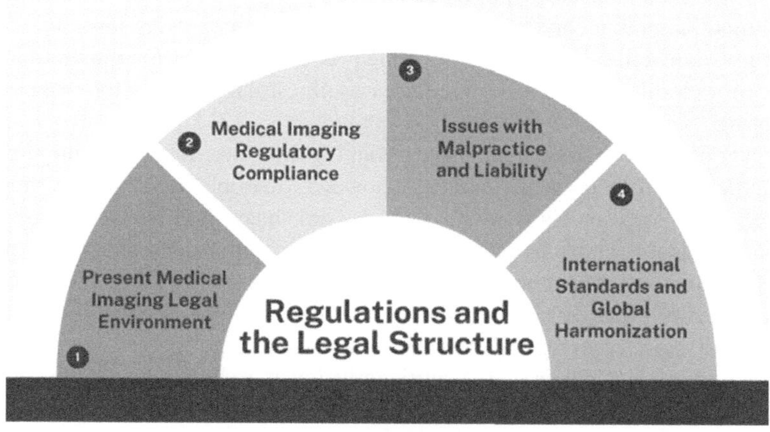

FIGURE 10.6 Legal frameworks shaping medical imaging

of HIPAA provides detailed instructions for protecting protected health information (PHI), which includes medical photographs [32, 33]. It makes sure that only those with the proper authorization may access this data and that patient agreement is sought before sharing or using it. Healthcare organizations are required under the Security Rule to put in place the necessary protections to secure electronic PHI, including medical pictures, against any risks to the availability, confidentiality, and integrity of the data [34]. In addition, medical imaging restrictions are not limited to HIPAA. Standards for radiography procedures and image interpretation are established by the American College of Radiography (ACR) [35]. Following the ACR criteria for image collection and interpretation places a strong emphasis on preserving imaging quality and making sure that facilities fulfill certain standards. Standards for picture quality control, equipment upkeep, and appropriate interpretation by licensed radiologists are all included in this [36].

Medical imaging equipment regulation is heavily influenced by the Food and Drug Administration (FDA) of the United States. Before imaging equipment is put on the market, the FDA verifies its efficacy and safety. To ensure that imaging equipment fulfills requirements and does not place patients or healthcare professionals in unnecessary danger, it is necessary to examine the quality, safety, and performance of these devices [37–39]. The Stark Law, which mostly addresses physician self-referral, is another important statute that regulates medical imaging. Under this rule, unless certain restrictions apply, healthcare practitioners are not allowed to recommend patients for certain designated health services—like advanced imaging—if they, or a member of their immediate family, have a financial relationship with the organization that is delivering the service. The objective is to avoid conflicts of interest and guarantee the reliability of imaging service referrals [40].

10.5.2 Medical Imaging Regulatory Compliance

Medical imaging administrative compliance may be a principal column, guaranteeing the most noteworthy measures of security, quality, and morale hone. It incorporates a set of multifaceted measures pertinent to healthcare organizations and symptomatic imaging centers to guarantee ideal operation and execution of imaging innovation while prioritizing security and quiet well-being.

One of the key angles of administrative compliance includes strict adherence to quality-control guidelines. This incorporates comprehensive conventions and controls executed in demonstrative imaging offices to guarantee the precision, exactness, and unwavering quality of symptomatic pictures. Quality-control measures incorporate customary gear calibration, schedule upkeep, and quality affirmation strategies to guarantee that imaging gadgets reliably deliver high-quality, clinically valuable pictures [41]. Compliance is generally subordinate to hardware determinations. Administrative organizations give exact benchmarks and suggestions relating to the working, security, and execution of imaging gear. These rules make beyond any doubt that the gear utilized in imaging operations fulfills the essential prerequisites in terms of proficiency, security, and picture quality. By following these rules, the plausibility of hardware disappointments or insufficiencies is diminished, guaranteeing that patients get adjusted analysis.

When it comes to medical imaging controls, radiation security rules are vital. These proposals administer the judicious and secure application of ionizing radiation, especially in methods like fluoroscopy and CT looks. Strategies to diminish radiation presentation to patients and healthcare suppliers while protecting the demonstrative exactness required for precise medical appraisals are included in compliance measures.

Compliance is additionally generally guaranteed by the accreditation measures set by regulatory organizations just as the Joint Commission and the American College of Radiology (ACR) [42]. Accreditation programs are given by these organizations, which confirm that imaging offices fulfill characterized quality necessities by implying strict criteria. Keeping up these accreditations appears to patients and partners that the office is committed to advertising first-rate imaging administrations in a secure and effective environment.

10.5.3 ISSUES WITH MALPRACTICE AND LIABILITY

For a thorough grasp of this discipline, it is imperative to look into the legal ramifications and potential liabilities inherent in medical imaging. The many facets of legal obligations, hazards, and changing malpractice concerns that healthcare providers working in the diagnostic imaging field must deal with are covered in this section.

Healthcare practitioners, particularly radiologists and imaging experts, have extensive and intricate legal responsibilities in the field of medical imaging. These professionals are trusted to accurately evaluate and analyze medical pictures to make a diagnosis. Notwithstanding, the subjective character of picture interpretation, in conjunction with the possible intricacies and fluctuations within patient circumstances, poses a range of obstacles and hazards [43]. The potential for misinterpreting imaging studies is one of the main causes of worry. Accurate diagnoses run the danger of being compromised by the subjective nature of picture analysis and the potential for subtle or confusing results. Errors or misinterpretations in imaging examinations may result in inappropriate actions or delayed, necessary treatments, which may cause harm to patients. Healthcare personnel may be subject to legal consequences in cases where misdiagnoses or insufficient interpretation result in patient damage. These may take the form of accusations of medical malpractice, citing carelessness, or a failure to interpret imaging data with the appropriate level of care. Patients may file lawsuits claiming they suffered harm, more medical costs, or psychological discomfort as a result of an improper or delayed diagnosis.

Given the need to strike a balance between professional accountability, patient welfare, and the difficulties involved in accurate diagnosis, the liability landscape in medical imaging is complicated. Since there is a need to strike a balance between the benefits and drawbacks of integrating advanced imaging technologies, the landscape of liability in medical imaging is complicated. The integration of these technologies creates new risks and challenges for accurate interpretation and diagnosis, in addition to complicated legal issues. The difficulties in accurately diagnosing patients, professional responsibility, and patient welfare underscore the need for ongoing vigilance, continuous education, and professional development in medical imaging [44]. Healthcare suppliers and offices ought to be aware of the nuances around obligation and negligence issues related to restorative imaging. Keeping up watchfulness, persistent instruction, and proficient development are vital to decreasing the risks of plausible misinterpretations or oversights in demonstrative imaging. To diminish any dangers and maintain high measures of care in therapeutic imaging methods, it also emphasizes the need for open communication with patients, straightforwardness, and the utilization of quality confirmation frameworks.

10.5.4 International Standards and Global Harmonization

Among the most important things in the sector are the efforts to standardize procedures and coordinate medical imaging techniques worldwide. The worldwide standards set by reputable organizations like the International Organization for Standardization (ISO) and the International Electrotechnical Commission (IEC) are thoroughly examined in this section. It investigates the activities pointed at harmonizing imaging strategies, standard hones, and measures universally to supply a uniform, prevalent healthcare conveyance around the globe. Setting and upholding international standards in a variety of sectors, including healthcare and medical imaging, is mostly the responsibility of the International Electrotechnical Commission (IEC) and the International Organization for Standardization (ISO) [45]. With an assortment of strategies, approaches, and innovations, these measures look to ensure adequacy, security, and compatibility.

These worldwide organizations provide standards and guidelines about a wide range of topics in medical imaging. These cover things like security safety measures, information groups, hardware specs, and indeed, how to require and assess pictures. For example, the ISO benchmarks may incorporate data coding and compatibility in therapeutic imaging, though the IEC indicates specific prerequisites for the usefulness and security of restorative electrical gear utilized in imaging forms. The exertion to form a common set of rules and strategies for medical imaging over national boundaries is the thrust for worldwide harmonization. Through harmonization, professionals will be able to take steady quality benchmarks notwithstanding where they work or live within the healthcare framework [46]. It moreover endeavors to ensure a reliable conclusion. To encourage the trade of best hones, investigate, and advancements in imaging innovation, endeavors toward worldwide harmonization are particularly imperative in building up associations and participation all through healthcare frameworks. This ensures that standardized strategies are available to and utilized by healthcare professionals all-inclusive, coming about in more tried and true and uniform demonstrative forms.

Moreover, standardization and harmonization endeavors are not as advantageous to healthcare experts but are also fundamental for understanding care. They play a basic part in advancing exact and reliable symptomatic hones, minimizing mistakes, and guaranteeing that patients get reliable, high-quality healthcare administrations, in any case of area or the restorative office to visit. The intrigue in around-the-world benchmarks and around-the-world harmonization in helpful imaging underscores the commitment to an around-the-world healthcare environment centered on passing on strong, standardized, and high-quality care [47]. It clears the way for a future where creative imaging progresses and sharpens and is reliably open and contributes to the progress of the healthcare movement on a worldwide scale.

10.6 FUTURE CONSIDERATIONS AND SUGGESTIONS

A thorough assessment of expected technological advances and approaches to modifying ethical frameworks to adapt to new technologies, and policy proposals to harmonize legal and ethical standards are all needed to envision the future of medical imaging. This section attempts to outline the future development of medical imaging, emphasizing the need for ethical compliance and offering suggested tactics for a coherent and forward-thinking future.

10.6.1 ANTICIPATED TECHNOLOGICAL DEVELOPMENTS IN MEDICAL IMAGING

Imagining the future of medical imaging requires anticipating technical advancements. Imaging technologies continue to advance at a rapid pace, with great promise. It is projected that there will be innovations in molecular imaging, improved artificial intelligence applications, and spectrum imaging.

Spectral imaging is a cutting-edge development that has the potential to revolutionize diagnostic skills. Multi-wavelength picture acquisition and processing is known as spectral imaging, and it offers extensive knowledge of tissue composition [48]. Radiologists can more accurately discriminate between healthy bone, lesions, and surrounding tissues when using this technique for bone imaging. The capacity of this technology to identify minute variations in tissue composition may help identify and accurately diagnose bone illnesses early on, therefore avoiding invasive operations or opening the door to earlier, more successful treatment plans. Through expanded effectiveness and precision, artificial intelligence (AI) is changing medical imaging. Profound learning and convolutional neural systems, for example, are AI-driven algorithms that can distinguish designs and anomalies that will be invisible to the human eye. To help radiologists spot breast cancer side effects in mammograms, AI-powered frameworks are being developed. These strategies move radiologists' capacity to recognize patients more rapidly and precisely by analyzing hundreds of pictures and learning from designs [49].

Also, headways in molecular imaging procedures like positron emission tomography (PET) imaging are one case of a molecular imaging device that gives more prominent information about ailments at the cellular and molecular level, conceivably changing early diagnosis and treatment strategies [50]. These strategies can distinguish cellular and molecular changes connected to a range of ailments, including cancer determination, arranging, and treatment arranging, when matched with certain radiotracers. The advancement of molecular imaging devices makes it conceivable to recognize and characterize illnesses early on, which opens the door to customized treatment and more exact and successful treatment. The goals of medical imaging advancements are to increase accuracy, optimize processes, and deliver successful, individualized treatment. These developments will revolutionize healthcare by facilitating earlier detection, accurate analysis, and tailored treatments for better outcomes and long-term success.

10.6.2 TECHNIQUES FOR ADAPTING NEW TECHNOLOGIES TO ETHICAL FRAMEWORKS

The integration of advanced medical imaging technologies necessitates the development of ethical frameworks, focusing on patient privacy, informed consent, and fairness to maintain ethical standards in healthcare. Medical privacy is becoming more complicated as a result of advanced technology producing and analyzing enormous volumes of medical data. To ensure confidentiality and authorized staff access, healthcare settings should cultivate a culture of data security and implement strong data encryption and access restrictions. It's imperative to guarantee informed consent for novel imaging technologies [51]. To enable patients to make knowledgeable decisions, healthcare practitioners must tell patients about the advantages, dangers, and available options for these operations. It's critical to communicate the limitations and capabilities of these technologies transparently.

The ethical ramifications of using new imaging technology should be explained to healthcare workers, with a focus on the value of patient privacy, informed consent, and equity. Programs for ongoing professional development should emphasize both ethical and technological issues to make sure that medical practitioners are aware of the possible risks associated with artificial intelligence, enhanced imaging, and data analytics. To resolve ethical issues with the use of new imaging techniques, transparent governance, and regulatory frameworks are essential. These frameworks need to be ethically sound and flexible enough to keep up with technological changes. Guidelines that support justice, equity, and accountability in the application of new imaging technologies must be developed via cooperation between healthcare institutions, governmental entities, and ethical review boards [52]. To shape the future of medical imaging practices, healthcare systems must embrace policies that combine technical breakthroughs with ethical concerns. Only then can new imaging technologies be successfully integrated while maintaining patient welfare.

10.6.3 POLICY SUGGESTIONS FOR HARMONIZING LAW AND ETHICS

To ensure the responsible, ethical, and compliant use of these cutting-edge instruments, legal and ethical norms must keep up with the rapid improvements in medical imaging technology. Policy suggestions play a critical role in developing complete guidelines. Policy proposals should govern the ethical use of AI in medical imaging, with particular attention to standards for algorithm deployment, validation, and training. In addition to addressing data privacy issues, they should place a strong emphasis on openness in AI decision-making and guarantee the explainability, accountability, and moral functioning of AI systems. Recommendations should specify the moral use of patient data in AI model training, guarantee encryption standards, and protect patient data from unwanted access. In light of new developments in imaging technology, proposals for amended legislation and regulations ought to give priority to patient rights. They have to place a strong emphasis on informed consent, making sure that patients are aware of and agree to novel modalities and AI applications [53]. To provide patients control over their data and preserve their autonomy, policies should specify their rights concerning ownership and access to their imaging data.

International regulatory bodies and healthcare organizations should collaborate to establish global ethical standards and legal frameworks for medical imaging. This will ensure a harmonized approach to ethical and legal considerations, transcending geographical boundaries. This will enable the sharing of best practices, knowledge exchange, and the creation of globally accepted ethical standards that promote the ethical and compliant use of advanced imaging technologies across diverse healthcare systems [54]. The goal of the policy proposals is to guarantee that healthcare organizations and regulatory agencies utilize cutting-edge medical imaging technology ethically and responsibly. These rules uphold moral principles and legal requirements, safeguard patient welfare and data privacy, and encourage the adoption of state-of-the-art imaging technology (Table 10.1).

10.7 CONCLUSIONS

The chapter "The Future of Medical Imaging: Ensuring Ethical and Legal Compliance" examines the intricate interplay in the area of medical imaging between ethical considerations, regulatory frameworks, and technical breakthroughs. It draws attention to the revolutionary potential of imaging technologies as well as the significance of patient privacy, legal compliance, and strong safeguards for sensitive medical data. The assessment framework offers a methodical strategy for addressing undesirable results and offers direction for fixing them. By emphasizing patient care, protecting privacy, and maintaining high standards of ethical and legal conduct, the chapter seeks to direct healthcare professionals toward a healthcare environment that strikes a balance between technology innovation, ethical integrity, and legal compliance.

REFERENCES

1. Towsley-Cook, D. M., & Young, T. A. (2007). *Ethical and Legal Issues for Imaging Professionals*. Elsevier Health Sciences.
2. Duquenoy, P., George, C., & Solomonides, A. (2008). What ELSE? Regulation and compliance in medical imaging and medical informatics. Medical Imaging and Informatics: 2nd International Conference, MIMI 2007, Beijing, China, August 14–16, 2007. Revised Selected Papers. Springer, Berlin Heidelberg, pp. 340–357.
3. Pesapane, F., Volonté, C., Codari, M., & Sardanelli, F. (2018). Artificial intelligence as a medical device in radiology: Ethical and regulatory issues in Europe and the United States. *Insights into Imaging, 9*(5), 745–753.
4. Lekadir, K., Osuala, R., Gallin, C., Lazrak, N., Kushibar, K., Tsakou, G., ... Martí-Bonmatí, L. (2021). FUTURE-AI: Guiding principles and consensus recommendations for trustworthy artificial intelligence in medical imaging. *arXiv Preprint ArXiv:2109.09658.*

5. Currie, G., & Hawk, K. E. (2021, March). Ethical and legal challenges of artificial intelligence in nuclear medicine. In Kirsten Bouchelouche, M. Michael Sathekge, *Seminars in Nuclear Medicine* (Vol. 51, No. 2, pp. 120–125). WB Saunders.

6. Suetens, P. (2017). *Fundamentals of Medical Imaging.* Cambridge University Press.

7. Krupinski, E. A. (2000). The importance of perception research in medical imaging. *Radiation Medicine, 18*(6), 329–334.

8. Alzubaidi, L., Fadhel, M. A., Al-Shamma, O., Zhang, J., Santamaría, J., Duan, Y., & Oleiwi, R. S. (2020). Towards a better understanding of transfer learning for medical imaging: A case study. *Applied Sciences, 10*(13), 4523.

9. Teodori, L., Crupi, A., Costa, A., Diaspro, A., Melzer, S., & Tarnok, A. (2017). Three-dimensional imaging technologies: A priority for the advancement of tissue engineering and a challenge for the imaging community. *Journal of Biophotonics, 10*(1), 24–45.

10. Mohan, A. T., & Saint-Cyr, M. (2016). Advances in imaging technologies for planning breast reconstruction. *Gland Surgery, 5*(2), 242.

11. Malladi, R., Kimmel, R., Adalsteinsson, D., Sapiro, G., Caselles, V., & Sethian, J. A. (1996, June). A geometric approach to segmentation and analysis of 3D medical images. In *Proceedings of the Workshop on Mathematical Methods in Biomedical Image Analysis* (pp. 244–252). IEEE.

12. Barragán-Montero, A., Javaid, U., Valdés, G., Nguyen, D., Desbordes, P., Macq, B., ... Lee, J. A. (2021). Artificial intelligence and machine learning for medical imaging: A technology review. *Physica Medica, 83*, 242–256.

13. Castiglioni, I., Rundo, L., Codari, M., Di Leo, G., Salvatore, C., Interlenghi, M., ... Sardanelli, F. (2021). AI applications to medical images: From machine learning to deep learning. *Physica Medica, 83*, 9–24.

14. Pesapane, F., Codari, M., & Sardanelli, F. (2018). Artificial intelligence in medical imaging: Threat or opportunity? Radiologists again at the forefront of innovation in medicine. *European Radiology Experimental, 2*(1), 1–10.

15. Lee, J. G., Jun, S., Cho, Y. W., Lee, H., Kim, G. B., Seo, J. B., & Kim, N. (2017). Deep learning in medical imaging: General overview. *Korean Journal of Radiology, 18*(4), 570–584.

16. Tabib, N. S. S., Madgwick, M., Sudhakar, P., Verstockt, B., Korcsmaros, T., & Vermeire, S. (2020). Big data in IBD: Big progress for clinical practice. *Gut, 69*(8), 1520–1532.

17. Dash, S., Shakyawar, S. K., Sharma, M., & Kaushik, S. (2019). Big data in healthcare: Management, analysis and future prospects. *Journal of Big Data, 6*(1), 1–25.

18. Viceconti, M., Hunter, P., & Hose, R. (2015). Big data, big knowledge: Big data for personalized healthcare. *IEEE Journal of Biomedical and Health Informatics, 19*(4), 1209–1215.

19. von Haxthausen, F., Böttger, S., Wulff, D., Hagenah, J., García-Vázquez, V., & Ipsen, S. (2021). Medical robotics for ultrasound imaging: Current systems and future trends. *Current Robotics Reports, 2*(1), 55–71.

20. Taylor, R. H., Menciassi, A., Fichtinger, G., Fiorini, P., & Dario, P. (2016). Medical robotics and computer-integrated surgery. In Bruno Siciliano, Oussama Khatib (eds.) *Springer Handbook of Robotics*, Springer International Publishing, (pp. 1657–1684).

21. Halder Roy, A., Ghosh, S., & Gupta, B. (2023). Robotics in medical domain: The future of surgery, healthcare and imaging. *Wireless Personal Communications, 132*(4), 2885–2903.

22. Safdar, N. M., Banja, J. D., & Meltzer, C. C. (2020). Ethical considerations in artificial intelligence. *European Journal of Radiology, 122*, 108768.

23. Salerno, S., Laghi, A., Cantone, M. C., Sartori, P., Pinto, A., & Frija, G. (2019). Overdiagnosis and overimaging: An ethical issue for radiological protection. *La Radiologia Medica, 124*(8), 714–720.

24. Towsley-Cook, D. M., & Young, T. A. (2007). *Ethical and Legal Issues for Imaging Professionals*. Elsevier Health Sciences.
25. Duquenoy, P., George, C., & Solomonides, A. (2008). Considering something 'ELSE': Ethical, legal and socio-economic factors in medical imaging and medical informatics. *Computer Methods and Programs in Biomedicine, 92*(3), 227–237.
26. Smith, L. A. C. (2006). The red-dot system in medical imaging: Ethical, legal and human rights considerations. *Radiographer, 53*(3), 4–6.
27. Berlin, L. (1994). Reporting the "missed" radiologic diagnosis: Medicolegal and ethical considerations. *Radiology, 192*(1), 183–187.
28. Illes, J., Desmond, J. E., Huang, L. F., Raffin, T. A., & Atlas, S. W. (2002). Ethical and practical considerations in managing incidental findings in functional magnetic resonance imaging. *Brain and Cognition, 50*(3), 358–365.
29. Malone, J. (2020). X-rays for medical imaging: Radiation protection, governance and ethics over 125 years. *Physica Medica, 79*, 47–64.
30. Jones, D. N., Benveniste, K. A., Schultz, T. J., Mandel, C. J., & Runciman, W. B. (2010). Establishing national medical imaging incident reporting systems: Issues and challenges. *Journal of the American College of Radiology, 7*(8), 582–592.
31. Reiner, B. I. (2009). The challenges, opportunities, and imperative of structured reporting in medical imaging. *Journal of Digital Imaging, 22*(6), 562–568.
32. Cao, F., Huang, H. K., & Zhou, X. Q. (2003). Medical image security in a HIPAA mandated PACS environment. *Computerized Medical Imaging and Graphics, 27*(2–3), 185–196.
33. Freymann, J. B., Kirby, J. S., Perry, J. H., Clunie, D. A., & Jaffe, C. C. (2012). Image data sharing for biomedical research—Meeting HIPAA requirements for de-identification. *Journal of Digital Imaging, 25*(1), 14–24.
34. Liu, B. J., Zhou, Z., & Huang, H. K. (2006). A HIPAA-compliant architecture for securing clinical images. *Journal of Digital Imaging, 19*(2), 172–180.
35. Norweck, J. T., Seibert, J. A., Andriole, K. P., Clunie, D. A., Curran, B. H., Flynn, M. J., ... Wyatt, M. (2013). ACR–AAPM–SIIM technical standard for electronic practice of medical imaging. *Journal of Digital Imaging, 26*(1), 38–52.
36. Amis Jr E. S., Butler, P. F. (2010). ACR white paper on radiation dose in medicine: Three years later. *Journal of the American College of Radiology, 7*(11), 865–870.
37. Kinch, M. S., & Woodard, P. K. (2017). Analysis of FDA-approved imaging agents. *Drug Discovery Today, 22*(7), 1077–1083.
38. Harrison, C. (2018). FDA backs clinician-free AI imaging diagnostic tools. *Nature Biotechnology, 36*, 673.
39. Gallas, B. D., Chan, H. P., D'Orsi, C. J., Dodd, L. E., Giger, M. L., Gur, D., ... Zuley, M. L. (2012). Evaluating imaging and computer-aided detection and diagnosis devices at the FDA. *Academic Radiology, 19*(4), 463–477.
40. Mitchell, J. M. (2007). The Prevalence of Physician Self-Referral Arrangements after Stark II: Evidence from advanced diagnostic imaging: Data from California suggest that physicians exploit exceptions in the Stark II law to continue to self-refer patients for imaging. *Health Affairs, 26*(3)(Suppl2), w415–w424.
41. Brenner, D. J., & Hricak, H. (2010). Radiation exposure from medical imaging: Time to regulate? *JAMA, 304*(2), 208–209.
42. Subhan, A. (2005). Regulatory compliance and quality assurance. *Journal of Clinical Engineering, 30*(4), 187–190.
43. Li, S., & Brantley, E. (2015). Malpractice liability risk and use of diagnostic imaging services: A systematic review of the literature. *Journal of the American College of Radiology, 12*(12), 1403–1412.

44. Whang, J. S., Baker, S. R., Patel, R., Luk, L., & Castro III A. (2013). The causes of medical malpractice suits against radiologists in the United States. *Radiology, 266*(2), 548–554.

45. Kaissis, G. A., Makowski, M. R., Rückert, D., & Braren, R. F. (2020). Secure, privacy-preserving and federated machine learning in medical imaging. *Nature Machine Intelligence, 2*(6), 305–311.

46. Skripcak, T., Belka, C., Bosch, W., Brink, C., Brunner, T., Budach, V., ... Baumann, M. (2014). Creating a data exchange strategy for radiotherapy research: Towards federated databases and anonymised public datasets. *Radiotherapy and Oncology, 113*(3), 303–309.

47. Regulla, D. F., & Eder, H. (2005). Patient exposure in medical X-ray imaging in Europe. *Radiation Protection Dosimetry, 114*(1–3), 11–25.

48. Tsapaki, V. (2020). Radiation dose optimization in diagnostic and interventional radiology: Current issues and future perspectives. *Physica Medica, 79*, 16–21.

49. Wang, Y., Zhu, H., Madabushi, R., Liu, Q., Huang, S. M., & Zineh, I. (2019). Model-informed drug development: Current US regulatory practice and future considerations. *Clinical Pharmacology and Therapeutics, 105*(4), 899–911.

50. Chamunyonga, C., Edwards, C., Caldwell, P., Rutledge, P., & Burbery, J. (2020). The impact of artificial intelligence and machine learning in radiation therapy: Considerations for future curriculum enhancement. *Journal of Medical Imaging and Radiation Sciences, 51*(2), 214–220.

51. Kouanou, A. T., Tchiotsop, D., Kengne, R., Zephirin, D. T., Armele, N. M. A., & Tchinda, R. (2018). An optimal big data workflow for biomedical image analysis. *Informatics in Medicine Unlocked, 11*, 68–74.

52. O'Sullivan, S., Nevejans, N., Allen, C., Blyth, A., Leonard, S., Pagallo, U., ... Ashrafian, H. (2019). Legal, regulatory, and ethical frameworks for development of standards in artificial intelligence (AI) and autonomous robotic surgery. *The International Journal of Medical Robotics and Computer Assisted Surgery, 15*(1), e1968.

53. Vlahou, A., Hallinan, D., Apweiler, R., Argiles, A., Beige, J., Benigni, A., ... Vanholder, R. (2021). Data sharing under the general data protection regulation: Time to harmonize law and research ethics? *Hypertension, 77*(4), 1029–1035.

54. Auffray, C., Balling, R., Barroso, I., Bencze, L., Benson, M., Bergeron, J., ... Zanetti, G. (2016). Making sense of big data in health research: Towards an EU action plan. *Genome Medicine, 8*(1), 1–13.

Index

For Product Safety Concerns and Information please contact our EU representative GPSR@taylorandfrancis.com Taylor & Francis Verlag GmbH, Kaufingerstraße 24, 80331 München, Germany